Licking Sweet Death

Energy and Information
to Stop Sugarcoating Your Addiction
to Processed Foods

Hugo Rodier, MD

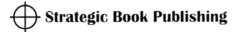 **Strategic Book Publishing**

Strategic Book Publishing
An imprint of Strategic Book Group
P.O. Box 333
Durham CT 06422
www.StrategicBookGroup.com

ISBN: 978-1-60860-475-3

Printed in the United States of America

Book Design: Rolando F. Santos

Contents

To all the parents who are struggling with their children's addictions, as well as their own, to candy, soda, white flour, and garbage food.

Introduction

Obesity and diabetes are literally changing the way we look and how our bodies function because of our addiction to refined sugars. We are poisoning our cells so that they are unable to optimally communicate with each other. Sadly, the statistics are well known; I am not going to bore you with them at this point.

What is really going on?

Have you heard about "insulin resistance"? It is simply a partial resistance to insulin at the cell membrane level of all fifty to one hundred trillion cells making up our bodies. And why are these membranes a bit resistant to insulin? The outer skin of every cell in our bodies—whether they are brain cells, heart cells, or the cells in our hangnails—are TOILing. The cell membranes are:

T – Toxic
O – Oxidized
I – Inflamed
L – Light, energy-, and/or love-deprived (mitochondrial dysfunction)

Cell membranes are delicate structures that must be flexible and soft, which is naturally the case when we eat the right proteins, sugars, and fats.[1] Since we are eating mostly refined/trans-hydrogenated fats, refined sugars, and proteins highly processed with steroids, antibiotics, hormones, and pesticides, our cell membranes are growing stiffer by TOILing,[2] or less responsive to the "messages of cell communication."

1

In other words, the more insulin resistance we have, the higher our body mass indexes (BMI)[3] and the higher the risk of death for us in the next five years.[4] Should we follow California's example and ban trans-fats altogether?[5] In my opinion, it is not a good idea to take away people's rights to poison themselves. It would be better to tax bad foods higher or eliminate taxes on healthy food.

Hormones—like insulin, neurotransmitters, enzymes, etc.—are nothing but molecules, or messengers, cells make to talk to one another. The whole network of cell communication should not have been divided into different systems. Now, it is widely accepted that this system, called the "psycho-neuro-immune-endocrine system," works as a single unit. Each messenger may function in any of the components of this system. For instance, one of the most powerful neurotransmitters, or messengers, that relay information back and forth in neurologic tissues, like serotonin or dopamine, is the thyroid hormone. Insulin has a powerful effect on our brains.

Our Cells, Energy, and Information

Each cell membrane of our fifty to one hundred trillion cells has "receptors" to which these messengers attach in a "lock-and-key" fashion. If the cell membrane is healthy, messages may enter the cell and be interpreted in the nucleus of the cell.

What is the main reason why cells communicate with one another? The answer is energy and information, or E&I for short.

If your religious beliefs are foremost in your mind, please, equate "energy/light" with God and "information/communication" with his Gospel. Many people feel that light is a two-sided coin: energy and information. After all, communication of information is achieved through energy, or light waves. From hereon, E&I will stand for energy and information.

Cells must communicate E&I to each other for our bodies to function as one single entity, or one consciousness. This is the message we get from the ages and pages of the human condition, recorded in the dustbin of history books and from thrilling modern research—particularly in physics. Cells communicate in order to process and consume E&I; these are the simple principles behind the laws of thermodynamics, the modus operandi of the whole universe.[6] It turns out that our cell membranes are key to the processing of E&I in cells.[7]

The E&I that comprise the whole universe are funneled to humans and the whole earth, for that matter, through the light of the sun. E&I end up fueling our whole bodies, particularly our hearts. Many people feel that it is not a metaphor that our hearts are the center of knowing, feeling, and our very consciousness, instead of the brain. In fact, our hearts have five thousand times more electromagnetism than the brain.[8]

Insulin Resistance = "Sweet Death"

Once we focus on E&I, the pillars of reality, we can see that these simple principles of thermodynamics not only rule the stars, the planets, and atoms, but living organisms. For humans, the most important messenger of E&I in our bodies is the hormone insulin. It brings E&I, or glucose (energy), to all cells for them to carry out whatever functions they specialize in. The main problems in our society — obesity and diabetes — are simply insulin resistance issues or dysfunctional cell communication of E&I. Actor Paul Newman, as Luke in the movie *Cool Hand Luke*, would have agreed: "What we got here . . . is a failure . . . to communicate."

Think about it: if cell membranes develop resistance to only insulin, they are discriminating against insulin. Why would they block insulin, and yet easily allow other messages of cell communication to freely enter the cell? If you have insulin resistance, you have resistance to practically all other messages, because your cell membranes are TOILing. You have thyroid resistance, adrenal hormones resistance, neurotransmitter resistance, etc.

In practical terms, detecting early signs of insulin resistance may lead to efforts to prevent the onset of "diabesity,"[9] or the "sweet death," that is ravaging our society.

Everything is Light

Light/E&I is what moves our world, enlightens our understanding and our souls, and quickens our bodies. Solar E&I is the basis of life on Earth. Through photosynthesis, plants absorb solar E&I. We eat the plants and the animals that eat plants. Think

3

of food as nothing but E&I. We also absorb solar E&I directly through the skin with the help of vitamin D.

Light/E&I from the sun fuel practically all activities on Earth. Our industries run on E&I; so do our buildings and our entire civilizations. Oil for gasoline is nothing but stored solar E&I, and oil also fuels our motivation to wage wars.

If we look at any issue in our society, we can discern the concepts of E&I at play. Take, for instance, immigration of Mexicans to the United States. They are immigrating in search of better E&I. Misguided food subsidy bills have made corn, rice, wheat, soy, and cotton very cheap in the United States, making it possible to flood our markets with junk food. This is one of the factors behind the epidemic of obesity in the United States.

In addition, these agricultural policies have contributed to cheap junk food being dumped on other countries like Mexico, where farmers are not able to compete with subsidized produce. This contributes to unemployment in their country, which puts pressure on them to end up dislocated to menial work in the United States.[10] Ironically, most of them end up in the harvest of the very subsidized United States products that compromised their Mexican sources of E&I in the first place.

Whether a factory makes paper clips, computers, or clothing, they need E&I to do so. These industries, and every facet of our lives, need E&I to get these jobs done. Industries also need a system to eliminate the garbage that they produce. Environmental pollution is nothing more than combustion problems from our less-than-ideal energy sources.

Our bodies are the same: we metabolize (E&I processing) and catabolize (get rid of garbage, or detoxify). We need cell communication to get all of these processes done. Simply put, we need energy—the male principle—and communication of information—the female principle. Let us not fight as to whom/what is more important, although I may end up in the doghouse if I don't say that the feminine principle is to rule again. (By the way, if you do not "communicate" in a relationship, you are going to have pretty "bad energy" at home.)

The Ancients

Since the dawn of mankind, we have known, either through meditation, revelation, scientific inquiry, aliens, angels, or demons (pick the one you prefer), that everything in the universe consists of E&I. Whether you believe in evolution, the Big Bang Theory, or Intelligent Design, you may concede that these systems have a common denominator: light, or E&I. "Let there be light" is the common ground. Hopefully, we will agree on this and not fight about which is the correct one. In my opinion, to do so may be an egocentric endeavor that stifles the best way of knowing: through the heart.

Modern physics focuses on these simple principles of E&I as the cornerstone of the universe. You may always ask your teenager about any issue, including this one. Teens know everything, especially that their lives depend on their cell phones, text messages, and their e-mails, to communicate information, which relies on energy to operate their gadgets.

Any philosophy, belief, or religious faith you may bring up is likely to be based on energy/spirit, and communication of information, or revelation. Judeo-Christian thought is a good example. The Egyptian god of writing and communication, Thoth, is a man with the head of an Ibis. He holds in his hand the Ankh, a key-like object with a closed loop for a handle. This represents "creation-destruction," which needs E&I to recreate the universe and everything therein, including our bodies.

The ancient Ouroboros symbol (a snake eating its own tail) represents the same concept. It is not a coincidence that a dove, the Judeo-Christian symbol of communication of divine knowledge, is found in the middle of the circle. A "feathered serpent" has symbolized Jesus, and many other Abatars throughout history. By the way, you will find many comments alluding to spiritual issues in this book. Hopefully, this is not offensive to you; the fact that 57 percent of Americans feel that God is able to heal the sick through prayer and divine intervention suggests that spiritual issues may be openly discussed in a health book.[11]

Energy, Information, and Food

Our bodies need a constant intake of E&I, or food, in order to maintain the circle of creation-destruction. Did you know that the lining of your stomach is totally new every thirty-six hours? Your skin is brand new every week. Your household dust is three-quarters dead skin. So, where do we get new cells from to renew these tissues?

Think of food as a practical source of E&I. Just like any engine (and I do not think we are like machines), we need fuel and an efficient way to get rid of the products of combustion. Imagine pumping bad fuel into your car's engine and having a pair of socks stuck in the exhaust pipe. Your car wouldn't get very good gas mileage, would it?

Eating poorly and having poor "energy" from emotional/spiritual/mental relationships provides poor fuel for our cells or sub-par levels of energy. [12] Our cells need E&I to communicate E&I, and to detoxify. If these problems continue for very long, entire tissues (collections of cells) and organs (collections of tissues) begin to malfunction. Even our deoxyribonucleic acid (DNA) for gene expression runs on E&I. Adapting to life's stresses and changes, or allostasis, is critical for survival—a process that needs the right E&I. [13]

It does not get any simpler than this: cell membranes are TOILing. This is why cells cannot communicate information effectively, resulting in significant deficiencies in E&I production and consumption.

Occam's Razor

Could it really be this simple? Stephen Wolfram's book, *A New Kind of Science*,[14] reassures us that simple concepts underlie the seemingly complex vastness of reality. The most complicated structures are born of simple patterns that may easily be discerned by a well-programmed computer.

The *J. Science* agrees:

"It is a mistake to imagine that complex disease may not be solved by simple approaches or that their causes are not simple. The grave danger is that terms such as 'multi-factorial' or 'complex' may justify the belief that solutions will come only from large and expensive managed projects rather than from simpler approaches."[15]

"Occam's razor" is a physics principle; "whenever one is confronted with many answers to a problem, the simplest one is the correct one." Sherlock Holmes would agree. While it is true that we are likely to run into "further light and knowledge" in the future, and that a true and rigorous scientific approach demands that we never contemplate any answers as final but mere approximations to truth, I will go out on a limb and agree with Wolfram and many others who feel that the final answers will involve E&I.

Once we grasp that E&I are the foundations of the universe, we may see that environmental pollution is nothing more than byproducts of energy-making industries. The toxins, or garbage, that industries produce are also called free radicals or oxidants. These environmental toxins are contributing to cell membrane dysfunction. Remember the "T" in TOILing. Our ability to detoxify them through our liver, kidneys, skin, and bowel detoxification pathways depends on good nutrition, or E&I, to fuel those cells' and organs' functions.

Solutions?

Don't hold your breath waiting for governments to start cleaning up our environment anytime soon. As problematic as pesticides, plastics, dioxin, heavy metals, chlorinated and fluoridated compounds are there is something much more toxic in the environment: refined sugars. Government policies subsidizing crops like corn, wheat, and soy have contributed to the flood of cheap, addicting foods that flood our markets and make fruits and vegetables less accessible. In my opinion, the number one toxic agent contributing to cell membrane breakdown of communication and energy production is the refined garbage foods we eat.

The simple principles that govern the stars, the atoms, and our societies are also the reason why "food is the best medicine." If you change the way you eat and improve your detoxification pathways (fix constipation, for example), your "engine" will work better; you will have better cell communication of E&I and, in turn, better health.

Some may say that our genes lock us into a hopeless creation-destruction cycle that perpetuates poor regeneration of cells and tissues. While this is true in rather rare diseases, it is not true for the common chronic diseases that are ravaging our societies. In other words, insulin resistance, diabetes, arthritis, high cholesterol, high blood pressure, heart attacks, asthma, colitis, cancer, Alzheimer's disease, Parkinson's disease, etc., may be controlled with diet. Genes are also influenced by E&I communication principles. [16] This is the message of hope in the new fields, or nutrigenomics and nutrigenetics.

In *Licking Sweet Death,* you will find simple answers to the cell communication of E&I problems we are having. Perhaps the most important solution is to own up to our addiction to refined food and to the factors that fuel such an addiction. One of the answers has been around for a long time: "Eat your vegetables!" I can still hear Grandma yelling at me. Unfortunately, today's grandmothers are, for the most part, treating our kids with candy.

Other solutions that will be discussed are well known to you, such as the mind-body-spirit connection, exercise, and supplements. However, none of these things do much good until we understand *why* we are so addicted to the refined fats, sugars, and proteins that are causing our cell membranes to TOIL.

Pharmaceutical drugs will always be part of the solutions. Unfortunately, they are often tried without addressing the simple principles you will read about in this book, like encouraging healthy lifestyles:

> "Clinical research involving pharmaceutical agents needs to focus more on the differential responses within diverse patient populations. This philosophy should be extended to the public to encourage healthy lifestyles rather than depending on the quick fix of drugs as panacea." [17]

We need a concerted public health approach to look at the forces that have contributed to the present state of affairs that is breaking our health care system. Only a society-wide frontal attack on the problem of obesity and insulin resistance can solve these vexing problems that, as you will see in this book, are the roots of most of our chronic health problems bankrupting our country (other than our wars for oil and corrupt corporatism of course). Truly, we face a sweet death, since obesity and diabetes significantly shorten our lifespan and increase disability. [18]

It is up to us, to our loved ones, our patients/clients, and our friends to assume responsibility for our own health. Our government is failing to control this runaway train. I am trying to *communicate* with you to invite you to empower yourself with *information.*

May the *force/energy* be with you . . .

—Hugo Rodier, MD

P.S. 1

When an ancient Egyptian woman kicked the bucket, they weighed her heart opposite a feather on a scale. If the heart were heavier than the feather, the god, Ammut, would eat it. And that is as far as the beloved departed got. I hope your heart passes this test as you read this book. Please don't be offended by my "lightheartedness." My definition of being professional does not exclude humor. Remember, "Humor is the best medicine." Freud said a lot of dumb things, but there was a pony under the pile he left: "When confronted with unrelenting suffering, the only sane response is humor."

P.S. 2

This is a work of integration, or consilience.[19] Consilience is the unity of all knowledge, which I pursue to the best of my limited abilities. I suffer from an ancient malady, "the Ionian Enchantment." An old fart named Thalus, who lived on the island of Miletus in the Mediterranean Sea, first documented this problem. The Ionian Enchantment is the delight in the pursuit of unification or integration of all knowledge, which I try to bring to the field of health and medicine.

I would like to believe I am a "synthesizer," but I pale in comparison to synthesizers like Nobel Prize winner Murray Gell-Mann who loved taking a "crude look at the whole." Some of you will conclude I am taking "a crude look at the hole in my head"; being a generalist and a synthesizer is both an advantage and a weakness. The fact that I am pushing the envelope in medical circles means I am not limited by the present paradigms that ignore E&I. While some folks will say I lack the depth of a specialist who may dismiss my generalist's views. To them, I simply say that a specialist is often one who knows a whole lot about very little.

No doubt many of the ideas in this book, even though they are backed up by solid research, will be categorized as "alternative." I feel this would be sad and helpful only to those who maintain that anything about health must be of a pharmaceutical nature.

My "disease" is very similar to what Tantalus was afflicted with, that is, the love of simplicity in unity. This leads the afflicted to an exhilarating rush of fulfillment and clarity when all things appear to fit so well, in a coherent whole. These are the reasons why you will find this book sprinkled with literature, movies, physics, theology, anthropology, science, politics, economics, arts, computer science, mathematics, mythology, (my editor advised me to leave out sex . . .), and the ideas of my most favorite philosophers, Calvin and Hobbes, that is, the six-year-old boy and his stuffed tiger.

P.S. 3

I have included technical references and information that non-medical people may find boring and over-their-heads. In my opinion, the concepts are easy to understand once you catch on to the simple ideas herein discussed.

As awkward as it seems, the references are numbered in an additive fashion. They go up to 2102, not a small number. I wish readers to see that the worn-out refrain that "alternative medicine has no evidence to back it up" is false and likely a mantra perpetuated by those who do not want competition against their established chemical approach to health care. In other words, I just want to loudly proclaim that a whole lot of evidence is not being made public for political and economic reasons. By the end of this book, I am sure you will add that said evidence is not widely circulated for monetary reasons.

"Medicine, the Arts, and the Humanities"[20]

"Medicine and scientific developments rely on multidisciplinary involvement of science and humanities. The arts and humanities can also contribute ways to re-conceptualizing medicine itself . . . Medicine and health are human concerns in the widest sense . . . The humanities can foster a depth of humane understanding, knowledge and experience."

"The medical humanities encompass history, literature, philosophy, ethics, theology, sociology, anthropology, and law. They value the aesthetic as well as reason, focus on meaning as well as emotion and explore ambiguity, uncertainty, and complexity, as well as theoretical lucidity. They offer understanding through synthesis as well as analysis. The humanities develop analysis of personal and professional values and the capacity for empathy and teamwork."

"Often, more than the body or mind is broken: patients' understanding of themselves is also disturbed . . . A sound grounding in the arts and humanities can enable an effectively critical, humane and ethical response . . . [but] caution against pitfalls into which medical ethics has fallen: narrowing, specialization and professionalism which could result in the elimination of 'radically different approaches to the big questions and issues of life.'"

Part I

No More Sugarcoating the Problem

Before we talk about how we may lick this sweet death, we have to discuss how we got into this predicament. Do you prefer a more positive approach? Okay, I am positive we are in deep trouble. Let's see if we can find some humor in what's really dragging us down.

Chapter 1

Sweet Death: A Failure to Communicate

We face a deadly epidemic of diabetes and obesity in the world, especially in the United States—the land of plenty. Some are proposing that our species name, Homo sapiens, be changed to "Homo obesus."[21] . In my opinion, the reason why we are struggling with these problems is often missing from those lectures: we are addicted to refined sugars and we are not addressing the factors that lead to such addiction.

You already know how bad things are[22] just by looking out the door, or worse: by looking in the mirror. Do you really need all the stats to get the point? You and I are sick of hearing about the statistics and all the intellectualizing that goes along with them. The main "numbers" we will focus on will be the inches around your waist and the economic incentives to keep you addicted to sugar.

Industries thrive by making larger clothing, furniture, etc. [23] Big Food and Big Pharma are given carte blanche and subsidies[24] by Big Government to pursue profits ahead of our health in the interest of "keeping the economy going." ("Big Food" and "Big Pharma" refer to the Darwinian conglomerate of corporations bent on pursuing profits in the food processing and pharmaceutical industries, at the expense of social wellbeing. "Big Government" refers to government institutions that lose sight of serving people in their efforts to maximize corporate interests.) Obesity and diabetes consume most of our health care dollars[25] after the expensive services we use for the last few months of people's lives. Our health care system would collapse if we all were to lose weight overnight.

I will ask you to think a little bit about these issues; "this will hurt a little."

> "Obesity seems to be perpetuated by a series of vicious cycles, which, in combination with increasing obesogenic environments, accelerate weight gain and represent a major challenge for weight management."[26]

You will get dizzy with all the "vicious cycles" you will find in this book, which are perpetuating our metabolic dysfunction epidemic called sweet death; "Insulin resistance is [truly] a secret killer."[27] About half of us struggle with insulin resistance, which, henceforth will be noted as "IR" to save you and I a lot of time. Since insulin is not entering our cells very well, our pancreases make more insulin to compensate. Basically, with "Insulin resistance and hyperinsulinemia: you can't have one without the other."[28] High insulin levels also increase inflammation or TOILing—another vicious cycle.

Drowning in a sea of refined sugar we put ourselves at risk of becoming diabetics.[29] This is why there has been a 70 percent increase in diabetes in the last thirty years [30] and a 100 percent increase in the last decade.[31] These statistics point to an environmental predominance in the factors leading to this condition, *not* genetics, or else we would have to conclude that our genes are mutating right before our eyes. We will discuss our strained "jeans" in more detail later on.

Shortly after graduating from medical school at the University of Utah in 1984, I was dumbstruck when I saw a little girl with type 2 adult-onset, or non-insulin-dependent diabetes. I had been taught that this type of diabetes was only found in older adults. I called my pediatric professor who sadly informed me that he was also starting to see this problem in children. Up until that time, children were known to have only type 1 diabetes, which is caused by a lack of insulin. Some researchers have proposed that we designate the patients who have both poor insulin secretion and IR as type 1-and-a-half diabetes.[32] The line between type 1 and type 2 is not that firm; some docs feel that type 2 patients do better when they are treated with insulin intensively when they are first diagnosed.

I will never forget the face of that child, who is now a young woman with many health problems. Type 2 diabetes is now 95 percent of diabetes and it is literally exploding in our children because of obesity.[33] This is why we don't call it "adult-onset diabetes" anymore. We estimate that one-fourth of children, and one-third of the population at large, has a pre-diabetic condition which will ultimately lead to diabetes if nothing is done about it.[34]

Poor E&I Processing: The Metabolic Syndrome

The metabolic syndrome, a combination of obesity, high blood pressure, high cholesterol, and diabetes afflicts about one-fifth of adults.[35] Treating the metabolic syndrome, which is reaching epidemic proportions, must be done on an individual basis, instead of a cookie-cutter approach.[36] As you will see later on, these are all problems of E&I at the cellular level. These problems are so common that insurance companies now have an ICD-9 code to track and bill for this syndrome. It will soon overtake smoking as the number one risk factor for heart disease in the United States.[37]

But, again, the problem is more profound than what sterile, numbing, and confusing statistics may show. We see the real face of this epidemic in the derrieres staring back in the mirror and in our fellowmen suffering under the strain of E&I communication issues. Surely all the numbers you have seen will be worse and more daunting by the time you finish reading this book. The most important thing is to realize that we are threatened by a sweet death of terrifying proportions. We will need to act with courage and determination to rescue our children from this cataclysmic problem; they are the most affected. Can we do something for adults? Maybe, if they are open-minded to the new ideas they are about to read.

It is not worthwhile to dwell on blaming each other about the roots of this sweet death. But it may be helpful to take a look at what we stand for, to change those factors, and move on and let bygones be bygones. Any historical analysis will point to E&I issues that have been mismanaged.

Are You at Risk of a Sweet Death?

The often-quoted mathematical formula known as the Basal Metabolic Index (BMI) is not the best measurement of obesity and predictor of coronary vascular disease.[38] You may need an advanced math degree to figure out how to use it. Besides, the BMI fails in muscle-bound people with high muscle mass, like me. The new concept of "normal weight obesity" illustrates the point that the BMI is not the best way to assess patients, since it is possible to have a high percentage of body fat with a normal BMI and a significant increase in the risk of heart disease.[39] The BMI also seems to fail to tract obesity trends in children and adolescents from 1999 to 2006, despite the obvious epidemic of obesity we see with the naked eye.[40]

The Waist Circumference (WC), or the famous beer-belly, seems to be a better indicator as it is the most practical; the waist should be measured at each doctor's visit.[41] Any man with a WC over forty inches and any woman over thirty-five inches are suffering from a degree of inflammation,[42] metabolic dysfunction, or IR.[43] However, problems may be seen as early as thirty-one-and-a-half inches for a woman and thirty-seven inches for a man. A rough estimate is that the WC should be half of one's height.[44] Short people like me don't find this very fair . . .

The WC is even useful in teenagers;[45] it should be standardized for their age to increase its use in screening.[46] WC also applies to children, albeit, in smaller, but proportional waist sizes. Any child with a WC above the ninetieth percentile has IR,[47] which increases his or her risk of cardiovascular diseases as they grow older.[48] Facial fat, or chubby cheeks, correlate well with abdominal fat.[49]

The WC is such a compelling way to predict a shorter lifespan[50] and so easy to carry out that Japan has instituted laws to get people between forty and seventy-four years of age to shrink their waist below thirty-three-and-a-half inches for men and approximately thirty-five-and-a-half inches for women. Those who fail the test will be given dietary instructions. If they do not shrink enough, people will be asked to attend special classes to meet their goal of reducing the overweight population by 10 percent in the next four years, and by 25 percent in the next seven years.[51]

Some doctors feel that measuring the height of the belly in a patient with a BMI of over 40 kilograms while lying down is better than measuring the waist circumference. More studies are needed to confirm their observations.[52]

The waist-to-hip ratio requires a little math, but it is probably the best way to see where you are at. However, it is not as simple as just measuring your waist. The waist-to-hip ratio is certainly much more practical than the complicated BMI. This ratio should be under 0.8. A ratio above 0.8 signals that the waist is larger than it should be. This is why "apple-shaped" people have the most problems.[53]

Skinfold measurement is as good as waist measurements covered above. A doctor will pinch you with calipers to determine how much fat you have under the skin.[54] Usually, the doctor will pinch the skin over your triceps. Personally, I would rather pinch your chubby cheeks. Since calipers are required, I feel skinfold measurements are not the most effective way to see how your metabolism is working. Maybe this test would make more sense if you are an athlete.

There are also blood tests to measure serum glucose and other parameters. Soon, nanotechnology[55] and hair analysis[56] will give us more accurate and faster results to see just where your butt sits (as opposed to "where you stand"). These and many other tests will be discussed in depth latter, after laying the groundwork for how they work. But, the WC and the waist-to-hip ratio may be quickly assessed during your next doctor's office visit; your primary care provider may determine whether you are at risk of developing metabolic problems before you are actually diagnosed to have metabolic problems through blood testing. If your body is starting to look like you have not missed too many meals, you are likely to have some degree of IR.

But, really, you know you are in trouble when you cannot live without refined sugar. In other words, if you act like a sugar addict, you probably have already started down the slippery path to sweet death. You might as well call yourself a "sugar-holic." After all, alcohol is nothing but fermented sugar. Perhaps this analogy is a bit strained, but when we see that alcohol, refined sugars, opioids, endorphins, and drugs like Valium share the same receptors with sugar at the cellular level in the brain, we may understand why it is so hard to pry the Twinkies from some of our friends' "cold, dead hands."

We will see below that the E&I stored in toxins, drugs, and refined foods are contributing to our addiction to sugar. We will also see why the politics, economics, and social pressures in our society have caused and perpetuated this problem.

Failure to Communicate

IR is the cornerstone of the metabolic syndrome, as you may recall from the discussion on metabolomics, cell membranes, and cell communication in the introduction. As we age, our cell membranes gradually lose their ability to receive insulin. This natural process may be accelerated by cell membranes TOILing. In other words, our ability to produce, metabolize, and share E&I may be compromised at a faster rate as we age, if we do not watch what we eat, and if we are not mindful of environmental and emotional toxins that surround us.

Of course, genetic tendencies play a role in IR (see chapter 2), but this factor has been overemphasized by scientists, researchers, doctors and, of course, Big Pharma, in order to shift blame to the consumer and persuade us to "pay no attention to the man behind the curtain," that is, environmental factors that often are influenced by the bottom line. By that, I not only mean our fat butts, but the profits that are made from perpetuating the status quo, which benefits the purveyors of refined foods and environmental pollution.

Note that emphasizing non-genetic factors in this book does not negate the fact that nature and nurture work in tandem. By emphasizing the environment and our foods, I merely aim to balance this equation.

IR results from a loss of flexibility of our cell membranes. Later, we will see that a lack of flexibility in our emotional lives also contributes to IR. To overcome this partial IR, the pancreas secretes more insulin, causing its levels to climb in the blood-stream.[57] Higher insulin levels may cause all kinds of problems, since insulin becomes an inflammatory agent at levels above normal. Insulin's job is to take glucose/sugar from the bloodstream into our cells; less insulin secretion causes glucose to build up in the bloodstream,[58] triggering more inflammation and oxidation, or TOILing in every cell—particularly those lining the arterial walls. When cell membranes TOIL, cell communication of E&I is not optimal.

Since all fifty to one hundred trillion cells in our bodies need E&I to do their jobs, IR signals a defect in these, the most basic of mechanisms; this translates into just about every chronic condition or disease we know. For example, the cholesterol story, to which we devote about one-tenth of commercials on TV: it turns out that refined foods also increase toxic fats in the bloodstream,[59] like very-low-density lipoprotein (VLDL), which in turn worsens cell membrane IR.[60] IR handicaps our livers' ability to keep cholesterol healthy and un-oxidized.[61] This is one of the many vicious cycles we will study in depth later in the chapter on heart problems.

Chapter 2

Jeans Too Tight

Most people wear their "jeans" too tight. I don't mean to be insensitive, but our genes drive only 15 percent of obesity and IR. Yet, most obese people blame their parents for their weight issues while claiming to eat a very good diet.[62] As we will see below, some of them are, indeed, eating very good food and still cannot lose weight. No doubt some of them have genetic tendencies influencing their metabolism.[63]

However, most people would do well to look in the mirror and acknowledge the addiction they have to refined foods—particularly sugar. In my opinion, it is best to face these problems straight on, since more tangential and perhaps more "sugarcoated" approaches have failed. (Paying people to lose weight only lasts as long as the money does.[64]) Even so, some doctors argue that most patients don't want to be reminded that they are obese. How will they get better if we continue to sugarcoat the problem?

The emperor is naked and his butt is too big.

Most people still believe that fats are bad for them (more below), which makes them eat more refined sugars, often found in processed foods right along with trans-hydrogenated fats, furthering cell membrane TOILing and DNA dysfunction. It is essential to get the right fats in the diet for optimal DNA function.[65] In other words, bad diets compound any genetic tendency we may have to IR. Conversely, good diets and even exercise trump "obesity genes."[66]

The article, "Nutrigenomics and Nutrigenetics: The Emerging Faces of Nutrition,"[67] tells us that we may control how our genes work through good nutrition.

> "The recognition that nutrients have the ability to interact and modulate molecular mechanisms underlying an organism's physiological functions has prompted a revolution in the field of nutrition . . . Nutrigenomics (diet influences gene function) and nutrigenetics (genes determine how food affects us) provide the necessary stepping stones to achieve the ambitious goal of optimizing an individual's health via nutritional intervention . . . The drastically different responses between individuals to a given diet clearly highlights the limitations of population-based nutritional recommendations."

Here is the rest of that article. Don't be lazy; give it a try:

> "Nutrigenomics and nutrigenetics optimize health through the personalization of diet, provide powerful approaches to unravel the complex relationship between nutritional molecules, genetic polymorphisms, and the biological system as a whole."
>
> "It is the integration of these technologies that provides the optimal means to unravel the effects of a biological challenge on an organism; thus, the concepts of systems biology, or integrated metabolism."
>
> "Whereas pharmaceuticals have a targeted approach aimed at restoring health, diet is a multi-parametric approach to preserve and/or optimize health. Indeed, the diet is compromised of a multitude of nutritional and chemical molecules each capable of regulating disparate biological processes, and thus cannot use an approach similar to the pharmaceutical industry, i.e., the "one drug one target" paradigm. Hence, nutrition is a true integrative science that is well positioned to benefit from the exploitation of novel technologies capable of assessing biological networks rather than single endpoints."

23

"Unlike the pharmaceutical industry, which aims to target a specific dysfunctional gene to improve health, the nutritional industry must manage health through a complex mixture of nutritional molecules. Thus, in comparison with a medical compound, consuming a diet drastically increases the number of molecular endpoints that are capable of influencing phenotype, and thereby places the field of nutrition in a prime position to benefit from the technological innovations brought forth by the post-genomic era."

"Nutrition in the twenty-first century is poised to be an exciting and highly relevant field of research, as each new day is accompanied by advances in our understanding of how the interactions between lifestyle and genotype contribute to health and disease, taking us one step closer to achieving the highly desirable goal of personalized nutrition."

"Nutrigenomics describes the use of functional genomics tools to probe a biological system following a nutritional stimulus that will permit an increased understanding of how nutritional molecules affect metabolic pathways and homeostatic control. Nutrigenetics aims to understand how the genetic makeup of an individual coordinates their response to diet, and thus considers underlying genetics polymorphisms."

"Complex cell and molecular biology coupled with biochemistry and genetics are required if the ambitious goals of nutrigenomics are to be realized."

"Studies aimed at elucidating the molecular mechanisms promoting cardiovascular disease have often used classical biomarkers, such as cholesterol, or CRP (marker of inflammation). Inasmuch as these studies are constantly improving the validity and accuracy of our knowledge of these diseases, they all suffer from a similar inherent quandary: these studies have been designed using current dogma . . . Nutrigenomics technologies resolve this tunnel vision by providing a means to identify previously unrecognized molecular points."

Polyunsaturated Fatty Acids (PUFA) are an example of how food influences genetic expression. They are involved in DNA gene expression regulation, energy production, inflammatory processes, growth, neurologic development, lean and fat mass development, reproduction, immunity, infections, and the incidence of virtually all chronic diseases and degenerative diseases, including cancer, atherosclerosis, stroke, arthritis, diabetes, osteoporosis, neurodegenerative, and skin diseases.

Many of us have do have a genetic disposition to IR,[68] particularly if short thighs are involved.[69] The Neuromedin B gene has been linked to a predisposition to eating behavior that leads to obesity.[70] Still, a common problem in genetics is to blame a disease on one single gene. We often see magazine articles with catchy titles, such as "Gene for Shopping Discovered."

Fortunately, modern genetics is corroborating the intuitive truth that many genes are likely involved in the development of any disease. For example, we now know that the risk of developing type 2 diabetes is increased by 20 percent in people who have at least six genes that contribute to IR. These genes include the ability to pump zinc into pancreatic cells to maximize their insulin-producing action and genes that have also been linked to cancer.[71]

Another gene on chromosome 16 partly influences how bad your sweet tooth may be. The FTO obesity gene variant seems to play a role in the control of food intake and food choices.[72] This may be why some people need to eat more sugar than others to taste sweetness. However, they really don't have to eat junk food to satisfy their sweet tooth; Mother Nature's sugars can do that.[73]

Even so, nutrigenomics is the final word for each of us as individuals.[74] I come from an obese family. My relatives are dark and short; they look like little cannonballs rolling around (don't tell them I said that). I don't look like that, yet, because I eat well and I work out one hour a day—a worthwhile prize to pay for vanity and/or health.

One of the main points this book tries to make is that diseases share common and simple mechanisms. Genetics is one of those mechanisms. There are DNA variances that are shared by seven six common diseases: bipolar disorder, heart disease, Crohn's colitis, high blood pressure, rheumatoid arthritis, and diabetes.[75] This tells me that those DNA variants likely act on the same pathways of E&I underlying these diseases.

25

Marie Antoinette

Marie Antoinette was oblivious to the revolution pummeling France; she buried her-soon-to-be detached head in the grounds around her "cottage," behind Versailles. When she was told that the people were starving because there was no bread, she declared, "Let them eat brioche!" She assumed that the townsfolk could afford cake or brioche since everyone in court around her did. But refined foods were a rare treat for the commoners, from whom most of us descend. We simply have not had the time to adapt to refined foods. Nutrigenetics is the field that tells us what foods are best for us, according to what our ancestors have been eating. Refined foods have not been available to us in such enormous quantities until the 1950s and 1960s.

If we are not mindful of our genetic pull, we might just lose our own heads in a sweet death.

Cavemen and Modern Diets

The article, "Genotype, Obesity and Cardiovascular Disease: Has Technical and Social Advancement Outstripped Evolution?"[76] reviews the concepts that our hunter-gatherer genotype (genetic tendencies) is ill-suited for our sedentary Western lifestyle. For a significant number of people, sticking to the Paleolithic diet is the best advice to prevent many of the chronic problems we are seeing today.[77] This diet consists of fresh fruits, vegetables, nuts, and lean meats but no grains or legumes. In contrast, our modern diets are high in refined sugars and processed animal fats, which generated more free radicals or oxidants that may cause TOILing to our cells and our DNA, thereby triggering IR. This has been referred as Glucose-Induced Genotoxicity (GIGT),[78] another vicious cycle. Get used to them.

The book, *The Paleo Diet*,[79] by Loren Cordain documents this genetic concept. Hunter-gatherer populations don't have metabolic syndrome problems or IR.[80] This diet has no milk, either. Can you imagine some caveman trying to milk a woolly mammoth? Paleolithic people didn't domesticate animals nor did they have time to plant crops. Their genes adapted to survival by selecting out IR.

If we are getting too much food or glucose, our cell membranes become resistant to avoid "revving up our engines," or overstimulating our metabolisms. Engines run better when they are cool. Overheating decreases their longevity and performance. The very genes that enhanced survival in starving populations are now deleterious: they result in a tendency to obesity.

Too Efficient

Our thrifty genotype, or genetic disposition to use as little energy as possible, has contributed to the epidemic of obesity. Survivors of historical upheavals tend to be those who get by with as little food as possible. They are genetically favored to avoid excessive feedings, which IR facilitates. Latinos, Asians, and African-Americans seem to be thriftier in their ability to get by with less food.[81] The metabolic syndrome afflicts 14 percent of African-American men and 27 percent of Latino women.[82] Also, most people gain 3 to 5 kilograms per decade, perhaps in anticipation of aging to guarantee survival in potentially leaner times.

How can we overcome these issues? Solutions "need to be culturally sensitive, integrated, and multi-disciplinary and involve individual and community interventions."[83] But, facing our addiction to sugar and the factors that lead up to it are still the main ways to overcome our sweet deaths once and for all.

Ancient Chinese Wisdom

There are those who feel it is better to be a vegetarian. This is the message contained in the book, *The China Study*,[84] by T. Colin Campbell and Thomas M. Campbell, II. While it is true that animal meat presents its own problems, some people are not genetically amenable to eliminating it from their diets. Besides, a self-sustained lifestyle practically demands that animals be part of said diet. Still, a vegetarian lifestyle is often associated with less chronic diseases like arthritis, or heart attacks.

Should you be a vegetarian? Only if you want to; you may want to check your genetic makeup to know for sure. This is what the science of nutrigenetics is about. What our ancestors ate for thousands of years will have a significant influence on how we should eat ourselves to maximize health.

Animal food may be seen as foreign molecules in some people, which may trigger an immune reaction; animal allergens may challenge the ability of the immune system to discriminate between foreign and self proteins.[85] In other words, animal proteins stress the immune system more. This may lead to practically all diseases.

In my opinion, a more practical way to see if you should eat like a "caveman" or become a vegetarian is to try both diets for a while. See what your waist, weight, and your cholesterol and insulin levels do. The proof of the pudding is in the eating.

Perhaps one of the most interesting points in *The China Study* is the "revelation" that we have been conditioned to think that proteins only come from animals. This is not true. In fact, you may get plenty of protein from fruits, vegetables, nuts, grains, and legumes. Ask yourself why we have been "brainwashed" to equate proteins with only animal sources.

Should We Eat a High-Protein or a High-Carbohydrate Diet?

This question is practically the same as wondering whether we should all become vegetarians or not. Should we eat more grains and legumes like *The China Study* suggests, or should we eat lean meats instead, with lots of fruits, nuts, and vegetables like *The Paleo Diet* suggests? As always, things are never either/ or or black and white. Again, you could do genetic testing to see what diet is best for you, but these tests are expensive and difficult to obtain. Besides, we are too mixed genetically. Our gene pool has no lifeguard. We are marrying people from all corners of the globe, which results in fewer and fewer people having only a single racial background. Most people are "Heins 57," including myself.

Don't take me wrong. I believe in the strength of the hybrid and I am proud of my mixed heritage. My father was French; my mother is a mixture of Basque, Spanish, and Chilean Indian. The milkman was Italian.

So what is the best diet for most of us? In my opinion, it is the low-glycemic index diet. This diet recommends that we make fruits, vegetables, and nuts the base of the food pyramid. All foods have glucose, but some have more than others. If you look at the Paleolithic and the vegetarian diets again, you will see that they both agree that we do well on fruits, vegetables, and nuts as the common denominator. Any diet for any racial background will do best to follow the same pattern. After we fill up like that, we may eat the lean meats, legumes, and grains. Hopefully, getting full on the lower glycemic foods keeps us from grabbing that donut you see at the office; more on the glycemic diet below.

Try eating this way and you will soon see what meals help you feel better. The quality of our bowel movements should also be a big tip. If meats tend to constipate you, take that as an answer. If you pursue a vegetarian lifestyle, make sure you supplement B vitamins; they are vital for DNA copying, liver detoxification, neurotransmitters' synthesis, etc. Perhaps the best practical approach is to eat vegetable-based protein; it is much easier for insulin to handle, even while in utero. Pregnant women would do well to limit their animal protein intake in order to reduce their baby's chances of developing IR. [86]

Micromanaging

The debate pitting high-protein diets against high-carbohydrate (or carb, for short) diets is distracting us from modern concepts that emphasize the "micronutrient" content of foods, such as the amount of antioxidants, minerals, vitamins, etc. Instead, we focus on the "macronutrients," like fats, carbs, and proteins. An approach that maximizes micronutrients in the diet seems more realistic, especially when the emphasis on macronutrients has proven unsuccessful. The more refined sugars we eat, the less micronutrients we have in our diets, and the more sweet death we see. Our cellular processes are highly dependent on micronutrients; a lack thereof, no matter what kind of diet we eat, will favor cellular membrane TOILing.

High-protein or high-carb diets are confusing a lot of people, particularly consumers who end up being preyed upon by food commercials trying to maximize sales of gimmicky diets. The misunderstandings are compounded by evidence supporting both types of diets. But, remember "nutrigenetics," which tells

29

us that certain people have been selected through centuries to eat like their ancestors.

Through trial and error, we may determine which diet is best for us. Since this may prove a bit cumbersome, most people give up and simply eat what is convenient. And, thanks to Big Food, or the corporations that make processed foods, what is most convenient and cheaper are mostly refined foods devoid of micronutrients, due to the harvesting, processing, and marketing of foods that are driven by profit maximization—not health.

> P.S. If you are going to eat a low-fat diet, don't eliminate the veggie-based fats (nuts, olives, avocados, etc.) and eat a lot of fish. Low-fat diets do not reduce the risk of diabetes.[87]

Back to Genetics

Contrary to most people's beliefs, type 1 diabetes is not just due to our genes. The article, "Nutritional Risk Predictors of Beta Cell Autoimmunity and Type 1 Diabetes at a Young Age,"[88] tells us that even type 1 insulin-dependent diabetes is only 5 percent genetics. Twins have only a 13 to 33 percent chance of both of them developing type 1diabetes. In other words, diabetes of any type is mostly an environmental problem, with genetics playing a secondary role. In fact, many docs feel that type 1 diabetes is mostly a result of inflammation; I would also add TOILing throughout the body, which affects the beta cells, or insulin-producing cells, in the pancreas.

Why would TOILing be confined to only a few cells? In the early stages, TOILing affects the most sensitive cells, that is, the ones that are more genetically susceptible. In later stages, if you haven't corrected the nutrition, environmental, and emotional factors that lead to TOILing, all cells in our bodies are affected. So, ultimately, insulin-producing pancreatic beta cells *and* body cells are TOILing enough to produce problems at the sending and receiving ends of cell communication.

This is probably why breastfeeding and the micronutrients nicotinamide (part of the B complex of vitamins), zinc, and vitamins C, D, and E have been reported as possibly protecting children against type 1 diabetes in (they decrease TOILing), whereas nitroso compounds in processed meats, cow milk, sugar, and excessive coffee increase the risk of type 1 diabetes.[89]

Mutants?

Did our genes start mutating thirty years ago when the epidemic of obesity/diabetes began? Of course not; the way we eat, pollutants in the environment, and our stressful lifestyles are affecting our genetic function. These stressors cause us to secrete more cortisol, which triggers more IR. We must not shift the blame from the real cause: environmental and lifestyle factors, which contribute 85 percent to obesity.[90] Even though one may have thrifty genes, the environment is still the major cause for tendencies to gain weight.[91] In fact, "even with a family history of diabetes, the risk reduction [is] 88 percent . . . most diabetes is preventable, irrespective of genetic background."[92]

Mommy's Uterus is "Environment," Not Genetics

A common misconception is that any tendency seen at birth is only the result of genetic factors. But the fetal exposure to Mom's diet is really an *environmental* factor. We know that what Mom eats, particularly in the third trimester, will significantly influence how the fetus will develop its fat thermostat in the brain (more below). In other words, Mom eating a poor diet may set the thermostat in the fetal brain so that her child may always have problems with weight issues.[93] Additionally, maternal obesity has been shown to increase the risk of IR in their children before they turn nine years of age.[94]

Children under two years of age, who are a bit skinny due to in utero undernourishment, tend to have more Impaired Glucose Tolerance, a test marker of pre-diabetes.[95] Babies who are born weighing very little have more IR—not, coincidentally, higher blood pressure.[96] Babies weighing more than 4 kilograms at birth are also more at risk of becoming obese as they grow.[97]

Moms with diabetes and obesity tend to have kids with higher risks of diabetes and neural tube defects.[98] Also, stem cells from a mother may pass through the umbilical cord to her baby, thus facilitating the function of beta cells in the baby's pancreas; this passage of stem cells influences the future risk of type 1 diabetes in that mother's child.[99]

The older Mom's uterus is, or the more children she has had (or the greater chances of TOILing in the cells of the uterus), the greater the body mass and percentage of body fat that her off-spring will have as they age.[100] Fortunately, the IR seen in children who develop in a deficient uterus and placenta may be ameliorated by breastfeeding.[101]

Mothers who have IR and/or are obese while pregnant (see gestational diabetes below) bear children with three times a higher risk of birth defects[102] and developing IR as they age.[103] Children born of type 1 diabetes mothers are more likely to develop type 2 diabetes and pre-diabetes when they grow older.[104] It is not clear to me whether this is a genetic or an environmental effect while in the uterus of a type 1 diabetic mother.

Interestingly, a mom's diet may play a role in determining a baby's gender; eating breakfast regularly and having a hearty appetite seem to increase the odds of having a boy.[105]

Shangri-La

Imagine a village so high in the Himalayas that no outsider has ever visited. The people there are very happy; they're isolated from the maddening world. Pretend that one day you manage to climb your way up to that Shangri-La. Strolling down Main Street, you see nothing but McDonald's restaurants, Taco Bells, Pizza Huts, and convenience stores filled with junk food. People pour out of these joints to greet you. They are shocked to see you and you are shocked to learn that they have been eating like that for millennia. Now, tell me, what do you think these villagers look like? Are they obese or unhealthy-looking?

I would guess they look quite healthy and trim.

If they have been eating like that for millennia, the E&I their food contains has thoroughly shaped the E&I stored in their genes, thereby adapting to that environment. They may not look exactly like us, but they will have adapted to that kind of food. We have only been eating badly for a few decades—not long enough for our genes to adapt.

White Food Makes You Fat

Refined grains are high in processed sugars and they lack enough fiber to optimize the absorption of glucose from the intestines in a controlled manner. This factor alone is enough to make us gain weight with "white food." But the plot sickens, my friends. It turns out that foods low in B vitamins, like refined grains, mess up DNA processing, or methylation, which is vital for many functions, such as detoxification, neurotransmitter synthesis, etc. We will discuss in more detail how these functions have a lot to do with metabolic issues in future chapters.

For, now, suffice it to say that we all "methylate" differently,[106] which becomes a factor in how we metabolize E&I. In other words, our DNA methylation varies from person to person. A relative lack of B vitamins may be a sufficient enough reason for some of us to gain weight. This is why supplementing B vitamins like folic acid, B-12, choline, and betaine may lower the risk of becoming obese.[107]

Better yet, try to quit your addiction to white bread, noodles, cookies, and pasta . . .

Chapter 3

Calories In = Calories Out?

The old worn-out dogma "calories in = calories out" is widely trumpeted as an established truth[108] despite very good evidence that it doesn't work all the time.[109] Granted, this approach gets you in the ballpark, but not to home plate in a significant percentage of people. Less calories and more exercise is effective for most people,[110] but not for very long. When we rely exclusively on calories in = calories out to maintain our weight, most people fail in less than twelve months,[111] unless they have an iron will—a rare commodity in our pampered societies. Calories in = calories out ignores the fact that many people do not seem to obey such overly simplified concept.[112] Many other factors contributing to our metabolism are ignored by this old refrain, including genetic tendencies.

What is Your Gas Mileage?

In the article, "Why Obese Patients Don't Lose Weight with Low Calorie Diets,"[113] the author postulates that it is because these patients have "metabolic adaptations induced by negative energy balances that are not captured by the present paradigm [of caloric intake.]" Also, we see here that the majority of patients with weight issues are not very candid about what they really eat.

34

This is why I insist that patients tell me the truth, after assuring them I am not going to put them in the corner with a dunce cap on.

The article, "Personal Metabolomics as a Next Generation Nutritional Assessment,"[114] tells us that we are different in our ability to metabolize nutrients and calories. We readily concede that two cars can vary in their ability to burn gas or their efficiency with gas mileage. People also obey the rules of thermodynamics that govern all engines and, for that matter, the whole universe. As a society, becoming more sedentary has altered our ability to deal with energy balances in our bodies.[115] People get different benefits from different intensities of exercise, which is further influenced by vitamin D levels in the blood,[116] and many other factors. The most important thing about our "gas mileage" is that the more we exercise, the less IR we have.[117]

Twin Studies

A study of identical twins in the Czech Republic gave twins the same amounts of calories in their diets, but they lost weight at different rates.[118] The same point was documented in a study in Quebec; twins on the same diet also lost different amounts of weight. The twins with the Gln27Glu gene gained more weight; presumably, this gene controls how we manage the calories we consume.

Calories and Our Genes

In Spain, researchers found that people with the PLIN4(A) gene cannot lose weight on restrictive diets. This gene seems to influence metabolic rates.[119]

Genetic differences also determine how we taste foods; some people have a sweet tooth that causes them to get pleasure only from high sugar diets.[120] Unfortunately, many of us have nuclear receptors (PPAR) that augment the predisposition to develop diabetes when we eat more refined sugars.[121] These receptors are found in all cells, especially in adipocytes, or fat cells. This is why PPAR drugs that treat diabetes and also essential fatty acids, like fish oil, work through these receptors to regulate our metabolism

35

and reduce IR.[122]

The calpain-10 gene has been found to be involved in the higher risk of diabetes seen in Mexicans and Pima Indians, all of whom are notoriously consuming excessive amounts of processed foods and refined flours. When the calpain-10 gene and susceptible PPAR receptors are found together, the risk of diabetes goes up twentyfold.[123]

Micronutrient, Macronutrients, and Calories

A study that compared low glycemic index foods (more on this below) with the typical low-fat diet that most doctors recommend showed that by carefully calculating the same amount of calories in both diets, both groups lost more or less the same amount of weight. But those on the low-glycemic index diet lowered their cholesterol more, had less IR, their caramelized hemoglobin was lower (test to measure degree of IR), as were their inflammatory markers like CRP; they also had lower blood pressure readings[124] and thinner blood, meaning it was less likely to clot.[125]

Drugs for cholesterol (statin), diabetes (metformin), and high blood pressure (ACE I) would not have matched such results. Why did the study show such dramatic differences between the two diets, even though both had the same amount of calories? Maybe the dogma of calories in = calories out is not the final word . . .

The key difference lies in the micronutrient and toxin content of the diets, not in their calories.[126] Of course, the more processed diets have more calories and less micronutrients, the latter being essential to keep cell membranes from TOILing and developing IR.[127] In other words, the content of micronutrients in the foods we eat often is forgotten when we emphasize macronutrients (fats, sugars, and proteins), and the calories contained therein. This concept is called "xenohormesis,"[128] which we will discuss later.

The fact that eating a boiled potato raises blood sugar levels higher than eating the same amount of calories from table sugar is an example that calories or energy are only one aspect of food content. The other is the information content.[129]

Food = Energy and Information (E&I)

Low-glycemic index diets require lower levels of insulin to metabolize; this affects short-term appetite sensations. In other words, the higher the amount of sugar in our diets, the hungrier we are after finishing those meals.[130] This is great news for Big Food: their processed foods are not only addicting, but also keep people eating more and more of their junk because they are not "filling." These types of foods cause IR to go up in brain neurons and in the rest of our cells in our bodies. Unfortunately, IR from high glycemic index foods is more pronounced in the hypothalamus of the brain, which governs our appetite and emotions. This means that the higher the amount of sugar in the diet, the more addicted to it we become. We will talk more about this in the section on our brain thermostat.[131]

Food is communicating information and providing energy to fuel our metabolism in all cells of our body. When we only focus on the fats, proteins, and sugars in the diet and ignore the information contained in the micronutrients therein (minerals, vitamins, pholyphenols, etc.), we may understand why so many studies contradict one another when they analyze the benefits of diets high in protein or high in carbs. So, instead of worrying so much about calories and the percentages of fats or carbs or proteins in your food, make sure you are getting plenty of micronutrients; they are highest in fresh fruits, vegetables, and nuts. After covering your bases with those foods, have fun with lean meats, legumes, and whole grains.

Not surprisingly, counting calories on a low-fat diet high in processed carbs makes us more inflamed. In contrast, a low-fat diet free of processed carbs, eaten "ad libitum," or whenever we feel hungry, lowers inflammation and people lose more weight. Remember that eating too much animal fat "activates a pro-inflammatory response and induces resistance in the hypothalamus."[132]

What is Your "Type?"

Our genes, waist sizes, potential for IR, intestinal health, detoxification pathways, and the quantity of fiber in our diets are some of the factors that determine how we respond to different diets, like high-protein or high-carb diets.[133] Remember nutrigenomics and nutrigenetics and how our metabolism differs from person to person.[134] These concepts are very likely to change the way dietetics are being taught in our colleges.

The Human Genome Project, a massive undertaking to map every gene in our DNA was completed in 2000; it found that we have approximately thirty thousand genes, but we produce one hundred thousand proteins. How can we explain this discrepancy, since each gene codes for one protein? The answer is simple: each gene is modified by the food we eat, which makes our genes copy more and different proteins from each gene. This is the central concept of nutrigenomics.[135]

Translating genes into working proteins makes up our "phenotype," or what our bodies are really like in function and structure beyond the DNA code. The code in our genes is known as the "genotype." When the genotype is translated into actual cell messengers or proteins, it gives rise to our phenotype. We are not just a blueprint in our DNA, but a working copy of said DNA.[136] The science of translating genes into proteins is also known as "proteomics." How we copy our genes into proteins has enormous implications for our metabolisms and cell communication in this modern "era of metabolism."[137] For example, a defect in a gene, or how that gene is copied, may cause problems with the way we process fats, which in turn may affect our metabolism.[138] This is why we now have lots of "Evidence of different metabolic phenotypes in humans."[139]

Ready to Abandon the "Calories" Dogma?

I am guessing many of you would still answer "no." I don't blame you. The doctrine of calories in = calories out has ruled modern science for quite a while. Why should you abandon it on the strength of the evidence presented by one single doc in some obscure suburb in Salt Lake City, Utah? Perhaps you need more evidence, and from more than just one doc. But, in my experience, old paradigms have more to do with emotional, social, political, and economic benefits than the evidence itself.[140] Even so, I would like to show you more scientific evidence to back up these concepts.

The Harvard Medical School symposium, "Science-Based Solutions to Obesity: What is the Role of Academia, Government, and Industry,"[141] concluded that some foods promote obesity more than others. Research has shown that "although optimal amounts and sources of protein cannot be determined at this time, evidence suggests a potential benefit of partially replaced refined carbs with protein sources low in sugar.[142] The article, "A High Protein Diet Induces Sustained Reductions in Appetite Ad Libitum Caloric Intake, and Body Weight Despite Compensatory Changes in Diurnal Plasma Leptin and Ghrelin Concentrations," at the same symposium, tells us that ad libidum means that you can eat anything that is not nailed down, without counting calories, as long as you are eating non-processed, low sugar, and low-fat foods—like vegetables, fruits, nuts, lean meats (especially fish), legumes, and whole grains. The way our bodies oxidate or process carbs makes it so that an ad libitum approach is healthier.[143]

In my opinion, only those who are addicted to bad food need a "caloric" line in the sand to stop eating. It would be better to quit the addiction, fix the thermostat, and "obey your hunger" with healthy foods.

Another article, "The Satiating Power of Protein—A Key to Obesity Prevention," documents that a high-protein breakfast is better than a high-carb one, because the former promotes a decrease in the hormone, ghrelin. Ghrelin is produced by the stomach after eating and reduces gastric emptying.[144] It gives us a feeling of being full longer after a meal. People with anorexia nervosa seem to have a defect in the regulatory function of ghrelin.[145] These concepts may be a bit too technical for you; just remember that skipping breakfast increases your risk of obesity by 455 percent; eating breakfast reduces your chances of becoming obese by 40 percent.

Ghrelin not only regulates our metabolisms, but also regulates how men's gonads function. There is an "integrative control of energy balance and gonadal function." Perhaps this is the reason why "the way to a man's heart is through his stomach."[146] (Read the reference before you send me a letter accusing me of sexism.)

The "Polypill" and the "Polymeal"

Medical doctors have been somewhat critical of a nutritional and herbal approach, thereby ignoring the E&I foods provide for our cells. The herbal approach, in particular, has been criticized for allegedly containing unreliable and not enough active substances. But, how useless can they be, when one-third of pharmaceutical drugs have been derived from food and herbs?

For example, statin drugs prescribed to reduce cholesterol levels were extracted from fermented red rice, which has been shown to be as good as the statins.[147] In fact, red rice lowers the mortality risk by 43 percent in patients who have already had a heart attack.[148] Pharmaceuticals took the chemical in fermented red rice that inhibits the liver enzyme HMG coenzyme reductase; it regulates inflammation and oxidation of lipids in the liver. According to many researchers, the red rice is less problematic because other antioxidants and micronutrients in red rice not only mitigate potential problems, but also help keep cholesterol from oxidizing.

The problem is that statin drugs, with this concentrated chemical, may harm the liver and muscles; the isolated chemical is not balanced by the discarded micronutrients found in fermented red rice. The pharmaceutical approach has typically ignored the combinations of nutrients found in whole foods and herbs in favor of a more concentrated and potent isolation of the most active substances shown to produce specific outcomes, like lowering cholesterol.

This is why I have been very interested in the new pharmaceutical trend that lumps several drugs together to treat the most common problems with one "polypill," especially when it comes to metabolic diseases (high blood pressure, diabetes, high cholesterol). It seems to me that Big Pharma is trying to put Humpty Dumpty back together again by recreating the holistic approach Mother Nature felt was best for us. Still, I don't think this trend will convince most people that it has been a mistake to separate and isolate the most active ingredients out of food and herbs, while throwing away the other balancing micronutrients. The arrogant belief that we may top Mother Nature is not going away anytime soon.

In response to the polypill concept, the article, "The Polymeal: A More Natural, Safer and Probably Tastier (than the Polypill) Strategy to Reduce Cardiovascular Disease by More than 75 Percent,"[149] thankfully gave us a better perspective. The "polymeal," which consists of wine, fish, dark chocolate, fruits, vegetables, garlic, and almonds reduced heart disease by 75 percent. Can you imagine how much a drug would cost if it promised to reduce heart disease by 75 percent? It turns out that the polymeal is just as good to lower cholesterol as any statin drug.[150] Does it make you wonder why you have not heard these facts before?

Don't "Catch" a Big Butt

We have more than one quadrillion organisms like bacteria, viruses, parasites, and fungal agents living inside our intestines. Each one of these organisms behaves much like any of our body cells; this means that these "foreigners" outnumber our body cells about ten-to-one. They constitute the majority of the genetic messages of E&I we carry. Most of them, especially the bacteria in our intestines, are healthy and work symbiotically with us.

But sometimes the friendly intestinal flora mutates to protect itself, adapt, and survive any hostile environment we may create for them by the way we eat or by the drugs and chemicals we take. For example, acid-blocking drugs like the purple pill,[151] chlorinated water, and antibiotics are notorious for negatively affecting our intestinal flora's health. Sometimes, toxic organisms in our food or our environment invade our intestines, precipitating infections in the gastrointestinal (GI) tract, which trigger an imbalance in the delicate ecology of the intestines. This may also happen to pregnant women[152] who, in turn, may influence the delicate ecology of their babies' intestinal flora.

Living in close proximity to pets and farm animals, eating refined foods high in processed sugars, and pesticides and who-knows-what other chemicals also create imbalances in our intestinal flora. Said imbalance may have serious consequences, not only in our intestines, but, in the rest of our bodies, since our intestinal flora is where most of our immune system is found. These friendly probiotics also play a huge role in our metabolisms and

41

they have just as much of a detoxification function as the liver.

In other words, our intestinal flora affects our ability to regulate E&I out of the food we consume.[153] This function is optimized by carb-restricted diets; they reduce our chances of developing the metabolic syndrome.[154] Because probiotics determine how we handle the E&I contained in food, it is logical to assume that "there are a number of chronic diseases for which there is tantalizing, piece-meal, reasonable evidence of microbial factors playing some kind of role."[155]

It seems a bit fantastic to say that intestinal flora can make us obese and increase the risk of type 1 diabetes.[156] This is why I will present several articles on this point in detail. You may want to explore them on your own to thoroughly understand "infectobesity," or the relationship between pathogens (disease-causing organisms, including bacteria and viruses) and weight gain.

Feed Me, Wilbur!

Cravings for chocolate and other sweets sometimes feel like they are coming from deep within your gut, right? Exactly. Researchers have discovered that bacteria living in our guts dictate what we are to eat. These little bugs love sugar and chocolate. Of course, *you* got them hooked on sugar. The actual study that backs up this fact was delayed for a year because the authors needed to find eleven "weird" men who did not eat chocolate to serve as controls for the study.[157]

The infectious paradigm is quite strong: it always surfaces when dealing with complex problems in order to blame something or someone outside of ourselves. For instance, we now blame H. pylori for ulcers and the human papillomavirus (HPV) for cervical cancer. We forget that Louis Pasteur felt that it was "not the germ, but the (TOILing) terrain" that renders the tissues more susceptible to infections. While I agree that bugs are playing a role in infectobesity, I feel that the choice is still ours to make: do we want to fight the addiction, no matter its roots, or are we just looking for excuses to look the other way?

Infectodiabetes?

We have known for some time that viruses may be associated with diabetes type I. Now we have reports that viruses not only may be involved in obesity, but also with type II diabetes. The human herpesvirus-8 (HHV-8) has been implicated in African-Americans who develop ketosis-prone diabetes—the kind that causes marked metabolic disturbances that may be fatal.[158]

According to researchers at Louisiana State University, one may even "catch" obesity through the adenovirus-36, which allegedly causes our stem cells to be more prone to becoming fat cells. Apparently, obese people are more likely to have been infected with this common cold virus that also causes pink-eye.[159] Talk about "seeing red" when we are told we need to lose weight . . .

Treating Infectobesity

The concept of rebalancing our gut flora to improve our metabolisms is sure to get a lot of attention in the future.[160] Becoming more aware of the negative consequences of overusing antibiotics is going to help; half of them are being given to cattle and poultry to increase productivity. Unfortunately, antibiotics affect their gut flora and, in turn, their metabolisms.[161] Poultry and beef are then "tastier" because they have more fat. Eating cattle treated with antibiotics no doubt has significant health consequences for us. We are also exposed to their mutated intestinal organisms, like the friendly bacteria E. coli, which periodically mutates into what we call E. coli 057. This strain is highly virulent, with devastating consequences like community infections, particularly in those who hang out at fast food joints.[162]

Rather than embarking on a potentially harmful path of prescribing antibiotics blindly to try to correct the intestinal flora imbalance, I feel it would be best to strengthen our friendly bacteria by taking probiotic supplements.[163] The yogurt industry is trying to cash in on these studies, offering friendly bacteria in their products. But they don't add enough probiotics to make a significant difference.[164] Besides, the dairy in yogurt has been found to be rather irritating to our intestines (see below)—never mind the preservatives and the high fructose corn syrup (HFCS) they throw in. Ironically, the fluoroquinolone family of antibiotics, which is often used for intestinal problems, may cause higher sugar levels in the blood.[165]

Since we love to use antibiotics for any medical problems that we don't understand very well, I am sure someone will eventually try to use antibiotics to see if they can help with weight loss. This may have unintended consequences, since antibiotics also kill friendly bacteria in the intestines. Talk about "friendly fire." Our friendly bacteria are the best defense we have to keep the bad guys from influencing our metabolisms and causing many other health problems, like infections, arthritic pain, auto-immune disorders, colitis, asthma, ulcers, etc. After all, it is not the invading organism that causes problems, but the quality of the terrain, or the "common soil," composing our tissues. Remember Pasteur.

If we do embark on the use of antibiotics for infectobesity, it should be done within a comprehensive program that includes a proper diet, probiotics, digestive enzymes, lots of fiber, and addressing environmental and emotional issues in patients—for example, learning to handle stress, simplifying our lives so that our diminishing incomes go further, drinking filtered water, etc. If we were to only use an antibiotic, infectobesity would come right back when we stopped it, since we would not have addressed the real issues causing the predominance of unfriendly organisms in the intestines. We need to change the environment that allowed the flora imbalance to develop in the first place. Hopefully, we learned these basic principles after the catastrophic use of Phen-Fen.

Story Time

Eavesdropping on a phone call: "Hello, boss; I'm sorry, but I can't come to work today. I caught a cold yesterday and I woke up with a big butt. I have nothing to wear and I don't want to infect the rest of the office . . ."

Starving to Death to Live Longer?

Limiting caloric intake leads to less IR, lower temperature, better metabolism, better hormonal function, and lower mortality.[166] Unfortunately, it also leads to boredom and starvation. Let me ask you something: would you give up sex if it meant living longer? I didn't think so . . .

It turns out that caloric restriction to live longer has two flies in the ointment: (1) it is only seen in obese rats[167] and (2) the studies on increased longevity by skimping on food don't clarify what the precise amount of caloric intake should be or why we live longer. In my opinion, it is because our "furnaces" burns less intensely; we would then last longer, like any machine under the laws of thermodynamics. But is it worth it to starve to death in order to live longer?

Still, some researchers are very interested in the concept of restricting calories.[168] Realizing that not too many people will stick to such a restrictive approach with a diet called "alternate day calorie restriction," study participants were told to eat ad libitum every other day, while consuming 20 percent less calories on intervening days. The researchers saw that those valiant souls who stuck to the program had less TOILing, or oxidative stress, and anyone who had asthma had their symptoms improve.[169]

If you are wondering why their asthma improved, think of IR and TOILing affecting the lining cells of the bronchioles—the little tubes that take air to the lungs. You may think of the lining cells of these tubes being "leaky," which allows more toxins to enter the respiratory system, thus triggering asthma.

The sirtuin/SIR2 gene that controls some of the functions of the mitochondria regulates lifespan and mediates caloric restriction.[170] According to what kind of SIR2 gene function we have, caloric restriction will affect each of us differently, so that we age at different rates,[171] and prevent chronic diseases at different rates.[172] When you consider that disease is a function of "aging organs," or cells, or tissues, we may see that practically all diseases may be addressed by slowing down the aging process.[173]

We may think of TOIL as a function of the mitochondria overworking; this produces a lot of oxidants and inflammatory molecules. Other than tanking up on antioxidants to neutralize this process, it makes sense to give the mitochondria a rest.[174] Simply put, rather than working on cooling the engine down with anti-oxidants, we could work on running the engine cooler and less often.

A "starvation hormone" has been discovered that plays a role in the shift seen in our metabolisms after a period of fasting and in those fed a refined low-carb diet.[175] Mice fed a high-fat, refined low-carb diet for thirty days turned up a gene encoding for liver-derived fibroblast growth factor FGF21; it helps burn more fat.[176] I think the diet itself is doable, but the starving part is not persua-sive enough. I ask again: is it worth focusing on caloric restriction and leave our addicting behaviors unexamined?

Long Live Bacchus

The concept of restricting calories is not likely to satisfy too many people. I would rather you ate a lot of grapes and never go hungry. A study in rats found that resveratrol, the main anti-oxidant in wine and grapes, reduces the protein SIRT-1; it fools the body into acting as if calories were being restricted, thus in-creasing their life span by 70 percent.[177] The rats were given the equivalent of resveratrol found in one thousand bottles of wine a day. Resveratrol has also been found to reduce the fat-storing function in fat cells, especially when given in conjunction with soy protein/genistein.[178]

Not surprisingly, resveratrol has been found to improve per-oxisome proliferator activated receptors (PPAR) on our cell mem-branes.[179] This means that TOILing is reduced; insulin sensitivity and lower IR follow. The PPARs are the main target of a whole group of diabetic pharmaceutical products and omega oils. Res-veratrol also improves the function of our NOS (Nitric Oxide Syn-thase) network of inflammation, particularly in our circulatory system. This means that resveratrol lowers the risk of clotting.[180]

A pharmaceutical company is trying to develop an improved version of resveratrol named SRT501. It is to be used in the treat-ment of diabetes. Also, they hope SRT501 can help people with MELAS syndrome, a disorder of mitochondrial function.[181] That resveratrol is an antioxidant, and it works in the mitochondria, are more clues that cell TOILing is involved.

Another study found that resveratrol protects animals from obesity and diabetes.[182] The authors suggested that humans try 5 milligrams of resveratrol, or 200 milligrams twice a day to increase their metabolisms.[183]

Some of you may just settle for the one thousand bottles of wine and forget the capsules of resveratrol altogether.

Our Broken Thermostats

We have a "thermostat" in the hypothalamus of the brain; it controls our appetite, according to our metabolic needs and diets. This thermostat is disrupted in people with metabolic problems. This is why most of them find it extremely hard to lose weight and maintain any loss. Consuming processed foods high in trans-hydrogenated, saturated fats and HFCS cause our thermostats to be set at a point where only increasing amounts of these empty foods will satiate us. When defective, glucose-sensing neurons making up the propiomelanocortin center of the brain contribute to the development of type 2 diabetes.[184] Sugar also causes a blunting effect on the sympathetic neural response of the brain in obese people with IR.[185]

Poor diets also reset the thermostat to a point where our biologic clocks are disturbed; we end up feeling compelled to eat junk food in the middle of the night.[186] In other words, micronutrients in food significantly affect how our thermostats set our metabolic rate.[187]

If we compared an addicted person to one who is not, we would find that their satiating point is set differently, regardless of the calories consumed.[188] This is yet another reason why the advice to count calories does not work well in some people. I am sure you have noticed that by now. How many times have you lost weight, only to regain it? Yet, many professionals continue to hammer the dogma of counting calories. While it is true that we are eating more calories than ever before, and that we should reduce said amounts, it is also true that the addiction problem and the changes in our thermostats have been largely ignored. What we truly need are "better strategies against obesity."[189]

After many years of advising my patients and searching through medical literature, I feel we must incorporate the latest findings in science in order to truly help people. Basically, you will see better results by abandoning the compulsive counting of calories and concentrate on fixing our thermostats in our brains. Counting calories is so cumbersome that few people stick to it; if they do, it's not for very long. If you still find people counting calories after one year, they are likely to be a bit compulsive and not very flexible. They probably do not enjoy eating. Why would you want to limit what a healthy body is urging you to do—that is, to eat? Why would you want to stop eating when you are still hungry? Would you not drink until you quench your thirst?

It is only when the brain thermostat is broken that you need to count calories. You may not know when to stop eating because you are addicted to bad food. A study of obese people undergoing magnetic resonance imaging (MRI) of their brains showed that their thermostats were underfunctioning.[190] Fortunately, eating the right foods will fix your thermostat; then, you simply "obey your hunger." Researchers at Brigham Young University documented this concept.[191]

The same university published a report about intuitive eating.[192] I would not trust anybody's intuition when the specter of addiction to refined sugars is present. In other words, I could not trust the intuition of an addict. Could you? Are they following their intuition, or their addiction? Are we mature and strong enough to tell the difference? Only we can answer truthfully for ourselves.

Sugar Addiction = Alcohol Addiction

For years I have been advising my patients not to count calories with dramatically positive results. I arrived at this simple conclusion through practical experience and by reading many medical journals and books on nutrition. The best article, the one that totally validated my semi-intuitive conclusion, was "The Influence of Food Portion Size and Energy Density on Energy Intake: Implications for Weight Management."[193] It simply says you can eat as much as you want, as long as you overcome your addiction to refined fats and sugars.

Okay, go ahead and continue to count calories: you will always need to do so if you do not stop the devastating addiction you have to refined sugars. Perhaps we have felt superior to our fellowmen's addictions to alcohol and other drugs. Before casting stones, it would be good to consider that his or her addiction to alcohol is fuelled by an addiction to fermented sugar. The mechanism of addiction to refined foods is much the same and the consequences, sweet death, may be as serious as you will soon learn.

Would you advise an alcoholic to count how many glasses he or she tips back before that person gets drunk? Isn't the counting of calories just as ridiculous if we do not focus on the addiction driving the overconsumption?

Oh, by the way, alcohol in moderation, that is, less than twelve ounces of wine, eight ounces of beer and two ounces of hard liquor a day[194] have enough antioxidants, like resvaratrol, to reduce IR; it does so through one of the gut hormones that talk to the brain thermostat, adiponectin.[195]

Don't Put Any Weight on Your Scale

Your weight is not the best way to tell how you are doing as far as your metabolism is concerned. Besides, our weight has become a huge emotional trigger, derailing many a resolution to lose weight, even in the most strong-willed. Focusing on our weight creates obsessive behavior and micromanaging that cannot be sustained, but only by those with Spartan characters.

Our waist circumferences are a better indicator of how our metabolisms are doing. When we fix our metabolisms, and when we overcome our addiction to refined foods, we gain more muscle and lose more fat. Since muscle weighs more than fat, it is conceivable that one may put on more weight. If we are not aware of this, we may become discouraged, especially when the weight loss appears to plateau. Many people give up eating healthier and exercising before they achieve their goal if they only focus on their weight.

Often, the ideal weight they shoot for is unrealistic and oblivious of the muscle gain that naturally occurs when we mature. If you are aiming to return to your high school weight, you will likely fail. Or worse, if you achieve that goal, you will look like you have been fighting cancer and you won't feel so good. Not achieving those unrealistic expectations often leads to the wrong conclusion: "I am condemned to be obese." Thus discouraged, people often go back to eating what is convenient. Sweet death, then, resumes its unrelenting course.

Story Time

I weigh twenty-five pounds more than I did in high school but I still wear the same pants size; I have a thirty-one-inch waist. At fifty-six years old, I personally think that I look better than that scrawny-looking teenager, shyly smiling for the prom picture with the rental tag still hanging from his tuxedo . . .

I advise you to throw away that little scale in the bathroom. Don't you trip on it every morning anyway? I guess you could renovate and expand your bathroom. Stop micromanaging and obsessing over your weight. You look like those weekend warrior-types who go out running, loaded up with a heart monitor, a scuba diving stopwatch, a belt to hold two bottles of water, and an iPod. Some crazy exercisers wear umbrella-types of hats and running shoes with lights that tell them how far they have run. How long do you guess this type of runner will keep up that routine?

Please, stop weighing yourself and concentrate on your waist size; it will shrink slowly, but surely, as you overcome your sugar addiction. Do you remember the commercial showing an overweight middle-aged male trotting around the weight room after weighing himself, only to get back on the scale after a few seconds? This is what happens when we focus on our weight, without understanding that it is not our weight—but our *waist*— that matters. Again, obsessing over our weight has diminishing returns. Emotions run high about weight; a perfect set up to give up trying when we don't see the weight drop when and as we think it should.

Better Motivation

If you understand the simple principles outlined in this book, you will be motivated to shrink your waist for your health. Then, you will patiently buy new pants every once in a while. Your weight will go down as an afterthought, or as a welcome "side effect" of focusing on your health. Your waist may be carrying too much visceral adipose tissue (VAT), not-so-affectionately also known as a "beer-belly" or a "breadbasket."[196] Skinny people may be hiding fat on the inside of the abdomen, which also increases the risk of endocrine disruption.[197] Not surprisingly, VAT is strongly associated with inflammation and oxidation[198]—integral components of the mechanisms of Toiling.

VAT should be an essential part of evaluating people's tendencies to develop the metabolic syndrome,[199] especially when VAT has been associated with diabetes and heart disease.[200] VAT should be discussed as much as we talk about our weight,[201] if not emphasized as the number one way to evaluate our metabolic function. Eating a diet high in vegetable protein and loaded with micronutrients—as opposed to processed, white, astronaut food—will help us reduce our VATs.[202]

Instead of sticking to the old refrain, "calories in, calories out," we need to consider the efficiency of each patient's metabolism, or what is now being called "personal metabolomics";[203] VAT is a reflection of our own personal metabolisms.

Now, please, skip the following part if you feel your sexuality is best discussed in church, a view I deeply respect.

Sexual Motivation

As your health improves, your libido will get stronger, like everything else. You will look better to your partner and to yourself. Hopefully, both of you have agreed to improve your lives at the same time, thus accruing the benefits of being healthy together. This will strengthen your relationship and decrease the chances that you split up in the future.

In my opinion, it is not healthy to separate our sex lives from our emotional, and/or spiritual lives. I think our libidos are God-given impulses to not only procreate, but to cement our relation-

51

ships within the bounds of mutual respect, honesty, and consent. To deprive ourselves of our sexualities in order to "save energy" — to channel it for individual "enlightenment" — seems, to me, rather selfish and contradictory to what I believe to be true: the more love we give, the more we receive. In fact, ancient traditions, especially in the Orient, maintain that our sexuality, when engaged correctly, enhances our spiritual lives and quickens our understanding of enlightenment. Look no further than the *Kama Sutra* for a more in-depth perusal of these themes.

I am trying to tell you that a very good motivator to decrease our VATs and adopt a healthy lifestyle is the goal of thoroughly enjoying our sexual lives within the bounds that you and your partner has set for yourselves. If this is shocking to you, check your testosterone levels, whether you are a man or a woman, and delve into your childhood, looking for clues that your sexuality may have been derailed by some traumatic event. These comments should at least put a smile on your face and justify those "naughty thoughts" you and your partner delight in, instead of putting you off.

Again, if your religious faith is your spiritual barometer, I hereby reiterate my desire to avoid offending you. I am no sexual expert, but fifty-six years of living, reading many books and articles on this subject, my clinical experience and my many years of spiritual training in practically all philosophies and religions, gives me the boldness to put my neck out like this. Ultimately, I have heard that small voice within my heart, assuring me that these ideas are okay, at least for me.

Ask yourself if it is worth it to you to munch on that Twinkie. Would you rather munch on almonds or a pear, so that you can get better sex later? The answer may well depend on your level of maturity, which dictates whether you may postpone small pleasures in order to get more pleasure, spiritual or physical, down the road.

Later in this book, you will see that testosterone issues, in both men and women, are linked to IR.

Fixing Our Thermostats: The Second Brain

One of the most dramatic discoveries in biology in the last decade is the fact that our VATs put out hormones that talk to the brain to regulate our appetites. The article, "To Eat or Not to Eat: How the Gut Talks to the Brain,"[204] discusses the hormonal connection between the gut and the brain. Also, the environment in our intestines influences our brains on what to eat, how much, and how often. As mentioned above, this is one of the reasons why the failing and oversimplified refrain of "calories in, calories out" does not work for everyone. The *New England Journal of Medicine* wisely concludes that:

> "It is unlikely that any one molecule or derivative will provide a magic bullet to induce and maintain weight loss. Successful treatment for obesity may be possible only by simultaneously targeting the interlocking, redundant systems that drive food intake and act to resist the loss of body fat."

The article, "The Gut Yields Clues to Obesity, Therapies,"[205] confirms that many hormones from our VATs have a significant impact on how our thermostats work. VAT and bad fats in the diet also put a bit of bother on the hypothalamic-pituitary-adrenal (HPA) axis, which compounds the negative effect on the brain thermostat.[206]

As you read on, you will see that the hormone oxyntomodulin, from the gut, is but one of the many hormones that continue to be discovered with a role on how much we eat.[207] Ultimately, the hormonal messages from the gut to the thermostat must be corrected for people to lose weight.[208]

MRI studies have shown that sweets have a significant impact on our thermostats in the hypothalamus and on how our gut hormones function. When we stop eating processed foods, we begin to heal this brain-gut connection, especially when we eat good amounts of essential fatty acids, since these micronutrients are vital for the health of all organs, especially the ones mentioned above. Besides, our brains are made up of 80 percent fat (I know some people whose brains are 100 percent fat . . .).

By now you may be able to guess which hormone from the gut has the most devastating effect on this brain-gut connection. Eating food high in sugar triggers the release of too much insulin; this is the most serious hormonal imbalance that messes up our brain thermostats.[209] In my opinion, this is the main cause of obesity.[210]

Supplements?

I generally do not recommend any supplements until I see that my patients are committed to changing their diets. I think that recommending supplements too early may enable some people to continue eating poorly and avoid overcoming their addictions. Some patients are very interested in solutions outside of themselves—the "quick fix" that will allow them to leave their cozy lifestyles undisturbed. Sadly, some practitioners are all too eager to comply and talk about supplementation without attempting to motivate patients to first change their diets. This understandable attitude is often the subtle result of being engaged in the sales of said supplements. Opponents of non-pharmaceutical approaches use this practice to cast aspersions at the entire nutritional medicine field. This is why, as a professor, I have never sold any items to my patients.

However, having said all of that, I do recommend some key nutrients in high doses; again, only *after* my patients have committed to overcoming their sugar addictions.

There are several things one may take to improve the function of our thermostat. The amino acid L-carnitine, 1 to 2 grams a day is indispensable for essential fatty acids to be incorporated into our cell membranes, particularly in the hypothalamus. Carnitine also functions as a vitamin that is essential for our metabolisms.[211]

Taking 600 milligrams a day of the antioxidant, alpha lipoic acid (ALA), has been show to help fix our thermostats, too. It decreases our appetites, specifically by working on the mitochondria of the cells that make up the hypothalamic thermostat. Additionally, ALA increases the metabolism in our "peripheral muscles," thus burning more energy.[212] I say "peripheral muscles" to differentiate them from the excessive muscle some of us have "centrally," that is, in the brain. ALA also increases our storages of the vital antioxidant glutathione.[213]

Pinoleic acid from Korean pine nuts is also helpful. People may reduce their food intake by 36 percent with pinoleic acid.[214] This substance encourages better function of hormones from intestines and their action in the brain. The hormones CCK and GLP-1 are 60 and 25 percent higher respectively in people taking pinoleic acid just four hours after ingestion; patients' desires to eat dropped 29 and 36 percent respectively. Also, people's blood pressure[215] and their bad low-density lipoprotein (LDL) cholesterol dropped.[216] As you will soon see, the common denominator to these problems is our E&I, and cell communication, or IR.

I also recommend (to those who can afford it) several other items to help them improve their metabolism: vitamin D3, DHEA, Korean ginseng, iodine, resveratrol, Guar gum fiber, chromium,[217] and green tea.[218] In subsequent chapters, we will discuss why these items help in detail and provide you with references to justify their use.

"The Right Brain Hypothesis for Obesity"[219]

The right front part of the brain is called the prefrontal cortex (PFC); it's involved in cognitive control of food intake, especially under conflicting situations, when inappropriate responses need to be inhibited. The PFC is also involved in self-image, self-recognition, spontaneous physical activity, the drive to move, sedentary behavior, apathy, disturbed sensitivity to several body signals, lack of embarrassment, and central fatigue. All of these functions seem to be impaired in obese patients. This may also explain why obese patients don't stick with weight loss programs. For example, obese people often display poor compliance in breast cancer screening programs, even though they are more at risk.

"Reflective eating," that is, eating with awareness of the damage or healing food brings to us, and self-awareness may be altered in the PFC. This problem has also been associated with weight gain, changes in personality, and dementia. *Great,* you're probably thinking now. *That's just what we need: to be crazy about bad food.*

The hormones leptin and insulin target the PFC; when they

are not functioning optimally, they may alter our metabolisms by influencing how our thermostats work. Also, the HPA axis affects the PFC, according to the article "The Right Brain Hypothesis for Obesity"

"Stressors that are perceived as uncontrollable, such as those that arise from social conflict . . . shame, defeat, frustration, and fear of social rejection are commonly perceived... as unattainable success. This chronic psycho-social stress, characterized by threat to self-esteem and the anticipation of an impending and lasting challenge, may disinhibit reflexive circuits through a cortisol-induced right PFC dysfunction caused by a prolonged activation of the HPA axis."

In case you are wondering what can be done about all this, this article talks about placing magnets on that part of your head. Maybe McDonald's restaurants could put the magnets in their "Happy Meals," instead of the worthless toys they usually include in the boxes. It also reinforces previous research that shows that the brain controls incoming and outgoing neuro-hormonal signals that influence our glucose metabolisms, energy spending, and storage. The brain is insulin sensitive; eating garbage that causes too much of an insulin elevation through IR causes overeating, weight gain, and liver IR. As we have already seen, the risk of these disorders is strongly increased by environmental factors that favor weight gain, such as an abundance of highly palatable, calorie-dense foods and minimal physical activity.[220]

Bummer

Brace yourself for a discussion on a very disturbing point. The article, "Childhood Sexual Abuse and its Psychological Correlates in the Obese Female Patient,"[221] tells us that approximately 33 percent of women have been sexually abused in the United States—a disturbing figure that is likely much higher than boys being abused. Many of these victims end up with compromised thermostat functions in the brain, specifically, their HPA axes are disturbed. This can have serious consequences on their metabolisms, and also their psyches. Abused women seem to subconsciously gain weight to protect themselves from potential sexual predators.

If you cannot lose weight, despite your best efforts, please consider investigating your childhood, because 90 percent of abused women have blocked out those dreadful memories. Children do not have the emotional maturity to deal with these catastrophic events; they may choose not to think about unpleasant memories.[222] The extent of the problem may not be known since some families often choose not to report these "embarrassing" violations. It's a sad commentary on the state of our society.

Chapter 4

Sweeteners = Methadone?

Comparing sweeteners to methadone is a rather tortured analogy, but hear me out. I intend to make the case that artificial sweeteners merely prolong the addiction to refined sugars, often with the same serious consequences we see with the real processed refined sugar we are trying to avoid to cut down on calories. Some doctors use methadone to help patients withdraw from narcotics, notwithstanding the serious side effects that may be seen, including death. This is standard practice and here is where my analogy breaks down. Again, be patient and read on . . .

The amount of caloric sweeteners consumed per person, per year, in the United States has increased from 38 pounds in 1880, to 149 pounds, or one cup a day, in 2005. This increase mirrors the increase in refined sugars and our exploding epidemic of obesity and diabetes. Since so many people have bought into the lies perpetuated by the manufacturers and marketers of artificial sweeteners, a quick overview of how we stumbled across these sweet poisons will help you see that using them is much like going from the frying pan to the fire. If you wish to read a more detailed account of this problem, read the book from which I gleaned most of the following data, *Sweet Deception*, by Dr. Joseph Mercola.[223]

You will see that these toxins, even in small amounts, contribute to our cell membranes' toxicity, or TOILing, which compromise cell communication, increase IR, and affect our metabolisms. They seem to increase appetite as well.[224] The concept that small amounts of chemicals have a profound effect on our metabolisms has been named "xenohormesis."[225]

Since artificial sweeteners are marketed to avoid sugar and lose weight, the analogy of using the very toxic drug methadone to overcome an opioid addiction is not that far fetched.

Consider the Source

Artificial sweeteners were discovered by accident. Saccharin, the first sweetener we were lied to about, is a derivative of toluene—a clear liquid produced in the process of making gasoline from crude oil and in making carbon residues from coal. Toluene is used in paints, paint thinners, fingernail polish, lacquers, adhesives, and rubber. Of course, it is very toxic. An accidental spill on the hand of its discoverer turned out to taste sweet and, well, the rest is history.[226]

Monsanto, well known for its lies and dirty-dealing in pesticides, was founded just to promote saccharin in 1901. What was its main customer at the time? Some rinky-dink company called Coca-Cola. Monsanto has gone on to include pesticides in the genetic code of many crops; approximately 60 percent of food produced in the United States has pesticides altering the genes of these foods. Remember that Monsanto developed pesticides from leftover nerve gas from World Wars I and II. Suffice it to say that most governments and banks in Europe have voiced concerns about Monsanto's dealings with what we now call "genetically modified organisms," or GMOs.

Interestingly, pesticides have been shown to increase the risk of developing diabetes.[227] So, the artificial sweeteners we are using, while they cut down on calories, may be even more harmful than the sugar we are trying to avoid. The damage these poisons are causing to our metabolisms will become more obvious in the next few pages.

In 1912, saccharin was banned because of emerging data on its side effects and health risks. But saccharin was soon back on the market because the World Wars in 1914 and 1939 created shortages of sugar. Any reservations about saccharin were swept under the carpet despite data showing an association with cancer in laboratory animals, especially bladder tumors.[228] Saccharin was allowed to remain on the market only because the public could not do without its sweet fix. This is why saccharin had a label warning people that it can cause cancer in animals. However, this label was removed in 2001.

Animal Studies

The concept of animal testing is a very curious thing. It is widely used to test and approve pharmaceutical products; but critics dismiss it when it comes to testing potential toxins. Why this double standard? Many people think that animal testing results are a very good approximation of the toxicity of chemicals humans are exposed to. What is good for the goose is good for Gus and Gayle; animal studies do tell us something about ourselves:

> "In the absence of adequate data on humans, it is biologically possible and prudent to regard agents and mixtures for which there is sufficient evidence of carcinogenicity in experimental animals as if they presented a carcinogenic risk to humans."[229]

More Sweet Lies

Soon after saccharin, other artificial sweeteners began to appear. Cyclamate was accidentally discovered in 1937 by a researcher working on fever-lowering drugs. But the sweet byproduct of his work was also eventually banned. Studies on rats and dogs showed that cyclamate caused testicular atrophy and reduced sperm counts (same as other xenoestogens, like pesticides). The main reason cyclamate was banned, however, was because its consumption would have exceeded the acceptable daily intake of 300 milligrams per day. Cyclamate was the main ingredient of Sweet 'N Low®, which now is composed of saccharin and dextrose.

Alitame (Aclame™) was discovered in 1979. It is made from

the amino acids, L-aspartic and D-alanine. It appears safer than other sweetener to date, but it is closely related to aspartame (see below), which has been associated with significant deceptive practices. Besides, alitame has not been tested in combination with other sweeteners. To this day, alitame has not been approved for use in the United States, although it is being used in Australia, New Zealand, Mexico, and China.

Acesulfame-K (Ace-K, Sunnett®) was also discovered by accident, while researchers worked in the production of fertilizers. It contains methylene chloride, a known carcinogen, as well as the reason for headaches, mental confusion, depression, liver problems, kidney problems, bronchitis, nausea, lack of balance, and visual disturbances in many people. Note that these claims were found to not be significant enough by the FDA.[230]

Neotame is aspartame plus 3-di-methyl-butyl. The United States Environmental Protection Agency (EPA) lists the latter as one of the most toxic chemicals known. Yet, it was approved for general use in 2002 with the support of laboratory data produced by Monsanto. No independent laboratories have produced any data on neotame's safety.

Like Sweet 'N Low, other products are blends of artificial and natural sweeteners. They combine the artificial garbage described above, plus sucralose, xylitol, and HFCS. They are supposed to save you money, but they really don't. They do, however, hide the chemical aftertaste of the artificial ingredients. They also make it very convenient for marketers to come up with new products.

Artificial Sweet Politics: Aspartame[231]

Aspartame is best known as NutraSweet® and Equal®. It has been found to increase the risk of cancers, such as lymphoma and leukemia, in quantities equivalent to four or five servings of diet soda in a 150-pound person. The European Ramazzini Foundation of Oncology and Environmental Sciences conducted a study that showed the original 1970s research done by G.D. Searle & Company, which claimed aspartame to be safe, was actually flawed.[232] Donald Rumsfeld, former secretary of defense under former United States president George W. Bush, was the CEO at the time. Does that mean anything to you?

Searle only tested less than 688 rats that were sacrificed with less than two years of life. A new study tested 1,900 rats and checked them for problems after three years, or the human equivalent of fifty-three years, which is the average of when we start getting cancers like prostate cancer.[233] Searle, at the time, was also criticized by a United States Food and Drug Administration (FDA) report that stated that its studies were "poorly conceived, carelessly executed, or inaccurately analyzed or reported." The FDA also cited a lack of training by the scientists analyzing tissue samples was a "substantial" loss of information, because of tissue decomposition and inadequate monitoring of feeding doses.

A grand jury investigation in Chicago looked into these irregularities, plus Searle's "concealing of material facts and making false statements in reports of animal studies conducted to establish the safety of the drug, aldactone, and the food additive, aspartame." However, the grand jury was never convened because Samuel K. Skinner, then the United States attorney for the Chicago area, left that low-paying position to work for a high-paying law firm representing Searle. Do you smell a rat going through a revolving door?

The FDA didn't give up. It continued to question the data from Searle, even pointing out that there was an increase in brain tumors, too. An FDA board of scientists recommended withholding approval of aspartame, but a review of Searle's tumor slides by academicians paid by Searle showed that there were no problems with aspartame. Finally, in 1981, aspartame was deemed safe by the FDA's Arthur Hull Hayes, who left the agency the year after to work for Burson-Marsteller, the public agency handling Searle at the time.

Of a total of 166 studies on aspartame, seventy-four were financed by the industry. They cited no problems at all. Of the ninety-two independent studies, eighty-four identified adverse effects: "far too much to be a coincidence"; yet, studies financed by the industry keep coming out saying that aspartame is not a problem.[234]

When you realize that 10 percent of the aspartame you consume becomes methanol or wood alcohol, you may want to make some changes in your life. It turns out that one can of diet soda has

16 milligrams of methanol in it. The EPA has determined that this dangerous substance should not be consumed over 8 milligrams a day. Even at cold temperatures, methanol can also break down into formaldehyde, which may disrupt cellular and DNA function.[235] The World Health Organization (WHO) has determined that exposure to formaldehyde should not exceed 0.05 parts per million.[236]

Want to be pickled before you die? Take aspartame.

Part of the problem is that most studies on aspartame have only looked for tumors, without realizing that it is also a potent neurotoxin and endocrine disrupter. This is why many psychiatrists see more depression, attention deficit disorder (ADD) and panic disorders in people consuming aspartame. In addition to the lymphomas documented above, aspartame may cause headaches, depression, mental retardation (through phenylketonuria, or the PKU mechanism), seizures, and visual disturbances.

Leaky Brain

All these problems have one thing in common: disturbance of the blood brain barrier (BBB). As noted elsewhere, cells shrivel up and die when they are TOILing, thereby causing leakiness of the tissues they compose. This is also seen in the brain, where toxins now may leak through the previously thought impregnable BBB. A dramatic presentation of this problem is the often-documented phenomenon of inverted vision with aspartame. Some people have suffered from a total flipping of the visual field, so that they have the sensation of being upside down. Even more dramatic is the blindness reported.[237]

Other documented side effects of aspartame include: genetic damage, fatigue, chest pain, dizziness, sleeping problems, burning skin, musculo-skeletal problems, gastrointestinal symptoms, nausea, palpitations, lack of concentration, infertility, low birth weight, memory deficits, and dexterity impairment. All told, roughly one million people have experienced adverse reactions with aspartame.[238]

If you want to know more about aspartame, read the book, *Aspartame Disease: An Ignored Epidemic,* by Dr. H. J. Roberts.[239]

Splenda® and Equal®, Anyone?

After all that data about aspartame, do you really believe that Splenda and Equal are okay? If you do, I have some land in the Everglades I would like to sell you . . .

Splenda and Equal are sucralose, a chlorinated artificial sugar derivative up to six hundred times sweeter than sugar. It was also discovered by accident, while researchers were trying to come up with a new insecticide by using sulfuryl chloride. It took more than eleven years of twisting the FDA's arm to get Splenda approved in 1998. There are only six published human studies on sucralose; the longest one was only thirteen weeks, but McNeil, the makers of Splenda, reported an unpublished study that lasted six months. All these studies focused on Splenda's effects on diabetics, not the general population. In total, they involved 191 people—hardly a reassuring number of subjects.

Three animal studies lasted about two years, using approximately two hundred rats and a few dogs.[240] Yet, McNeil claims that "more than one hundred studies conducted over a twenty-year period" have established the safety of Splenda. These findings may be true, but said studies, if they exist, are unpublished and not available to the public. Furthermore, McNeil would have conducted almost all of those studies itself.

Do you still want to buy my land?

Despite clear evidence that chloride compounds are not safe, Splenda is now found in practically all processed foods. This has led to significant exposure, which has been linked, in the short term, to agitation, seizures, hallucinations, respiratory problems, irregular heartbeat, cough, shortness of breath, nausea, vomiting, diarrhea, abdominal pain, skin rashes, headaches, dizziness, paralysis of the face, tongue, and extremities, respiratory failure, ear, nose, and throat irritation, blurred vision, and pulmonary edema. Other than those setbacks, Splenda is quite safe . . .

In the long term, Splenda has been linked to the following problems in animals (mostly rats): lack of appetite, central nervous system disturbances, reduced growth rate, decreased red blood cells, shrunken thymus, decreased thyroid function, mineral losses, decreased urination, enlarged colon, enlarged liver and brain, shrunken ovaries, enlarged and calcified kidneys, increased adrenal cortical hemorrhaging, and increased cataracts.

Do you really want to continue eating this garbage?

Only 15 percent of Splenda is absorbed, leaving the rest to irritate your intestines. Irritable bowel syndrome (IBS), a problem that afflicts 25 percent of people in the United States, may well be caused or aggravated by artificial sweeteners. Add all the refined sugar, the trans-hydrogenated fatty acids, the ibuprofen-like drugs, etc, and you have yourself a real irritable tummy.

Splenda is glucuronidated, or detoxified in the liver, which means it is fat-soluble, thus contradicting McNeil's claims that it is only water-soluble. This is a major point in considering the safety of Splenda, which is described as eliminated by the gastro-intestinal system "without side effects." This has been shown to be false.[241] Splenda is furthermore metabolized into twenty-one compounds—most of them chlorine-based—thus creating a very acidic environment inside our intestines.[242] Can you imagine what these products are doing to our natural intestinal flora? Additionally, these byproducts have been shown to cause infertility, brain damage, liver toxicity, depletion of the antioxidant glutathione, genetic changes, and low birth weight in rats.[243]

A study conducted on eighteen pregnant rabbits showed disturbing results, which NcNeil blamed mostly on the effects of tube feeding. Most of the mommy rabbits aborted their fetuses and showed significant gastrointestinal disturbances; yet, NcNeil reported no effects whatsoever.[244] If it is so "safe" in rabbits, why has Splenda not been tested in pregnant women? Do you think it is safe in children? An independent study on mice by Japanese researchers found significant damage to intestinal organs and induced DNA damage, concluding that more extensive studies should be undertaken.[245]

Don't let the "ose" ending in sucralose fool you. This is not a natural sugar as the makers of Splenda would like you to believe. The Sugar Association and the makers of Equal (Merisant) sued McNeil for making these false claims. In 2007, the suit was settled for an undisclosed amount.[246]

But it is true that McNeil adds to Splenda dextrose and maltodextrin, or refined corn syrups, in starch form. It does this to make the chemicals more palatable, affordable, and easier to handle and bake with. The end result is a much more expensive sweetener. The bottom line is that Splenda is 99 percent sugar. So, it is a lie that Splenda has no calories and it is "sugar-free." You end up paying more for Splenda than you would have by buying straight sugar. Dr. Richard K. Bernstein, author of *Diabetes Solutions*,[247] urges people not to consume Splenda or any artificial sweeteners—period.

Do you think that the 250,000+ toxins released into the air and water around the sucralose plant in McIntosh, Ala., may be affecting the people living close by? The neighbors think so.

What About Stevia?

This natural sweetening herb is very safe; Mother Nature does a better job and without toxicity. Stevia reduces IR because it helps TOILing at the cell membrane level.[248] This is why it also lowers blood pressure[249] and reduces cavities. So, why have we not been using it in processed foods?

If you guessed that the artificial sweeteners have played dirty politics to keep it off the market, you are correct. The American Herbal Products Association (AHPA) and Lipton have not been able to compete with the armies of lawyers, public relations agents, and lobbyists on the payrolls of Pfizer, Monsanto, Johnson & Johnson, Abbot Laboratories, and Hoechst—until now. The AHPA and Lipton presented compelling evidence that Stevia has no safety issues in 1994, but the FDA turned down Stevia for consideration as a sweetener under "Generally Recognized as Safe" (GRAS) status, which allows for grandfathering of old sweeteners and other supplements.

Because of this, Stevia/Sucanat® could only be used as a sweetener if consumers add it to food or drinks themselves as a powder or pill to their homemade products. It could not be used in the production of industrialized foods, that is, until Coca-Cola decided to use Stevia in its Odwalla and Sprite drinks. The announcement was made December 21, 2008, but these drinks were to be available only in New York and Chicago.[250] Many countries have been using Stevia in their commercial products, most notably Japan, where they have reported no side effects from Stevia in the last thirty years.[251] The Japanese even use it in their version of Diet Coke™.

If you want more information on how to use Stevia, including your cooking and baking, get *The Stevia Cookbook*, by Dr. Ray Sahelian and Donna Gates.

Healthier Sweeteners, Yes, But . . .

Okay, you cannot lick your sugar addiction so you want safer sweeteners. They're available, *butt* (the extra "t" is intentional) . . . can you afford the extra calories? If you are really skinny, maybe you can get away with these unnecessary extra calories. However, most of us cannot afford this luxury, since we struggle with genetic tendencies to IR, especially as we age.

Raw organic honey has been shown to be quite safe and it has many health benefits to boot. However, most of the honey available is neither raw nor organic. To be considered raw, honey has to guarantee not to have been heated over 117 degrees Fahrenheit, which destroys a significant amount of micronutrients in the honey. Because of this, raw honey may be contaminated with bacteria. This is why pregnant and nursing women, and infants who are less than one year of age, must avoid it. Immunocompromised people, the elderly, and those taking statin drugs should avoid raw honey to lessen the risk of exposure to botulism. Only about one-third of honey available in the United States is considered natural. Most of it is likely produced by feeding bees HFCS. You may find natural honey at your local Farmers' Market. Honey also fights mutating bacteria in the intestines.[252]

Date sugar is 85 percent sucrose. It has minerals, betacarotene, B vitamins, folic acid, and fiber. It does not dissolve very well and you cannot bake with it. Most people use it by sprinkling it over recipes or to sweeten a smoothie. Date sugar has been shown to help children with ADD because of its high concentration of the amino acid tryptophan, which has a calming affect. Date sugar and honey are less processed, thus preferable to the more refined ones.

Barley malt is made from the sprouted grains of barley; it contains mostly maltose. It is not very good for cooking and it will spoil if it's not refrigerated. In the United States, barley malt is mostly camouflaged HFCS. The FDA does not appear to care about this deception because it believes HFCS is okay. Real barley malt is high in fiber; it helps relieve constipation and irritable bowel syndrome.

Brown rice syrup comes from fermenting brown rice, which involves significant processing that loses many micronutrients. Brown rice syrup is mostly maltose; it is less sweet than sugar. It may be used in most recipes but it is difficult to bake with.

Lo Han Kuo is the momordica fruit, which is in the same family as cucumbers and melons. It has a licorice flavor; this is the main reason it is not used very much. It is 250 times sweeter than sugar but without the calories. Mercola states in his book "sweet Deception" that Lo Han Kuo has been used in China as a cooling nutrient in many diseases and it has a very good safety record.

Maple syrup is sap from maple trees. It has lots of trace minerals and it is 90 percent sucrose. It should be refrigerated upon opening. Organic brands are more expensive; therefore better, since they avoid formaldehyde used in the processing of regular brands. Maple syrup may be used for baking.

Molasses is the leftovers from sugar refining out of sugarcane and sugar beets. As such, it contains all of the nutrients that the sugar industry discards to come up with the addicting sugar you crave. What a world we live in, huh? Molasses consists of 50 percent sugar; the other 50 percent is water, amino acids, and minerals. In fact, molasses is a very good source of the latter. The lighter molasses is, the more sugar it has.

Sucanat® comes from drying up the juice from sugarcane; it is much less processed and it still has molasses in it, but it is very expensive. Food companies use it to avoid labeling their products "sugar," thus violating an FDA regulation. This is another deception, since it is as toxic and addicting as sugar. It may be used in baking, but it burns more readily.

Turbinado sugar is regular sugar with a small amount of molasses added to call it "natural." Other products, like agave syrup, claim to be natural as well, but it is really high fructose inulin syrup, similar to HFCS, and just as toxic. The FDA is doing nothing about this garbage being sold as a healthy alternative, even in health food stores.

Fructo-oligo-saccharides (FOS) is a soluble fiber that feeds friendly bacteria and reduces IR.[253] But that is not what you may be getting when you buy products labeled with FOS as an ingredient, since it is often nothing but fructose—another blow to truth in labeling. Fructose, itself, is natural, but it is often highly processed and even replaced with outright HFCS in the refined products you buy.

Fruit juice concentrates are one of the best examples of deceptive labeling and nothing is being done about it. These concentrates are just sugar; they are just as toxic as the worst refined products you find. The companies using them have done such a great job marketing these products that I often find strong resistance from patients whose addiction to concentrated juices makes it hard to believe that they are not what they appear to be. These juices increase IR.[254]

IR is worsened by the lack of fiber in these juices, which makes the sugar in them more damaging, since fiber mitigates the high rise in sugar absorption from the intestines. These so-called natural juices are also pasteurized; this process destroys the enzymes and micronutrients found in fruits. Worst of all, they increase obesity in children, particularly those below the poverty line who love the sweet taste and partake of these juices as a misplaced effort to eat healthy.[255]

Perhaps this will convince you: a half a cup of whole orange segments has 59 calories and 14 grams of carbs, whereas a half a cup of orange concentrate has 226 calories, and 54 grams of carbs.

Sugar alcohols (polyols) are a mixture of sugar and alcohol; yet, they are labeled "sugar-free," despite having half the calories of sugar. Polyols are found in just about every product you buy—especially those chocolate bars trying to pass as healthy alternatives. It is true that sugar alcohols are found in low levels in fruits and vegetables, but in such company, they do not cause any problems. It is the highly processed polyols that are questionable, they may elevate fat levels in the blood that lead to bloating, diarrhea, dehydration, malnutrition, and even an increase in tumor formation. There is only one polyol that appears to be good for us: xylitol (see below). It has been shown to be low in the glycemic index, which means it is low in sugar.[256]

Another deceptive polyol is tagatose, or naturalose®. It tries to pass itself for natural fructose extracted from the heating of dairy—yet another deception designed to facilitate your sugar addiction. The health claims are equally false, but the indigestion it may cause is very real. Just as phony are the natural, sugar-free claims of shugr™, which is nothing but a mixture of the some of the sweeteners described above.

Perhaps the worst example of the marketing going on to maintain people's addictions is senomyx®, a chemical that fools your taste buds into thinking that what you are eating is more sweet and salty. Kraft, Nestle, Coca-Cola, and the Campbell Soup Company plan to use it. They will not be required to list senomyx on their labels by its name because only a tiny amount is required to fool you—in more ways than one. Your only warning on the label will be "artificial flavors."

The Big Bottom Line

Not convinced yet? Then you're really addicted, aren't you? Perhaps this will help you break away: artificial sweeteners, in general, increase the risk of cancer in humans by 30 percent if consumed over 1.7 grams per day.[257]

Unfortunately, artificial sweeteners have an impact on our thermostats in our brains and our cell membranes throughout our bodies. They perceive sweeteners as flat-out sugar. Consequently, one may avoid calories by eating sweeteners, but not the hormonal messages we discussed above, and the cell membrane toxicity caused by these agents. In other words, artificial sweeteners do not correct the obesity problem; they make it worse. The resulting TOILing leads to IR, metabolic problems, hormonal dysfunction, (thyroid, adrenals, etc.), poor brain-gut function, hypothalamus, and pre-frontal cortex dysfunction.

Artificial sweeteners are still seen as toxic agents by our bodies, much like the refined sugars you are trying to replace. Yes, they do not have the calories you fear, but they also lack the micronutrients you need to avoid oxidation, inflammation, toxicity, and lack of E&I at the cellular level. Have you ever seen people losing weight while using sweeteners? As you will see below, toxins, like artificial sweeteners, still cause people to gain weight. According to researchers at Purdue University, foods sweetened with no-calorie saccharin can lead to greater body-weight gain that would consuming the same food sweetened with high-calorie sugar."[258] This is the reason why even diet soda causes weight gain and IR.

Your consumption of sweeteners also tells me that you are still in the throws of a sugar addiction. If you just quit sugar, in a few weeks your taste buds and your thermostat will be functioning much better, so that you may taste the natural sugars in all foods. Eventually, consuming refined sugars will correctly be perceived as too sweet and too toxic. You will also fix your thermostat and will then be able to "obey your hunger." Please, believe me: quitting sugar will make it so that fruits, legumes, and whole grain breads will be sweet enough to satisfy your sugar cravings. Truly, using sweeteners is much like using methadone to quit a narcotic addiction; it just prolongs the addiction.

Chapter 5

Sweet Politics

We will not avoid a sweet death until we examine the politics and economics fueling the massive addictions we have to refined sugars. While I understand the wish to tread lightly around the powerbrokers of America, I feel the time is right to take back our health and face the "the man behind the curtain." Simply put, the economic unraveling of 2008 has also affected our health care industry, Big Food, Big Pharma, and the health insurance industry; the people running them (into the ground) went to the same business schools and pal around in the same circles.

Health issues need to rise above politics; health care does not obey the same principles that govern Darwinian Capitalism. Unfortunately, science often takes a backseat to narrow political interests.[259] For instance, a former surgeon general, Dr. Richard Carmona, was told by the Bush, Jr., administration to refrain from discussing stem cell research, mental health, emergency contraception, abstinence, and several other politicized issues: "I was blocked at every turn, told to stand down, that the decision has already been made,"[260] he said. We will now see that the same political pressures contribute to our country's sweet death. Unfortunately, the health care reform debate in the fall of 2009 does not appear to be interested in addressing it.

Our Fat in the Fire

Our addiction to sugar began to increase exponentially around thirty years ago when the federal government helped Big Pharma and Big Food in their campaigns to demonize fat, despite clear evidence that fat was not the cause of heart disease. The *New York Times Magazine* article, "What if Fat Doesn't Make You Fat,"[261] re-emphasized what the journal, *Science*, the most prestigious scientific journal in the world, revealed a few months before in the article, "Nutrition: The Soft Science of Dietary Fat."[262]

Fats were demonized for the benefit of certain special interests.[263] But the argument that good fats do not make us fat is very hard to swallow, thanks to the highly successful campaign referred to above. I still see patients worrying about the fat in olives, avocados, and nuts.

Around 1980, the National Institute of Health spent hundreds of millions of dollars on five studies that found no correlation between fat and heart disease. About the same time, Merk, the pharmaceutical company making lovastatin/mevacor—a drug extracted from fermented red rice—showed that their drug lowered cholesterol and reduced the incidence of heart disease. Their marketing department used this single study to convince the federal government that fat was the problem behind heart disease; never mind the millions of neutral dollars already spent in studies showing no correlation.

The feds felt that people would start consuming more fruits and vegetables to replace the demonized fat when they launched a massive campaign to warn Americans about fats' dangers. Phil Handler, then President of the National Academy of Science, did not agree with this approach:

> "What right has the federal government to propose that the American people conduct a vast nutritional experiment, with themselves as subject, on the strength of so very little evidence that it will do them any good?"[264]

Today we see more and more evidence that the "right fats"—like medium chain triglycerides, unsaturated fats, and omega three oils—in our diets prevent obesity, hypertension, IR, and

73

cholesterol problems:[265] the very diseases that are integral components of the metabolic syndrome. It's not fats in general that are bad; only saturated and trans-hydrogenated fats are, particularly fats from animals that have been exposed to antibiotics, steroids, pesticides, and growth-promoting hormones. Only the saturated and trans-hydrogenated fats have been shown to increase the risk of developing diabetes by increasing IR,[266] whereas the unsaturated fats—especially from vegetarian sources—reduce the risk of metabolic problems, including heart disease, substantially reducing the risk of death.[267]

Moreover, we have genetic tendencies in the production of more or less "brown fat," which helps the body handle calories better. The optimal expression of this gene seems to be programmed in the embryo's stem cells.[268] Still, mothers' healthy eating habits are likely to tip the scales in favor of brown fat formation.

The Results

The results of the "experiment" condemned by Handler are now clear: we have a massive epidemic of obesity and diabetes that seems to have started when the food industry took over the nutritional teaching in our country by spending $33 billion per year in advertisements to sell us processed food—mostly refined sugars and simple carbs—claiming that their "fat-free" products would be good for us.

All the while, farmers spent about $2 million a year back then, advertising their fresh and unprocessed produce. What do you think people will eat with this kind of unbalanced advertising saturating the airwaves? Cheaper junk food makes it even easier for poor people to perpetuate their dependence on processed food.

We cannot improve our food supply until we deal with the politics and economics driving this sweet death.

"The health food industry needs to take a leaf out of the junk food industry and promote its products more effectively."[269] Well, we tried. In the 1990s, the government and farmers launched a campaign to increase the consumption of fruits and vegetables in the United States. Their modest recommendation of eating five servings a day, which, according to the latest data should be *thir-*

teen servings a day, was a smashing success: Americans increased their intake from one-and-a-half to two servings of vegetables per day.

Go ahead and laugh, but I'm afraid this is not a joke. How badly are we doing when consumption went up only one-half a serving per day? What did we expect though, when we are up against $33 billion of yearly advertisements for foods that are leading us to our sweet deaths?

After that short-lived campaign, Americans went back to eating French fries and their ketchup, their average daily intake of fruits and vegetables. Americans are now eating less fat and more refined sugar than ever, which is the root of the diabetes/ obesity epidemic.[270] Of course, the Sugar Association of America disagrees with these facts.[271]

It is time to restore natural fats—like olives, nuts, fish, and vegetarian fats—into our diets.

Are There Beneficial Effects of Cholesterol-Lowering Drugs?

The evidence presented by the makers of lovastatin was used to assume that fat was the cause for heart disease. There is now irrefutable evidence that the beneficial effect of many drugs that help heart disease (and the same goes for fermented red rice and most herbs) is through the mechanism of lowering inflammation and oxidation with antioxidants.[272] In other words, the original cholesterol lowering drug, Mevacor®, was helping heart disease not so much through its cholesterol-lowering effect, but through its anti-inflammatory and antioxidant effects. This was confirmed by a study that showed these drugs work by lowering the C-Reactive Protein, CRP marker of inflammation, "regardless of the levels of LDL."[273]

"Big Food" Wants to Help Us

Companies processing food in the United States are now trying to recreate themselves as deeply caring about our health, much like the tobacco industry has done. But, the reality, according to the medical journal Lancet, is that:

75

"The majority of food companies are not fully engaged with the seriousness and urgency of today's health challenges… in failing to respond… companies appear to be distancing themselves from their responsibility for unhealthy consumer choices… Only a small minority of companies are engaging with the health agenda and rethinking their business strategy accordingly."[274]

The WHO recently suggested restricting added sugars to 10 percent of total calories consumed. Big Food complained that this was "too restrictive." Isn't it nice how the industry looks out for us? But, the final WHO report shows that the WHO caved in; it now only recommends to "restrict free sugars" without mentioning a specific percentage. What could the WHO do with a budget smaller than the combined budget of Coca-Cola and Pepsi?

Here is a sample of Big Food's business approach to our health.

Company Sales (United States Dollars in Billions) Advertising Expenses/Statements		
Coca Cola	$21	2.2 *"The company exists to benefit and refresh everyone it touches."*
CanAgra	$14.5	Not available *"We touch lives of many people. This brings with it a special responsibility, one we take to heart."*
Danone	$18	1.2 *"Help people around the world, live better and get more out of life through tastier, more varied and healthier food products, every day."*
Kraft	$32	1.6 *"Our vision is about meeting consumer's needs and making food an easier, healthier, more enjoyable part of life."*
PepsiCo	$29.3	1.7 *Our health and wellness initiatives strengthen our commitment to contribute to the well-being of our consumers."*

Company Sales (United States Dollars in Billions) Advertising Expenses/Statements		
Kroger	$51.1	0.667 *"Our mission is to be a leader in the distribution and merchandising of food, health, personal care and related consumable products and services."*
McDonald's	$51.3	0.723 *"McDonald's cares about the well-being issues that are so important to many of our customers."*

HFCS

The trend toward more refined foods laden with HFCS co-incided with a decrease in fiber intake and the beginning of the diabetes and obesity epidemic.[275] Protein, especially vegetarian-based, was never given a chance, despite clear evidence that protein lowers cholesterol levels.[276] HFCS is arguably the most powerful tool with which Big Food fueled the flames of our national addiction to sugar. Since it is cheaply produced, due to our own farming subsidy policies, HFCS is now found in practically all processed food.

Big Food continues to deny that HFCS has anything to do with our sweet death epidemic. Studies funded by the food industry pop up once in a while to reassure the public that we may continue eating this poison with impunity.[277] While it may be true that the calories in HFCS may not add up to obesity (which I doubt), Big Food fails to take into account the TOILing that HFCS triggers in the cell membrane and the marked metabolic/hormonal changes that result.[278]

Homo Economicus

It has become very clear to Americans that the health care industry, pharmaceuticals, insurance companies, and the food industry are engaging in practices that are just as questionable and, at times, just as illegal and immoral as the rest of the corporate world. It's useless to deny the obvious: people are heavily influenced by money. Our nation's founders were very aware of this issue. Thomas Jefferson was very vocal in his opposition to our penchant for elitism and its close partner, wealth. His buddy, John Adams, was more realistic about our human nature, arguing that we needed to manage it, regulate it, but not deny it. They argued until they died the same day on July 4—fifty years after the Declaration of Independence.[279]

Even though Jefferson's version of America ended up winning the day, the tension of their argument still rages in our country, as well as around the rest of the world. While both philosophies are equally worthy, my contention is that John Adams's viewpoint is often buried under a mountain on Jeffersonian idealism, which maintains that the poor shall inherit the Earth. As much as I get teary-eyed every time I am in Jefferson's rotunda in Washington, D.C., I feel that the present state of affairs in our country proves Adams correct: money and the elitism it begets are running our country. To deny this fact is a losing battle. But we don't have to let it ruin our lives.

It is a self-evident truth that we need money to provide for our basic necessities. Money is a symbol of the work we do. Money is a symbol of E&I (sound familiar?). Since the dawn of mankind, humans have conducted "business" to provide for themselves. Trading my chickens for the right to use your mill was the way we bartered in fairness. In fact, we are conducting business right now, you and I: you bought this book to pay for the E&I that I put into it.

Business is such a big part of our nature that some people feel Homo sapiens would be more accurately named "Homo economicus."[280] Adam Smith said "business is a grand and noble enterprise."[281] What is often forgotten is that Smith also said "most of the world troubles come from somebody not knowing when to stop and be content."[282] In my opinion, health care has become big business and the people running it started with the goal to do good but now are happy to do well.

Agribusiness

Agribusiness, or growing food in massive quantities by a few industrialized farmers, has become such a behemoth that we are hard-pressed to even think that we could feed ourselves cheaper and better with locally raised food. We have been brainwashed into relying solely on big chain grocery stores that, for the most part, provide us with processed food that is packaged and produced to last longer on shelves—not to maximize our health.[283] In addition, their approach takes money away from our communities to enrich distant and uncaring corporatists.

The results are pretty clear: devastating chronic illnesses that we are told cannot be managed but only with pharmaceutical products we see advertised on just about all TV programming.

Do you see a problem here?

Are TV and other media, which are owned by the same corporations that own Big Food and Big Pharma, going to tell you that you could avoid chronic health problems by eating better, cheaper, and more organic food that is raised locally by people like you? Are they going to emphasize in the nightly news, sponsored by these corporations, that many answers are simple and self-empowering?

Sugarcoating Bitter Politics

I highly recommend the book, *Food Politics: How the Food Industry Influences Nutrition and Health,* by Marion Nestle.[284] Many scientists favorably reviewed it.[285] Nestle tells us that the United States Department of Agriculture (USDA) should give up its roll of advising people on what to eat, since that role conflicts with its other job of promoting the interests of Big Food. She also corroborates what we already knew: there are many behind-the-scene deals made with politicians to encourage legislation to maximize Big Food's profits—*not* people's health.

A glaring example of this is the scheming by Big Food that led to a mountain of misinformation in the form of the Food Guide Pyramid. This is why Physicians for Social Responsibility (PSR), an organization I have personally joined, has called for the ousting of seven of thirteen federal committee members who were in charge of revising the Food Guide Pyramid because of their financial and organizational conflicts of interest.[286] PSR won the 1985 Nobel Peace Prize.

According to the Center for Responsible Politics, candidates for the United States congress and presidency received more than

$12 million between 1989 and 2000 from the sugar industry.[287] This is not surprising in light of the scandalous affairs in the corporate world discovered in 2002 and 2008, which highlighted the dearth of social responsibility in modern corporations. The food industry is no different.[288] Neither is the health industry, for that matter.

The United States government heavily subsidizes sugar production. About 42 percent of the money goes to 1 percent of growers—most of them in Florida. These farmers have donated so much to their politicians' campaigns that their Political Action Committee (PAC) donations rank tenth in the country. This buys them access to politicians.

A Little Gossip

A glaring example of this disturbing "access" issue is found in the 1998 book chronicling the politics surrounding the Monica Lewinsky scandal, *The Starr Report,* by the *Washington Post* and Kenneth W. Starr. When former President Bill Clinton was breaking up with Lewinsky in the oval office, a call came in from Alfonso "Alfy" Fanjul, a prominent sugar grower from Florida, who had access to Clinton's attention at such a delicate time and on a federal holiday, no less. Apparently, Fanjul was upset about the report that former Vice President Al Gore had recently spoken about heavily taxing sugar and eliminating the farm subsidies. Needless to say, neither took place after his phone call: money buys access.

. . . And it also buys the chance to build the greatest monopoly of Sugar Growers we have ever seen. Now that the Fanjul family is getting ready to take over United States Sugar, adding to their Domino Sugar, C&H Sugar, and many other international sugar companies, any sugar you put in your mouth will come from its sweet empire.[289]

Politics and Economics = E&I

Today it is cheaper for a family to eat at McDonald's than to buy fresh fruits and vegetables. Poor people don't have the money or the time to buy and cook fresh foods. The less education people have, the more influenced they are by food commercials, which makes people more susceptible to misinformation contained in said ads. Watch most people's carts at the grocery store: they are spilling over with foods in cans, bags, and boxes; these items are highly refined, high in calories, and low in micronutrients. This is why the lower the socioeconomic status, the higher the risk of type 2 diabetes.[290]

It is well known that nutritional research is influenced by Big Food's money. The *Journal of Nutrition Education and Behavior* acknowledges eight corporate sponsors. The *American Journal of Clinical Nutrition* lists twenty-eight companies supporting them, including Coca-Cola, Gerber, Nestle/Carnation, Monsanto, Procter & Gamble, Slim-Fast Foods Company, and the Sugar Association. This is the rule rather than the exemption when it comes to journals and dietetic associations. In fact, the Dairy Council and the Sugar Association of America sponsor the American Dietetic Association (ADA). The ADA acknowledges donations of $735,000 from groups and individuals contributing over $10,000 during the 1998 and 1999 fiscal years. About 8 percent of the ADA's annual budget comes from the Sugar Association.[291]

Could this be why the ADA "never criticizes the food industry?"[292] The ADA is definitely pro-Big Food. One of its main tenants is that "there is no such thing as good or bad food." The ADA routinely carries a page of federal nutrition news compiled by the Sugar Association of America.

Willie Nelson's Biofuel

"The stage is now set for direct competition for grain between the eight hundred million people who own automobiles and the world's two billion poorest people."[293]

We have all heard about Willie Nelson using leftover cooking oils from French fries to power the diesel engine in his bus. He motors down the road, stinking up the neighborhood, quite happy to be environmentally responsible. I wonder if he also uses weed fumes in his engine . . .

Food is E&I. Biofuels from food tap into foods' E&I. Since our societies also run on E&I, the future struggles for energy sources will make biofuels more and more attractive.[294] The politics of energy, food, and power will soon get more entangled as we leave the era of cheap food and fuels that only lasted fifty years. Ironically, food became very cheap after World War II because of cheap and abundant oil, which fueled corporate agriculture. But the honeymoon is over as we see the price of corn doubling and wheat futures at their highest in a decade.[295]

More people on the globe drive up demand for food and biofuels. In 2007, one-sixth of all the grains grown in the United States were used for "industrial corn" destined to be converted into ethanol. The amount of United States farmland dedicated to biofuels grew by 48 percent in 2006. As the price for a barrel of crude oil goes up, so will the price of biofuels and the price of food. I am sorry to say that subsidized cheap food may become even more attractive in the future (see below). In my opinion, the only way to avert these calamities is to demand that our politicians address our energy issues in a concerted fashion, much like the Marshall Plan to rebuild Europe after World War II. If we don't face the music, Willie Nelson's country Western, crying-in-your-beer songs will come in handy . . .

"Agriculture" of Obesity

The article, "The (Agri) Cultural Contradictions of Obesity,"[296] traces our sweet problems to our farm bill subsidy politics that lead to excessive production of corn by farmers who get about $22 billion per year in subsidies from the government. President Nixon restarted this policy in 1972 to rescue the Soviet Union from a terrible famine. In doing so, he repealed Roosevelt's New Deal laws that limited too much food production. These laws had been in the books to prevent rampant alcoholism (remember Prohibition?) since booze production was the cheapest way to process sugar from too much corn being harvested at the time.

Shhh! "Speak-easy": we don't want to upset the Sugar Association, nor John D. Rockefeller's heirs who surely remember the wheeling and dealing their ancestor used to demonize alcohol, then an important biofuel in early cars. Rockefeller wanted his Standard Oil petroleum to be the fuel of choice; he funded the movement that led to prohibition.

Today, corn and food processing have another outlet other

than alcohol. Turning pennies worth of corn into products or junk food full of HFCS takes care of the artificial abundance of corn and maximizes profits. The consequences of these practices are devastating: (1) abuse of political power to fund farmers, who fund politicians in return, (2) misery in Third World countries unable to compete with our subsidized farmers (3) and rampant obesity in our country, which is worse in our children. Their generation will be the first whose longevity is less than their parents.[297]

The article, "The Fat of the Land,"[298] makes the same points, adding that Dr. James Tillotson, a professor of Food Policy and International Business at Tuft University, has shown that United States public policy encourages obesity at the expense of sound nutritional practices by subsidizing wheat, soy and corn, while ignoring other crops like fruits, vegetables, and other grains.[299]

In June 2007, the American Medical Association (AMA) called for this sad state of affairs to be reversed, especially in school lunches and food assistance programs, which so far have reflected purchasing patterns that support agricultural businesses without regard for nutritional values. This is why school lunches are loaded with cheeseburgers, roast beef with gravy, and sausage-and-cheese pizza; low-fat and vegetarian options are virtually absent. The Salt Lake Tribune reported that

> "WIC [Special Supplemental Nutrition Program for Women, Infants, and Children] programs operate much like Dairy Queen, dumping 24 quarts of milk and 4 pounds of cheese on recipients every month. A woman looking for vegetables will not qualify for a single carrot unless she is breastfeeding. In that case, she will have to make two pounds of carrots last the whole month. She will get no other vegetables or fruits at all, except in WIC's small farmers' market program, which has limited availability."[300]

Marc Morial, president of the National Urban League, stated that since 1985 the actual price of fruits and vegetables has increased 40 percent while the price of sugar and fats has declined by 14 percent. He added, "Underserved communities cannot be denied access to the same healthy and affordable food that is available to more affluent Americans."

83

"The real scandal in Washington is the farm bill," he added. "Senators take millions from corporations that produce fatty foods. Then, Congress buys these unhealthy products and dumps them on our school lunch programs. Companies get rich and kids get fat."[301]

Tyson Foods, Smithfield Foods, and other meat providers have made millions of dollars through this aberration in our farm bill. They perpetuate these gains by regularly contributing thousands of dollars to members of the House and Senate Agriculture Committees and other members of Congress who continue to vote for farm bills favoring meat, corn, wheat, and other crops, like soy.

Soy is used to produce most of the trans-hydrogenated fats used in refined foods. Together with wheat, these foods comprise the bulk of cheap food, which is most of what poor families can afford. These problems are compounded by Big Food's toxic practices, such as coating French fries with sugar and beef flavoring.

Crop subsidies are projected to grow to $190 billion by 2012. Maybe *this* is the apocalyptic vision of the Mayans? In my opinion, this is "corporate welfare" for giant farms, grain brokers, food processors, fast food chains, and prepackaged food companies. But if we so much as dare ask to have some poor soul's medical expenses subsidized, the cry of "welfare state" goes out. No, I am not a communist. I just feel that we could do business with more of a social conscience.[302]

"The fat of the land" also reports that HFCS consumption has grown 1,000 percent since it was created in 1970. The human body processes fructose differently than glucose; the latter releases insulin, which promotes satiety. Fructose does not, since it is processed in the liver. This is why people keep eating it, since they don't feel full. HFCS products also taste sweeter and children soon become addicted because their still-developing brains are more sensitive, according to "The Fat of the Land":

> "We may be damaging the neuronal circuitry in the brain during this highly plastic period of development... People consume more calories when sweetened products are offered as liquids than when they are offered as solids."

Corporate Welfare vs. Our Farmers

The article, "You Are What you Grow,"[303] adds a very interesting twist to our chaotic sweet death politics: our farm subsidies are said to have put two million farmers out of work in Mexico, thus compounding the plight of poor people because their staple food, tortillas, are then more expensive. Many of these displaced farmers end up immigrating to the United States to harvest the very products that caused their unemployment. The author concludes by saying that the United States farm bill must become a food bill.

As much as we feel bad for Mexican farmers, read what Steven L. Hopp, professor of Environmental Studies at Emery and Henry College, has to say about United States farmers:

> "Doesn't the Federal farm bill help out [our] . . . poor farmers? No. It used to, but ever since its inception just after the Depression, the farm bill has slowly been altered by agribusiness lobbyists. It is now largely corporate welfare. The formula for subsidies is based on crop type and volume: from 1995 to 2003, three-fourths of all disbursements went to the top-grossing 10 percent of growers. In 1999, over 70 percent of subsidies went for just two commodity crops: corn and soybeans. These supports promote industrial-scale production, not small diversified farms, and in fact create an environment of competition in which subsidized commodity producers get help crowding the little guys out of business. It is this, rather than any improved efficiency or productiveness, that has allowed corporations to take over farming in the United States, leaving [less] than one-third of our farms still run by families."

But those family-owned farms are the ones more likely to use sustainable techniques, protect the environment, maintain green spaces, use crop rotations, and management for pest and weed controls, and apply fewer chemicals. They are doing exactly what 80 percent of United States consumers prefer to support, while out tax dollars do the opposite."[304]

In chapter 30, we will discuss the inroads that enlightened

politicians and Big Food representatives are beginning to make toward fixing this Faustian bargain. This will benefit consumers throughout the world and make it more likely that they, too, will have a place at the table. After all, immigration, politics, and money are all E&I issues.

How Does Big Food Respond?

Kellogg's reaction to studies condemning processed sugar exemplifies Big Food's reaction to these ideas:

> "We don't apologize for putting sugar in cereals. There is no scientific evidence to implicate sugar as an independent risk of any disease, except for cavities. The last word about sugar in cereals is that children like it."[305]

Great, now "Mickey" is supposed to be our main teacher of nutrition. What a disgrace; if you are not upset, your prefrontal cortex may already be caramelized to a crisp.

Many folks feel that our growing sweet deaths need to be checked by government and industry, both of which could be more socially responsible. I feel that only a public campaign, such as we saw against the tobacco industry, is going to reverse the tide of cookies, Twinkies, and candy bars threatening our well being in catastrophic proportions.[306] "It's our lifestyle and high energy foods. It is one of the greatest challenges in public health of this century. We need a public health approach—and the need is urgent."[307]

Speaking of tobacco, let us not forget that litigation against Phillip Morris led the company to diversify its portfolios by buying Kraft Foods. Changing its name to Altria has not totally diverted our attention to these telling facts. It is my opinion that the tobacco people knew a thing or two about addicting customers to their products, which they vehemently deny, even in the face of mounting evidence proving their guilt. Is it too farfetched to believe that they may have transferred those practices to their new commercial interests? It is well known that monosodium glutamate (MSG), AGE products (Advanced Glycosyated End products are derivatives of cooking refined sugars at high temperature), and who knows what else they put in refined foods cause significant addiction to refined foods.

Sweet Intrigues

Given all the money, power, and politics at stake, it is not surprising that articles are starting to emerge opining that the obesity epidemic is a fabrication. Alex Avery of the Hudson Institute, a think tank in Washington, D.C., feels that the data pointing to an obesity epidemic is flawed. I question his objectivity and I wonder if the Hudson Institute is one of many public relations institutions bought and paid for by Big Food. Consider that Avery has also written the articles, "McDiet: Losing Weight on Fast Food," "Farmed Salmons Are Safe," and "Fear Not the Farms and the Fertilizers."

Because of all of these forces at play, I believe we should instill a "Twinkie tax." Candies and junk food should be heavily taxed, just like tobacco, to discourage consumption and fund the devastating negative consequences on our health. Governor David Patterson of New York has proposed an 18 percent sales tax on soft drinks and other non-diet sugary beverages to help raise $400 million a year.[308] Or, if you don't like taxes, we could stop taxing good food like fruits, vegetables, legumes, whole grains, and lean meats but retain taxes on processed and packaged foods.

I was very disappointed when a Utah doctor successfully campaigned against the Twinkie tax at the 2006 AMA meeting in Las Vegas, Nev., arguing that the Twinkie tax "made a lot of people uncomfortable."

Dear colleague, who was made "uncomfortable"? Who do you work for? Who are you protecting—your patients, or your friends at the Alta Club in Salt Lake City, Utah?

Sweet Food Stamps

Another political problem is the food stamps program. Sadly, the majority of recipients cash in their stamps for junk food, thus displacing more wholesome fruits, vegetables, nuts, etc.[309] In my opinion, and I know this is not politically correct, food stamps should be limited to good foods only. If my tax money is going to help those who are less fortunate than me, I think my voice should carry some weight: we are paying for the rope that hangs them, as well as ourselves. We all end up paying more for chronic health care, even for those who don't have insurance; they end up overburdening our emergency rooms.

Salus Populi

Lawyers are predicting a wave of lawsuits against the food industry for its role in the epidemic of obesity in our country through deceptive and manipulative marketing techniques.[310] I believe Big Food will win those lawsuits for two reasons: one, we cannot compete with the armies of lawyers and public relations people it hires to protect its interests. Two, it is ultimately our responsibility to eat good food, no matter the challenges. Blaming others, instead of looking deep within ourselves, is never going to succeed.

Will things be different in the near future? Since "the business of America is business," it will be a while before we strike at the root of these problems. However, there is hope. Gus Schumaker, a former under secretary of agriculture under George W. Bush, used to be Kellogg's CEO. At first blush, I thought that this was an example of the infamous "revolving door," whereby the government and corporations hire each other's former employees to have some influence in each other's policies. Schumaker may well have been representing Kellogg's best interests while he worked for Bush. However, today, he is singing a different tune:

> "Congress and the administration have a unique opportunity to begin reforms providing a sustainable, community linked food system... Will they take this opportunity to start or will it be business as usual?"[311]

Interestingly, his quote came out on the fourth of July. I believe the business of America should be the health of Americans. Take the ancient Roman law principle; "Salus populi suprema lex esto: the health of the people is the supreme law."[312] Sadly, so far our government (and I feel both major political parties are to blame) has chosen another Roman principle to guide its politics: "Bread and circus." As long as people get lots of food, preferably refined comfort foods and lots of cheap TV entertainment, sprinkled with mind-numbing junk food commercials, people think themselves to be free and will allow governments to do whatever they feel is in the best interest of politicians, thus perpetuating the myth of freedom and democracy. If we were truly a democratic and free people, we would be better informed and we would be compelled to put a stop to all these shenanigans, would we not?

Sweet Deal for Insurance Companies

No health-related book can be written without at least briefly touching on the politics of having almost fifty million uninsured people in the United States. We are the laughing stock of the in-dustrialized world because we are the only country that doesn't have enough social and community responsibility to cover its people's health expenses. Even though we spend about double the money other countries spend per person, per year, America is dead last in health parameters when compared to other rich countries.

From a purely economic perspective, we could save millions of dollars if we covered people's medical expenses before the un-insured are forced to wind up in the emergency room. Even hos-pitals, the bastions of capitalism in health care, are realizing it makes financial sense to care for the uninsured. In New York City, hospitals are saving about 50 percent in emergency room (ER) costs by providing free care clinics for "frequent fliers" without insurance. In one case, caring for a brittle diabetic woman in the ER cost $200,000 per year. With the clinic, the hospital cut that in half.[313]

At the risk of offending the 33 percent of people who approve of George W. Bush, I must report on his comments when asked about covering the uninsured in America: "There is health care in the United States. After all, people can go to the ER."[314] In my opinion, this comment not only reflects a lack of compassion, but also a staggering lack of insight into our health care crisis.

Our economic problems are significantly worsened by the politics of health care. While each of us has a polarizing opinion on this topic, we all agree that the status quo cannot be maintained. The ones that benefit from the chaotic way we now administer health care are the insurance companies, Big Food, and Big Pharma. Hopefully we will be able to discern the lies they plant in the media to shoot down any attempt to take any amount of power from them.

Not having health insurance may be devastating to families, especially where children are involved. The uninsured may not only lack treatments for acute conditions, but also miss out on preventive measures. The latter may mean that people are not educated about their lifestyles or their diets. The result is a higher risk of sweet death in the uninsured.

If you wish to read more about our health care crisis, these books were recently reviewed in the *Journal of the American Medical Association:*

1. *Medicine and the Market: Equity v. Choice* by Daniel Callahan and Angela A. Wasunna

2. *Cities and the Health of the Public* by Nicholas Freudenberg, Sandro Galea, and David Vlahov

3. *The Truth about Health Care: Why Reform is Not Working in America* by David Mechanic

4. *Medical Management of Vulnerable and Underserved Patients: Principles, Practice, and Populations*[315] by Talmadge King, Jr., Margaret Wheeler, Alicia Fernandez, Dean Schillinger, Andy Bindman, Kevin Grumbach, and Teresa Villela

Doctor or Politician?

No doubt some would prefer that I stayed in my office, arguing that my obstreperous discussion on politics and economics is unwarranted in a health book. I disagree,[316] and so does Dr. Edward Hill, the 2005 president of the American Medical Association. He stated that, "Public Health should be every physician's second specialty," at the 2005 Utah Medical Association Annual Meeting in Salt Lake City, Utah.

Aristotle would agree:

"A society's obligation to maintain and improve health is grounded in the ethical principle that a society is obligated to enable human beings to live flourishing and healthy lives... public policy should focus on people's capacity to function and improve meeting health needs... Health improvement and economic development are both linked to individual opportunities to exercise their free agency and participate in political and social decision-making."[317]

I leave you to ponder two things: Nestle's buying Jenny Craig[318] and a quote from Dr. Richard Feynman, a renowned Nobel Prize winner in physics:

"So I have just one wish for you, the good luck to be somewhere where you are free to maintain the kind of integrity I have described, and where you do not feel forced by a need to maintain your position in the organization, or financial support, or so on, to lose your integrity. May you have that freedom."[319]

Chapter 6

Fast(er) Food Nation

The campaign to demonize fats and steer the public to simple, cheap foods full of HFCS contributed to the chaotic way we are eating in our country. In my opinion, this is a moral, physical, and spiritual disaster that is bitterly exemplified when mothers plead with me to help them motivate their children to stop eating refined sugar. It breaks my heart to see the frustration in their loving eyes. What can I say? My own children are also being brainwashed by Big Food. I tell them about food politics and addiction issues, besides giving them the practical suggestions you will find below; I also tell them a story I am saving for the end of this book.

Eating at fast food joints is one of the most toxic things families can do. Parents often end up giving into their kids' whining for those addicting foods. Sadly, parents may also go there because it is cheaper (and faster) to eat there than at home. And, let's not forget that many parents, themselves, are also addicted to that fare.

We may even "super-size" these fast meals for only a few more pennies.[320] These outlets are so conveniently placed that their clustering has been associated with higher rates of obesity. Conversely, the presence of grocery stores, produce vendors, and farmers markets lower the incidence of obesity.[321]

Story Time (Warning: Potentially Offensive)

At least the McDonald brothers Mac and Dick had enough class and social responsibility as a "family restaurant" to choose Mac—not Dick—to name their bestseller sandwich, the "Big Mac."

By the way, the Big Mac celebrated its forty-fifth birthday in 2009; it is starting to outlive most people who eat it.

Over one-half of poor families' budgets are now consumed by the fast food industry.[322] In general, people who are eating at fast food joints are so busy and tired working at two or three low-paying jobs that they don't have the time, or the will, to exercise—making sweet death worse. They get fatter and have even more difficulty working out: another vicious cycle. Less than 2 percent of Americans work out five times a week.[323]

Fast foods have too much refined sugars. Sadly, even moderate elevations of blood sugar in normal people may place metabolic and oxidative stress on the pancreatic B-cells and cardiovascular system to increase the risk for diabetes and heart disease.[324] In practical terms, the more sugar we eat, the more obese we become.[325]

Hugo Size Me

I am not sure what to make of the name of the new super-sized soda at McDonald's. The "Hugo" has 410 calories and it's selling well—conveniently prized at eighty-nine cents in some markets. McDonald's needed to compete with 7-Eleven's big seller, the Big Gulp. McDonald's is, after all, a public company that needs to show profits to its stockholders; it knows that healthy menus just don't sell as well. McDonald's, like most fast food joints, has tried to make its menu healthier, but people buy one salad to ten cheeseburgers. In my opinion, it doesn't matter what the menus look like when people are already addicted to sugar. Would you expect alcoholics to buy more milk if you offer them cheap booze at the same time?

Many nutritionists are of the opinion that super-sized meals are the main reason behind the epidemic of sweet death. The numbers are there to justify that position. Portion sizes are two to five times bigger compared to the early 1980s. A small soda was 7 ounces in 1955; now it is 16 ounces and a child's soda is 12 ounces. What was considered a normal adult meal back then is now a child's meal. The original patty size for an adult's regular meal, plus the French fries, is now a child's Happy Meal.[326]

Isn't it ironic? Now our laptop computers, weighing in at 1.2 pounds, are heavier than our hamburgers . . .

I am sure that the super-sizing of meals is a big part of the problem. But, in my opinion, I think there is another factor that is more important: the disruption of our brain thermostats where we control our appetites. If they were functioning normally, we would be able to stop eating when we felt full, no matter the size of the meal.

If the thermostat in the brain is disturbed, we are not able to judge when to stop eating so many calories. One thing is to eat lots of calories. Another thing is to be healthy enough to know when you are overdoing it. The main question should be why we cannot stop eating all that junk. Shouldn't we feel full when we start to go over the satiety point? A healthy thermostat stops us from eating when we have consumed more than the amount of calories we need.

In response to the problematic existence of fast food joints, Los Angeles, Calif., imposed a moratorium on opening new facilities in July 2008.[327] Even though at first blush this sounds like a prudent thing to do, I am of the opinion that this is a bad move; it only creates heroes out of those constitutionally aggrieved patrons, who then make it a moral issue to stuff themselves with whatever they wish to eat to prove their point.

State of Denial

The word "addiction" is not well received by most people. Only those who are sufficiently self-aware accept this bittersweet truth about their sugar issues. For example, addicted behavior is readily seen in patients who cannot give up soda. "But, Doc, what am I going to drink?" You can see the fear and panic in their faces.

It turns out that "liquid candy," or soda, takes up 14 percent of the calories consumed by the average American. In 1970, when I was a senior in high school, Americans consumed one hundred liters a year. By 2000, that figure, and many people's figures, had doubled. In part, this is the result of eating 25 percent more calories than we did back then.

The sugar industry, under the name "Industry Trade Association"—which includes Coca-Cola, Pepsi, Proctor & Gamble, General Mills, Kraft, and Monsanto—has sponsored seven studies finding no problems with refined sugar. But when the studies are financed by independent sources (seventeen of them), they clearly document the damage inflicted by junk food.[328]

In 2001, NBC ran an exposé called, "Fleecing of America: Sugar." It documented that politicians were seeking $70 million (in addition to the existing $22 billion) to subsidize sugar-growing farmers. There is such an abundance of sugar in our country that farmers want to be subsidized to keep supplies low to drive up price. Of the proposed increase, $65 million was going to only one magnate in Florida. The money that farmers may be getting means that each family in the United States is contributing $26 per year to sugar farmers' subsidies. In other words, taxpayers are subsidizing the very industry that is making them sick. Then, we have to pay ever-spiraling health insurance premiums to treat the ravages created by sweet death. A *New York Times*[329] editorial opines that we should put a stop to these subsidies.

Monitoring Your Food

The commercialization of our diets by Big Food has produced many "studies" intended to maximize their profits, not our health. Since they often contradict each other, depending on what items the USDA has been paid to emphasize, the American public has very little confidence in any nutritional report. In fact, many people choose to ignore any report about foods. This situation is ideal for Big Food. Since people give up on figuring out what is true and what is propaganda, they end up eating what is convenient and what their addicted metabolisms "intuit" they must eat. When it comes to self-monitoring what we eat, we often undercount and under-report refined carbs in our diets.[330] So much for intuition when we are addicted . . .

Monitoring food labeling is not that helpful either. Labels are confusing and the serving sizes are getting bigger—a very good clue for people to eat more at a single seating.[331] Big Food has been caught lying about the contents in its products. Refined foods tend to have real fruit only 50 percent of the time, contrary to their package claims of 100 percent fruit content.[332] Are you surprised?

In the Netherlands, Big Food has started to monitor customers' reactions to food in order to maximize their sales. In so-called "restaurants of the future," your chair will measure your reactions to everything you put in your mouth, how fast you chew, and who knows what else. The data will be used to alter the lights, sounds, and even scents in the restaurant, in order to respond to the feedback that will cause you to consume the most food. These restaurants will even have "face readers," to analyze customers' reactions to the food being served in front of them.[333]

. . . A chair that senses how I react to a restaurant's food? It makes me want to pass gas sitting on it.

"Sugaraholics"

The extent of our addiction to sugar was painfully displayed when I went to the 2004 movie, "The Passion of Christ." It was sad to watch so many people load up on huge buckets of popcorn, soda, candy, nachos with artificial cheese, doughnuts, etc., to sit down to watch the torture of our greatest spiritual icon in our society. Just as sad is the fact that there are very few healthy snacks in theaters. Pop corn without the butter would be OK. I often get a taco salad with chicken; hold the sour cream and the salad dressing, and ask for extra avocado to replace them.

The addiction is so profound that MRIs of the brain show significant responses in the hypothalamus to ingestion of sweets.[334] Sugar addiction is so serious that it has been compared to alcohol addiction[335] and to the addiction physiology of uploads. In fact, refined sugars act exactly like uploads. Sugar hooks up to the same receptors for uploads in the brain,[336] as do drugs like Valium. A study showed that a sugar addiction in rats is as powerful as an addiction to heroin.[337]

Some of you may argue that you are not addicted to sugar. Fair enough. Could you prove it to yourself by refraining from it for a week? Hopefully, you can be honest with yourself, keeping in mind that most people hide the sweet truth when they talk to doctors.[338] How could we possibly lick our sugar addiction, or any addiction for that matter, if we do not own up to it?

Most people continue to eat lots of sugar because everybody else does it. They may even feel it is the "American thing to do." Okay, I can understand that; my response is to say that we do well to question whatever culture we belong to because bad habits and attitudes are often perpetuated by socialization. The Holy Book would agree.[339]

Why Do We Get Addicted to Anything?

When we are traumatized emotionally or physically early in our childhoods, we are left with a void that cannot be filled. Unless we revisit those events with the eyes of an adult, we will carry that baggage, or emotional imprinting/programming, for the rest of our lives.[340] We often try to fill that void with anything outside of ourselves, like junk food, that may hold a glimmer of hope of making those empty feelings go away.

The extra boost of energy and the calming effect of processed foods perpetuate our addiction; the strain on our adrenal glands, which loan us some energy from the future, may then continue unabated. Quick junk food shortcuts make our addiction to said food stronger. This is how we easily succumb to ads and the siren songs from anybody trying to satisfy their own agenda of gratification at the expense of our well being.

"Life is suffering," said the Buddha and the masked man in *The Princess Bride.* "Anyone who says otherwise is trying to sell you something," added Wesley, hiding behind the mask. It is "as you wish." Will you face those skeletons in the closet and face your suffering, or continue to fill the void with addictions?

We tend to overburden our intimate relationships, expecting them to heal our broken spirits; this leads to more heartbreak, over and over again. Most people go on to the next relationship, blaming the break-up on their sad luck of not being blessed with the good fortune of finding their soul mate. If they only found

97

the right partners, surely everything would be better, like the pop songs they load in their iPods suggest. In a way, it seems that we even have the ability to get addicted to toxic relationships.

Throw in the pressures of our rushed lifestyles, our "bread and circus" society, our polluted environments, our socioeconomic and agricultural policies, and you may see why our goose is cooked in very sweet sauce. Only restored self-respect and self-sufficiency can heal our broken hearts. Only then can we lick our addictions and fill those emotional holes that only love of self and love of others can fill. Only then may we forgive the hurt done to us in the past.

In my opinion, discovering that our egos or our thoughts are nothing but biologic tools to deal with our world around us—much like our eyesight and hearing—brings immense healing. We then may see that our wounded feelings are only on the surface. Our true spiritual nature cannot be harmed. Only putting off our egos may bring on this healing realization.

Of course, the addiction is also physiologic, as we have already discussed.

Is there a division between the mind and the body? No. We must consider all the angles that perpetuate our addictions and harness all of our resources to overcome them—even using pharmaceutical agents, if necessary.[341] In a society where we see way too many prescription drugs being abused and more and more illegal traffic of addicting drugs, our addiction to sugar is an integral part of the problem.

Birds of a Feather

Our friends' and loved ones' addictions may also influence our own behaviors. A study from the University of San Diego showed that our risk of obesity goes up more than 40 percent when those close to us have a lifestyle that increases their VAT. If we hang out with an obese friend, our risk of obesity goes up 57 percent; it goes up 40 percent if a sibling is obese and 37 percent if a spouse is obese. If we are really chummy with these contacts, the risk of obesity almost triples.[342]

Some people have wondered if hanging out with obese people may increase the risk of "catching obesity." Maybe so; we already saw how bugs in the intestines may mess up our metabolisms. Perhaps we infect others with those very organisms when we live close to them. In my opinion, the problem is more likely to be from our addictions getting reinforced by others who are just as addicted, if not more so. Do you feel like eating a salad when your honey is diving into a huge bowl of macaroni and cheese? Do you go jogging when your roommate would rather watch a reality show on TV?

However, hanging out with thinner people may be a bit of a problem since the obese may feel very self-conscious and thinner people may discriminate and look down on them. The end result is that the behavior of obese people is mutually reinforced.

Compounding the Addictions

Even seemingly unrelated products are aggravating the addictions driving our sweet deaths. Steroids fed to farm animals diminish our bodies' abilities to handle crabs.[343] The antibiotics that we feed animals also contribute to metabolic problems. Excessive coffee over stimulates the adrenal glands, worsening diabetic tendencies.[344] Lack of zinc in our diets, from eating few vegetables, causes our taste bud to under-function. People are then driven to eat more sugar because it is the only thing they are able to taste. This leads to even fewer vegetables in the diet, thus perpetuating a vicious cycle.[345]

Urban sprawl, the result of short-sighted energy policies cemented in the 1950s, makes us drive more and walk less, compounding the staggering inactivity and lack of exercise that afflicts our society.[346] "Years of Life Lost Due to Obesity" is a grim report on this sad state of affairs.[347] The Lancet estimates that correcting urban sprawl would result in people walking an extra fifteen to twenty minutes a day, enough to lose the one hundred extra kilocalories most people eat. Physical activity does not have to be exercising, but engaging in gardening, taking stairs rather than elevators, etc.

"Cities need to be built to human scale, not automobile scale . . . Building safe schools, bicycle trails and community projects . . . Physicians need to shift from an individualistic approach and ask what in the environment prevents people from incorporating activity into their lives and what changes to recommend to policy makers."[348]

My home state of Utah recently published statistics showing that walk able communities had a 39 percent obesity rate, whereas the cities suffering the most from urban sprawl had an obesity rate of 66 percent.[349] Of course, the latter cities tend to be blue collar, so, the income and education level of people are probably contributing to the difference in rates.

Our society's policies continue to increase the gap between the haves and have-nots, the latter already more at risk to become obese. The anger that fills our fellowmen who are not invited to the party causes more metabolic and health problems that poverty alone could explain.[350]

The United States is the industrialized country with the lowest rate of vacations taken each year; the French take the most. Our rushed lifestyles, a consequence of our national character of putting business ahead of everything else, often rob us of enough restorative sleep, causing significant metabolic changes and IR.[351] Children routinely sleep one to two hours less than the 9-12 hours they need.[352]

Sleep deprivation makes us crave sugary snacks more,[353] which increases IR, the BMI, and the risk of obesity.[354] Lack of sleep causes an inflammatory, or Toiling, state[355] that is aggravated by the increase in leptin levels seen with sleep deprivation. (Leptin is one of those hormones that go from the gut to the brain thermostat.)[356] Getting our "beauty sleep" takes on a new meaning. If we only sleep two to four hours each night, the risk of obesity increases by 73 percent; five hours a night decreases to 50 percent; and six hours per night goes down to 23 percent. These figures were disclosed at the 2004 Annual Meeting of the North American Association for the study of Obesity in Las Vegas, Nev. I wonder how many of the delegates stayed up partying all night as part of their "research"?

Rushed lifestyles also result in skipping breakfast, which is very stressful to our bodies. The added stress drives up insulin and cortisol levels in the bloodstream, increasing the risk of diabetes and obesity by 455 percent.[357] Having skipped breakfast, people are starving to death about the time they find themselves conveniently near fast food or vending machines. Speaking of "starving to death," each year in the United States approximately thirteen people are killed by vending machines in freak accidents. I wonder how many die from the junk in the machines in the long run . . .

It is very easy to eat poorly when caught up in this treadmill lifestyle perpetuated by our socioeconomic stress. We end up dragging ourselves home after frustrating commutes on crowded highways and freeways and breathing fumes that compromise our metabolisms. When we get home we want to drown our frustration in "comfort food." Most people end up gorging themselves for lunch or dinner, elevating their blood sugar excessively. We go to bed bloated, filled with poorly digested food that is low in fiber and high in sugar—the perfect recipe for disturbed sleep. It is also another vicious cycle perpetuating our addiction and our growing number of rings around our straining belly. Stuffing ourselves like that increases the risk of developing diabetes.[358]

Here is another vicious cycle: sleep apnea due to obesity causes IR[359] and metabolic problems drive sleep apnea.[360] This is enough to make you lose sleep. Sleep apnea, or snoring that causes a drop of oxygen levels, increases the risk of heart disease in type 2 diabetics,[361] raises the risk of metabolic problems five times,[362] and raises the risk of diabetes type 2 three times.[363]

Pollution and Addictions

"You have to be kidding!" This is the typical reaction I get when I point out that toxins in the environment are contributing to IR, our sweet deaths, and addictions.[364] For example, pollution in traffic worsens our TOILing thermostat cells in the brain. Toxins like Agent Orange, or dioxin, have been linked to diabetes[365]—the same as heavy metals like mercury and arsenic.[366] Unfortunately, all of us have these toxins in our bodies from being exposed to our industrialized environments.[367] Environmental pollution is such a serious problem that I have dedicated an entire chapter to it; I just wanted to give you a sampler to round out the discussion on the forces that contribute to our addictions.

Doctors in our Fast(er) Food Nation

The New England Journal of Medicine reported that

"Despite the evidence of benefit, dietary fiber ingestion by diabetics has not increased. In part, this failure is due to the lack of educational campaigns. Also, there is insufficient awareness on the part of physicians of the benefits of dietary treatment. Although dietitians do have an important role in patient care, the key to dietary changes is the repetition of dietary education by the Primary Care Provider at each visit. Doctors are too busy documenting their activities to invest the considerable effort required for dietary counseling. Insurance companies don't reimburse for such efforts."[368]

Two extremely important issues are highlighted in this article.

The first is the fiber problem. The shift to processed diets has been well correlated with a lack of fiber. The empty foods we are brainwashed to eat have very little fiber, if any. Most people eat only half of the 25 grams recommended. Fiber can overcome IR by delaying the absorption of sugar so that our bodies are not blasted by too much sugar being absorbed too quickly.[369] Fiber also decreases the release of insulin in the first half hour of a meal, even in normal people.[370] People who ate oligofructose, a type of soluble dietary fiber derived from chicory root, lost about 1 kilogram of body fat over a twelve-week period in the absence of dieting and exercise.[371] By the way, black, green, and mulberry teas also block the absorption of refined carbs;[372] there is more information on fiber in chapter 32.

The other point of the article is that doctors are "nutritionally deficient." Doctors' involvement in nutrition is often limited to offhanded remarks like "all you need is a balanced diet," despite the fact that they usually don't have the time to discuss what that means. Sometimes doctors confuse patients with unrealistic plans about their diets, particularly in diabetes. It is best to frame nutrition through patients' perspectives and give them more personal freedom. In other words, empower patients to treat themselves after they are given sound and unbiased advice.[373]

In my opinion, doctors often buy into the calories in =calories out paradigm; adding unrealistic discussions on portions sizes, percentages of fats, sugars, and proteins only serve to pacify the obvious need to do something quick without a good understanding of the complex issues driving our addiction to sweets.

Jail Food

The prophet, Daniel, wound up in jail where he was fed the king's meat and junk food.[374] After a while, he started to feel like trash; he asked to be feed "pulse," or a natural diet of fresh water, grains, and vegetables. "Come back in ten days and I bet I will look better," said Daniel. Sure enough, in ten days he was back to feeling and looking good. The rest is history, much like we will be if we continue to eat "jail food" that is being marketed so cheaply so that we feel rich and in control of our fates.

Remember "bread and circus"?

Chapter 7

Everything Has Sugar: The Glycemic Index

Have you ever wondered why you love some foods more than others? For example, we all love potatoes. I still have scars to show for misbehaving in the kitchen; I used to sneak a few spoonfuls of mashed potatoes while they were still on the stove, eliciting my mom's ire. All foods have sugar; we seem to like most the ones with a higher glycemic index. I am talking about natural sugars—not those that are processed, refined, or contaminated with HFCS.[375]

The glycemic index lists the sugar content of all foods;[376] it also recommends consuming foods lower in the index, especially if we have metabolic issues.[377] The index was determined by – measuring blood glucose at two-hour increments after consuming a test food (containing 50 grams of available carbs), relative to that of a control food(white bread or glucose.) Researchers found that mixing foods of different glycemic index results in slowing down glucose absorption. For instance, peanut butter—which is high in fat, fiber, and protein—slows down the absorption of the sugar found in bread. If you need to add honey or jam to your peanut butter sandwich, you are likely a bit addicted to sugar. If you were not, you would find such a treat too sweet. This is why I delight in organic almond butter on rye bread, without anything else added.

A high glycemic index diet increases IR and contributes to the poor control of sugar levels in diabetics.[378] Foods with the lowest glycemic index are high-protein foods like fruits, vegetables, nuts, and lean meats; after that come the complex/whole grain carbs, and then the simple/refined sugars and fats. Eating lower in the glycemic index helps us to lose weight in a more sustainable way, without starving, since the quality of foods is thereby emphasized more than the quantity.[379]

The ADA used to say that the glycemic index was bad science. Since the ADA has been proven wrong, I have not heard it apologize, nor embrace this concept. Why? In my opinion, it would not be good for Big Food, whose interests are intertwined with the ADA, to say that refined foods with high glycemic indexes are not good for us. How else would you explain the fact that the WHO and most of Europe, Canada, and Australia advocate the low-glycemic index diet while the United States does not?[380] At least the ADA has started to lump junk food in the "sometimes" category; I feel this is a timid approach that will not get the job done.

Dr. David Jenkins came up with the glycemic index concept a number of years ago. Even though he was initially ridiculed for it, he is now revered as a pioneer in the science of nutrition. I was immediately taken by his humor and wisdom when I met him at a conference in Vancouver, Canada. It wasn't hard for me to take his advice to leave the conference early to go running along the waterfront in Stanley Park with his simple and humble teachings resonating in my head.

When Sugar Levels Drop

The diagnosis of "Hypoglycemia" has been ridiculed by the medical profession for some time, despite the evidence that:

> "A high glycemic diet elicits a sequence of hormonal events that challenge the balance of glucose levels in the blood. After such a meal, insulin levels go up—higher than the response triggered by low glycemic meals. The high glycemic meal inhibits glucagon secretion [the hormone in charge of increasing blood glucose when we don't eat].

The resulting elevated ratio of insulin/glucagon inhibits metabolism, and promotes the storage of nutrients in the liver, muscles, and fat. About an hour after a high glycemic meal, blood glucose starts to fall, often below fasting levels, which inhibits the burning of fat tissue. [All these things] stimulate hunger and overeating, in the body's attempt to restore the concentration of metabolic fuels to normal." [381]

Some people get headaches, dizziness, heart palpitations, and several other symptoms when their levels of blood sugar drop too precipitously, due to the yo-yo effect of junk food consumption. This creates "mountains and valleys" of high and low sugar levels in the blood. Insulin climbs with each high glycemic meal and remains in the bloodstream long enough to trigger a drop in sugar levels. This drop triggers the release of hormones that increase sugar levels and cause the heart to race and the other "low sugar" symptoms. The hormones that come to the rescue are cortisol, adrenaline, glucagons, epinephrine, and growth hormone.

Unfortunately, to feel better, most people reach for refined sugars—just like an addict would reach for his or her "fix." Another vicious cycle gets started when:

"Insulin-induced hypoglycemia provokes prolonged overeating, persisting well after restoration of normal glucose levels. Furthermore, hyperinsulinemia and hypoglycemia may preferentially stimulate consumption of high-glycemic index foods, leading to cycles of hypoglycemia and overeating . . . [This is why] the concept of glycemic index has simple public health applications: increase consumption of fruits, vegetables, and legumes, grain products processed according to traditional methods rather that modern methods, and limit intake of potatoes and concentrated sugar." [382]

Reactive hypoglycemia is now considered a pre-diabetic condition because it signals that the thermostat is a bit dysfunctional, a sure sign of TOILing cell membranes. Long gone are the days when several colleagues yelled at my patients, trying to convince them that their welcome improvements of eating a low-glycemic index diet, and eating often, was merely a placebo and that the changes in their diets were too restrictive and unsustainable. I agreed with their last point: a healthy diet is unsustainable in our society, *unless* we face the music, look in the mirror, and brace ourselves to live above the maddening crowd.

And why do we have a hard time doing so? Could it be that money has something to do with it?

> "Regrettably, funding for nutrition research is not endless. Effective dietary change reduces the need for drugs and therefore gives no benefit to the pharmaceutical industry. Lower consumption of processed food does not benefit the food industry. Yet, there is much potential for gain for global health if we find the right nutritional way to address the risk of obesity and diabetes . . . We know the benefits of statin therapies (drugs to lower cholesterol) in coronary disease and can counsel patients accurately. When will we be able to offer nutritional advice with the same confidence?"[383]

The Lancet pulls no punches: "Effective dietary change reduces the need for drugs and therefore gives no benefit to the pharmaceutical industry. Lower consumption of processed food does not benefit the food industry." These are fighting words; Big Food and Big Pharma wouldn't like this sort of thing to spread around. It may make them "uncomfortable." Are you ready to fight for your health, for the health of your loved ones, and especially for the health of your children? I would like to hear your answer to this question.

Dynamic Action

Coincidentally, the foods that require the most energy to consume or the ones that end up providing fewer calories (some of the calories are used in the metabolizing of these foods) are low in the glycemic index. Proteins require 30 percent of the calories they contain to be used in their metabolism, thereby lowering the risk of obesity and IR. Complex carbs require 15 percent; simple carbs 10 percent; and fats 5 percent. This is called the specific dynamic action (SDA) of foods.[384] The practical point: eat more protein.

Sweet Death: A Burning Hell

Remember that inflammation "burns" our cell membranes, a process found in practically all diseases fueled by the high glycemic index meals we consume.[385] The degree of inflammation may be measured with several protein markers; the best know is the C-reactive protein (CRP), now routinely used to measure the degree of "burning" in cardiovascular diseases and in metabolic problems. The process of consuming energy or metabolism produces heat, or TOILing.[386] CRP is higher with a high glycemic diet;[387] a higher CRP has been found to be a predictor of diabetes in Japan.[388] Inflammation and oxidation are practically the same thing. There is also less oxidative damage when we eat low glycemic index meals[389] and the CRP levels drop when we lose weight.[390]

Dr. Atkins

Although many health professionals have warned us about sweet death beginning in our fifties and sixties, Dr. Robert Atkins is the best known out of those pioneering doctors. Even though his diet was poorly conceived (he claimed that all carb should be avoided and that all meat/fat was good), he was somewhat correct in saying that the main problem in nutrition is the excessive consumption of carb.[391] Still, avoiding *all* carbohydratesis clearly wrong and reminiscent of the ill-advised campaign to demonize all fats. It is not the carbs in fruits, vegetables, and whole grains that are problematic; it's the refined carbs.[392] In fact, whole grains reduce IR[393] and help with weight loss.[394]

Atkins also went wrong in advising people to eat toxic trans-hydrogenated and saturated fats, mostly from animal sources, to replace the loss of carbs he advised. Still, after one year, people consuming the Atkins diet lose the most weight[395] and reduce their cholesterol better than low-fat diets.[396] The problem is what happens *after* that year is up. No diet will succeed when we eliminate entire groups of foods.

Good and Bad Carbs

The article, "The Changing Roles of Dietary Carbohydrates: From Simple to Complex,"[397] tells us that "beginning in the 1970s, carbs were recommended as the preferred substitute for fat by the American Heart Association and others to lower cholesterol." But, the advice to restrict fat has led to increased triglycerides and lower good cholesterol, HDL, the very one that lowers inflammation and oxidation.[398]

People ended up consuming high amounts of simple carbs or refined sugars, white breads and pastas, instead of complex carbs found in fruits and vegetables. Eating like that leads to TOILing and IR: the excess insulin thus produced ends up in the liver, whose capacity to correctly handle cholesterol in our diets is then impaired.

Instead of worrying so much about fats in our diets, we would do best to worry about refined sugars because a low-glycemic index diet lowers cholesterol better than a low-fat diet.[399] Still, keep in mind that we do best by avoiding saturated, trans-hydrogenated fats found in animal products and processed foods.

Some worry that low-fat diets may raise triglycerides and decrease HDL because those diets tend to have more carbs. Again, this problem is avoided when the carbs are complex or high in fiber, like fruits, vegetables, nuts and whole grains. Because of the experiment to demonize fats, forty-seven million Americans now have the metabolic syndrome, which may be just as harmful as smoking tobacco.[400]

The above article on carbs also reviews the role of fiber in the metabolic syndrome. Simple carbs can be broken down into monosaccharides (glucose and fructose) and disaccharides (sucrose and lactose). Complex carbs have lots of fiber (soluble, insoluble, nondigestible, lignans, etc.) that slows down the absorption of complex carbs from the intestines, which results in less of a burden to insulin. Conversely, simple carbs are quickly absorbed; more insulin is then needed in a shorter period of time.

The most common soluble fibers are psyllium, beta glucan (oats, barley, and yeast), and pectin (fruit). Just 10 grams of psyllium a day reduces triglycerides by 4 percent and LDL by 7 percent. The Atkins diet is very low in fiber, whereas Dr. Dean

Ornish's diet (mostly vegetarian) is very high in fiber; Dr. Barry Sears' Zone Diet is intermediate. All three of these diets result in a loss of about 2 to 3 kilograms over a year. But, in my opinion, any diet will fail if the issue of sugar addiction is not addressed.

What About Fructose?

Fructose is a sugar mostly found in fruit; it is poorly absorbed from the intestines when it is consumed by itself, that is, in fruits. This means that fruits are not to be feared: we don't get acutely elevated sugar levels in the blood when we eat them.[401] In fact, fructose lowers the Glyco HB/A1C.[402] I feel bad for diabetics who are instructed to avoid fruits, yet they are allowed to eat refined sugars in "exchange diets." Right, let us condone their addiction to refined sugars and eliminate God-given sugars found in fruit . . . It is true that fruits raise blood sugar a bit more than other nutrients, but this is a short-term effect seen right after ingestion, which is mitigated by all the fiber fruits contain. Fiber delays the absorption of sugar from the intestines.

Even though blood sugar goes up a bit more after we first eat fruit, the average daily sugar blood level will not be any higher. Cell receptors are better able to carry out their duties; specifically, they are more sensitive to insulin when we consume fruits.[403] They will be a great treat for you, once you get off refined sugars.

The real problem with fructose is the processed HFCS, which is quickly absorbed and extremely toxic.[404] Fructose metabolism differs from sucrose and glucose. Most of it takes place in the liver where it is almost entirely detoxified unless the liver is over-whelmed by excessive toxins (see below). When this is the case, fructose is partially metabolized into intermediate molecules, like acetyl coenzyme A—a molecule involved in cholesterol process-ing. If fructose is not well detoxified in the liver, it raises trig-lyceride levels; but complex carbs do not.[405] Because of these issues, fructose has also been linked to nonalcoholic fatty liver disease.[406]

Again, do not interpret these facts to mean that fruits are bad for you. Remember that fruits have a lot of fiber so they qualify as complex carbs. HFCS is not a complex carb; it adds to liver overloading because it is not a natural substance. Besides, there is

110

evidence that our livers are quite forgiving; they can put up with 25 percent of calories from HFCS before they are overwhelmed.[407] I am not sure this gives me comfort because studies tend to look at the "average person." Are you an average person? Do you feel like gambling and running the risk you are affected by HFCS more dramatically?

In the long run, fruits provide the correct sugars for glycosylation of cell membranes and they have more micronutrients like antioxidants to keep our cell membranes from becoming oxidized and inflamed. This is why there is less TOILing in cell membranes with fruit consumption.[408] It has been shown that our metabolisms, insulin functions, and lipid profiles do not suffer with fruit.[409]

Story Time

One day, I was standing by a nurses' station at my local hospital in my warm-ups; I was ready to go for a run after tending to a few patients. An overweight doc volunteered some free advice: "Hugo, don't waste your heartbeats by running; they are numbered."

He's right that heartbeats are numbered, but he apparently failed to realize that the transient rise in heartbeats with exercise is offset by the lower heart rate I have the other twenty-three hours of the day. Do the math: higher sugar levels in the blood after eating fruit is a transient effect. The bottom line is that people end up with lower sugar levels the rest of the day because they are reducing IR.

Food and Our Paychecks

Before you go through the evidence below pointing to nutrition as the main solution to our E&I, metabolic, and cell communication problems, I have to tell you about an angry cardiologist who berated me in front of other docs, arguing that there was no evidence that nutrition is helpful. He felt that there was too much controversy in nutrition research to pay much attention. I didn't respond because it was obvious where his paycheck came from: he does research for the pharmaceutical companies.

He did have a point, though: there is a lot of confusion generated by Big Food in order to sell its garbage. The more confused people are about nutrition, the more they will react like my not-so-friendly cardiologist, and the more they will look like him, too: he is very obese.

I bet you have heard the campaign slogan: "Milk does a body good." Well, no, it does not. However, the milk industry continues to lie about the benefits of milk.[410] Another example of creating consumer confusion is that about half of products claiming to contain whole fruits in their products . . . don't have any fruit in them at all.[411]

Getting Too Full Too Fast

Eating too much processed food on the run as if there is no tomorrow worsens IR. It is much like overburdening a motor with too much work all at once, which I often do when I am making carrot juice with the puny little juicers I buy at Kmart.

Our gut gets used to a certain load and quality of food. This is how the seeds of IR and the metabolic syndrome are planted; over eating triggers an:

> "Immune response to food ... intestinal hormones play a central role in insulin secretion and insulin resistance. Excessive postprandial (after meal) glucose rise has harmful effects on the vessel wall endothelium via oxidative stress . . . Metabolic learning and the adaptation of the intestine to nutrition and luminal (inside intestine) factors may influence disease development . . . The metabolic syndrome starts with abnormal postprandial regulation as a consequence of overnutrition and low physical activity in an environment of stress and social frustration."[412]

Slow down when you eat; don't inhale your meal.[413] Chew your food at least twelve times before you swallow.

Stiffed by the Staff of Life

Some people maintain that all foods are created equal[414] and that calories are the only important factor in weight gain. They ignore the "information" part of food/light/energy. This approach seems to dismiss the glycemic index and ignore studies like the one showing that rye promotes more insulin sensitivity than wheat,[415] as do whole grains in general, compared to refined grains.[416] And wheat itself may be a problem: it may cause more TOILing, not only in the thermostat but in the intestines. About 12 percent of children with type 1 diabetes have a wheat allergy that compromises their intestines and increases inflammation.[417] In fact, type 1 diabetes and celiac disease seem to share genetic risk factors.[418]

Yet, we continue to subsidize wheat—not rye. Big Food uses wheat as bulk for all its packaged products. Wheat may be even more questionable for people who have the gene HLA-DQB1*0201. Carriers of this gene are predisposed to even more intestinal damage from wheat.[419] This problem causes more nutritional deficiencies that lead to TOILing. Unfortunately, this issue is rarely entertained in modern medicine.[420] Innovations and the dissemination of new knowledge take quite a long time to gain a foothold in the minds of most people.[421]

The Fattest People in the World

The Dutch are now the tallest people in the world.[422] Don't worry: Americans are still the widest. With our society being brainwashed to eat so poorly, it takes an iron will not to succumb to the $33 billion a year spent on ads by Big Food.

Greg Critser's book, *Fat Land: How Americans Became the Fattest People in the World*, was favorably reviewed by doctors.[423] In it, you will find the concepts discussed above in more detail, including an indictment of doctors who have not emphasized nutrition in their practices. It seems like more and more books about diet and the glycemic index continue to come out, instantly catching people's attention. But perhaps the most appalling evidence of misinformation specifically aimed at our children is the article that claimed that refined sugar does no harm to children and teenagers.[424] As you probably guessed, this article was supported by a grant from the Sugar Association of America.

My friends, "there was never a time when Americans so desperately need sound, unbiased advice on how to eat."[425]

Chapter 8

Whitewashing Bad Food

If you believe, like the ADA does, that all foods are good and that there are no politics in the food industry, you might want to skip this chapter so that you don't get an ulcer reading it.

Slamming a Sacred Cow

Science has repeatedly shown that dairy products are quite problematic. For the purposes of this book, let's focus on the fact that milk increases IR and cow insulin in cows' milk triggers an autoimmune reaction in the intestines to children's native insulin.[426] Despite these facts, the dairy industry is spending a lot of money on propaganda to convince us that "milk does a body good." It has even tried to tell us that milk helps with weight loss, which is not true.[427]

Amy Joy Lanou, author of the book, *Healthy Eating for Life for Children,* is the nutrition director for the Physicians Committee for Responsible Medicine. She reported on the study financed by the dairy industry used to advertise milk for weight loss: only five males completed the protocol on a restricted diet of about five hundred calories a day. The participants lost one pound per week, typical of such diets, while they consumed three to four servings of dairy a day.[428] Lanou also reminds us that milk is 55 percent sugar. This is why dairy calcium supplementation[429] and skim milk do not help lose weight.[430]

Milk is also the single largest source of saturated fat. Even ice cream is suspect: a waffle cone at Ben & Jerry's has 320 calories and one scoop of ice cream has 820 calories and 26 grams of fat; this is why ice cream is a "coronary in a cone."[431] You may want to switch to soy shakes, which are just as nutritious and do not cause IR.[432]

This book is not big enough to show you the many problems we may have when we consume dairy products. So, I will only present this quote from the American Journal of Preventive Medicine for you to "ruminate" on this issue:

> "High milk consumption has consistently not been associated with lower risk of fractures in large prospective studies, whereas increased risks of advanced or fatal prostate cancer have been observed in many studies."[433]

Breast cancer is also increased with milk.[434] In my opinion, milk does not do a body good—not when it is processed and pasteurized as much as it is. You will read even more about milk when we get to the biggest lie about it: osteoporosis.

Have a Cup of Joe, or Not

I wish I had clear and unambiguous data for you when it comes to coffee. Unfortunately, the data are mixed. After reviewing the article below, you may get a sense that coffee is likely okay (I think it is) if not abused. Coffee reminds me of alcohol; by now you know that alcohol is okay in moderation, that is, less than 12 ounces of wine, 8 ounces of beer, and 2 ounces of hard liquor a day. Even elderly people may safely follow these recommendations.[435] In fact, consumed in moderation, alcohol reduces IR[436]—like coffee does.[437] I believe this is the reason why alcohol reduces the risk of heart problems by 38 percent.[438]

But you will still hear about articles saying that coffee may worsen our risk of pre-diabetes.[439] Coffee also has been reported to increase insulin levels after a meal, but not the fasting levels of sugar. One researcher showed that sugar after meals may actually improve by 20 percent if diabetics get off coffee altogether.[440]

I feel the problem is drinking too much coffee, particularly if your liver does not detoxify it very well. Coffee, in excess, increases the risk of non-fatal heart attacks if the person has a slow CYP1A2 allele, or gene, which impairs coffee metabolism in the liver.[441] So, it's not just the coffee itself, but how we handle it in the liver; again, it is the same with alcohol. For example, I will be drunk under the table after one glass of wine while you may prop me up after drinking enough to float a battleship.

Weak adrenal glands, perhaps from genetics or too much trauma—emotional and/or physical—also has a lot to do on how you handle coffee. Then, people with a tendency of TOILing in the cell membranes lining their esophagus and stomach may get symptoms of reflux, and even gastritis with too much coffee. I am one of them; so, I am forced to limit my coffee to one cup a day. My dad died from a bleeding ulcer. I am afraid I inherited his poor tendency to molt the lining of my stomach, which, by the way, is brand new every thirty-six hours.

Compounding the coffee problem is the possible factor of having an addicting personality, which would make it very hard to stop at one or two cups a day because caffeine has an addictive potential. Again, this is the same as alcohol. The AMA recommends that you limit your alcohol intake to one or two drinks a day. Also, don't start drinking if you don't do so now; you don't know how you will react when faced with the potential of developing an addiction. I would advise you to do the same with coffee. A moderate amount has been defined as less than four cups a day. This seems excessive to me; I limit myself to one cup a day with a meal, and never in the morning or late at night.

Get yourself a cup of Joe, or not, and read the highlights of one of the best articles I have seen on coffee: "Is Coffee a Functional Food?"[442]

Coffee has a lot of antioxidants (flavonoids, phenolic compounds, theobromine, xanthine, nicotinic acid, trigonelline, quinolinic acid, tannic acid, pyrogallic acid, and hydroxycinnamic acids). This is why coffee is the single most important source of antioxidants in the United States—a reflection of how low the American diet is in fruits and vegetables[443] Note that coffee's maximum antioxidant activity is maximized when it is roasted medium.

117

Other drinks have antioxidants, too. The most are found in green and black tea, then, in descending order, coffee, Coca-Cola, red wine, carrot juice, apricot nectar, and white wine. Coke is on the list because the company adds teobromines, caffeine, and vitamins. Too bad it also adds HFCS, artificial sweeteners, preservatives, colorings, and acid.

A few quick brew facts to wake you up:[444]

- Unfiltered Italian coffee raises glutathione levels (the strongest antioxidant).
- Coffee decreases the absorption of potassium, magnesium, and manganese.
- The average caffeine content is 58 to 259 milligrams per serving.
- Coffee is best decaffeinated through the supercritical CO2 method. Arabian coffee is 70 percent caffeine free. Ethiopian Coffea arabica is 94 percent caffeine-free.
- Coffee decreases early morning drive sleepiness for about thirty minutes following no sleep and two hours after sleep restriction.
- Coffee reduces breast cancer risk, except in obese women. It decreases liver cirrhosis, pancreatitis gall bladder stones, asthma, and sugar levels after a meal. It also decreases the risk of diabetes and the risk of cardiovascular events.
- Coffee increases body temperature, energy expenditure, testosterone, potency, and sexual activity in elderly women.
- It improves mood, lowers risk of suicide, increases speed of processing information, and improves cognitive performance. Coffee induces better neurologic outcomes, ADD improvement, and lowers risk of Parkinson's disease and Alzheimer's disease. It also improves the dopamine system, which may be useful in alcohol and drug addiction.
- Cappuccino may be used to treat the dry mouth as seen with tricyclic antidepressants.
- However, problems may be seen after four cups a day: withdrawal syndrome, short sleep, increase in blood pressure, increased inflammation, and lower infant birth weight. Additionally, coffee decreases the oxidation of LDL lipids.[445]

Story Time

The first day of spring in 2008 found me sitting outside of my neighborhood Starbucks. I was enjoying the first timid rays of the season—drinking my black coffee and reading the *New York Times*. I could hear people ordering their drinks at the drive-through window from their cars. All of them wanted the fancy, expensive drinks full of sugar that take a long time to make. Nobody ordered the house coffee I prefer. It became obvious they were after the sugar, not so much the coffee. Now, I know, "to each his own," but I am just wondering about why all of them "preferred" the sugar-added coffee. If it were just a matter of taste, wouldn't *some* people have ordered straight black coffee? I did not conduct a scientific poll that day, nor do I claim statistical certainty; mine is just a pedestrian observation that will likely be dismissed by those who may be addicted to sugar. Those that are not addicted, and those who are slowly becoming aware of their sugar addiction, will see these silly statements for what they are: a reason to give us pause.

"Chocoholics"

I used to be one myself. In fact, I survived my medical internship and residency on Tab and peanut M&Ms. Do you know someone who doesn't like chocolate? There is no question that chocolate is the "food of the Gods." Studies on how good chocolate is for us are a dime a dozen. In general, they show that chocolate lowers IR, blood pressure,[446] and the risk of heart disease,[447] probably by decreasing the TOILing of the arterial lining;[448] neurologic problems are also improved.[449] One study showed that dark chocolate, the equivalent of one-and-a-half Hershey kisses, when consumed consistently, lowers blood pressure about 3 points. The polyphenols in dark chocolate have been shown to be critical micronutrients to maintain our nitric oxide systems of arterial wall inflammation in healthy balance.[450]

Now that you are feeling really good about chocolate, I am going to pop your bubble.

Everybody gets really excited when these types of pro-chocolate articles come out and, sometimes, those whom are teetering on the fence about their health begin to eat chocolate—or increase their daily "dose." Sadly, the people who comment on these wonderful and accurate findings leave out some vital information to bring perspective to the chocolate issue:

One, they say nothing about TOILing, E&I issues, or cell communication being improved with any antioxidant that we may be lacking due to overconsumption of junk food.

Two, they don't clarify that what people are really addicted to is not the chocolate. And what might that be? Dairy and refined sugar, the very items chocoholics really crave, but not the chocolate itself. Most chocolates that are mass-produced are heavy on these sweet additions because very few consumers buy the real chocolate. Why not? It is too bitter for most people, especially those whose taste is ruined by sweet death. I have never met a true chocolate addict and I doubt I ever will. You see, it is very hard to be addicted to healthy food. Have you ever tasted true, unadulterated chocolate? If you have, I am sure you can put it aside after only a bite or two; you are done eating it and you don't go around looking for your next fix.

Three, they seldom point people to the real chocolates, like Lindt, which contains 85 percent cocoa. There are several other high-end chocolates that are the real thing. Knock yourself out *if* they are, indeed, real chocolates. I keep a few bars of Lindt on my coffee table to munch on with pine nuts or almonds while I watch the Yankees lose.

Liquid Candy

Soda is so toxic that dentists are now advising people to drink it through a straw. They feel this simple intervention makes soda miss your teeth and go directly to the back of the throat, thereby preserving your pearly whites' integrity.[451] Talk about passing the buck. What about the damage to softer and more delicate tissues than your teeth, like your throat and the whole digestive tract?

This is the "last straw": You best get a straw long enough to come out your rear end.

It turns out that oral health has been linked to more diabetes and diabetes, itself, increases oral health problems.[452]

Sure, your teeth are the first to suffer; but the increase in acidity and reflux caused by soda doesn't just end in discomfort and maybe ulcers: we may get esophageal cancer from it.[453] And this is well before soda is absorbed into our bodies.

Soda and refined sugars have been linked to practically all diseases. For example, drinking soda raises the risk of developing gout by 85 percent.[454] Any drink containing fructose can trigger gout attacks.[455] (A good drink to lower the risk of gout is coffee.[456])

HFCS in pop increases the risk of obesity and diabetes, even though the total number of calories from solid food is decreased in the average drinker;[457] yet another fact demonstrating how our thermostats are altered by liquid candy. One or more sodas a day raises the risk of becoming diabetic by 83 percent.[458] Any sugar-sweetened drink on the market is likely to increase the risk of developing type 2 diabetes, especially in ethnic minorities, like African-American women.[459]

A recent study[460] showed that one serving of liquid candy a day also raises the risk of developing the metabolic syndrome by 48 percent. This means that our cholesterol, blood sugar levels, and blood pressure go up, together with the risk of clotting too much, while we watch rings piling up around our waist. Interestingly, it doesn't make any difference whether soda is regular or diet: both raise the risks of sweet death.[461] Why? Think of "T" for toxicity.

Soda is not only a direct cause of the metabolic problems, but also a marker for the poor eating habits of people who drink it everyday. Researchers have been "surprised by the magnitude of the association." They felt that maybe soda decreases satiety while one eats a meal because one ends up eating more. Or perhaps soda might get people used to a sweeter taste and "into the snacking mode."

The study above followed 2,400 middle-aged people who drank soda for four years, after which Harvard researchers noted that the risk of becoming obese was 31 percent higher. Their triglycerides went up 25 percent, low good cholesterol was 32 percent more common, and patients showed a trend toward higher blood pressure. In my opinion, the most shocking news about this report was the American Heart Association's (AHA) comment that diet soda "remains a good option."[462] We can only hope that the small dip in sales (2.3 percent) in 2007 will become a trend[463] that shows that some people were not fooled by the AHA's reassurance. But don't hold your breath; wait until you see how most people reacted to the Harvard study . . .

The best article on liquid candy that I have come across is called, "Intake of Sugar-Sweetened Beverages and Weight Gain."[464] It is a Harvard review of thirty studies between 1966 and 2005 showing that monitoring a school where soda was limited resulted in significant weight loss in students in twelve months. They also noted that the average American gets 16 percent of daily calories from soda—the largest source of refined sugars. The consumption of soda and sweetened fruit drinks has increased 81 percent in twenty years. One can of soda increases the chances of gaining fifteen pounds in one year. Their conclusions are sobering:

> "Sugar-sweetened beverages, particularly soda, provide little nutritional benefit and increase weight gain and probably the risk of diabetes, fractures, and dental cavities. Given that global incidence rates of overweight and obesity are on the rise, particularly among children and adolescents, it is imperative that current public health strategies include education about beverage intake. Consumption of sugar-sweetened beverages such as soda and fruit drinks should be discouraged, and efforts to promote the consumption of other beverages such as water should be a priority."[465]

Any sweetened beverage increases the BMI[466] and the risk of becoming diabetic.[467] They also increase hunger; yet, they are often marketed to help people lose weight.[468] Undeterred, the American Beverage Association continues to fund studies saying that soda has nothing to do with children's obesity.[469] The president of the association, Susan Neely, said:

> "The assertions defy the existing body of scientific evidence, as well as common sense . . . It is scientifically implausible to suggest that diet soft drinks, a beverage that is 99 percent water-cause weight gain or elevate blood pressure."[470]

Poor Neely. She is blinded to modern research showing that diet soda does, indeed, cause weight gain (a JAMA report, no less)[471] because of where her bread is buttered.

"Cokeaholics"

The strength of the addiction to liquid candy was clearly demonstrated by the dozens of hate-filled letters to the editor in the *Salt Lake Tribune* after it reported on the Harvard study on soda,[472] discussed above. Cokeaholics are so deluded and addicted that they even called this Ivy League research "junk science." Even Rush Limbaugh denounced the results, commenting that people have a right to eat and drink whatever they want. I agree: they also have a right to die of sweet death; just don't expect me to pay for the health devastation that comes from this addiction. Ironically, Limbaugh has had a history of addictions and his waistline is as ample as his political pronouncements (I just lost all the Red States . . .).

In my clinic, I try to pry soda from my patients' hands. You can see the panic in their faces every time I wrestle with them about this ("Doc, what am I going to drink?!"). Watching their addiction to soda, I am reminded of Charles Heston, a former president of the National Rifle Association (NRA), who, while visiting Salt Lake City, Utah, said you will d have to pry my gun from my "cold, dead hands." Well, I may have to pry your Coke from your cold, dead hands, too, if you persist on killing yourself with this sweet death.

Chapter 9

Doctors: Are They Minding the Store?

The *Salt Lake Tribune* published an ad for an orthopedic surgeon offering free information on shoulder surgery. If you went to his clinic to hear about it, you would get a heaping serving of cake and ice cream, which he would hold in his outstretched hand while innocently smiling at the camera.[473]

What is it going to take to raise awareness in the public and in doctors? Government involvement? Perhaps; but the government seems to be in bed with Big Food and Big Pharma. Yes, we need a public health effort, but most of all we need the will to educate ourselves. We desperately need to take a good look at the man in the mirror. Still, many people think that the key to change is a doctor teaching nutrition at each visit.[474] Unfortunately, most doctors still focus on treating the devastating consequences of this sweet death, not on preventing it. A simple blood test would do:

> "Increased awareness of risk factors such as obesity and impaired glucose tolerance is needed among primary care doctors . . . who tend not to accept a role in the prevention of diabetes."[475]

> "The most efficient way of managing the metabolic syndrome and its complications is to prevent it from developing in the first place. Prevention has yielded a 25 to 60 percent

risk reduction, especially for diabetes, but an even more promising reduction of cardiovascular risk."[476]

Overburdened Doctors

I will never forget the comments made at a medical meeting some years ago. We were discussing new testing to pick up diabetics a lot earlier, even before patients develop the disease. I caught a lot of flack for proposing to call the problem "pre-diabetes" back then, which is now an accepted term. These are some of the comments I heard at that meeting:

- "We should not scare patients."
- "Insurance companies won't pay for the visit."
- "I don't have the time to look for diabetes in normal people. I am too busy taking care of patients who already have it."

Most doctors are not aware that the early signs of diabetes may be diagnosed ten to fifteen years before the fasting blood glucose test goes over 126. A simple screen with a two-hour glucose-tolerance challenge may pick up the problem in time to reverse the disease process. Yet, this simple procedure is not followed as often as desirable.[477]

I don't blame my colleagues. If you only knew how rampant burnout is in our profession. Many of these honest, dedicated professionals are disillusioned with the way we are practicing medicine in our country—perhaps as much as you are. Yet, a lot of them are caught in this web, much like "hamsters on a treadmill,"[478] because most of them depend on the check that somebody is signing for them.

But there are still some docs who may be so busy carrying out the message pounded into them by Big Pharma that their non-pharmaceutical skills, like communicating with patients and discussing lifestyle changes, have atrophied. This is not what most of them envisioned doing when they entered medical school. I know this t because I am on the Admissions Committee at the University of Utah School of Medicine; this honorable assignment allows me to read the essays young aspiring doctors write when applying to our institution.

More so, a vending machine could be passing out pills in clinics and hospitals because patients now come in nearly demanding that they get the new and improved pills they saw on TV while they were watching "The Biggest Loser."

Besides, some HMO suit is likely standing outside the door with a stop clock, recording how long the doc takes with each patient. Docs end up quickly prescribing one drug for each complaint voiced by their patients, which is exactly what docs are advised to do in "education programs" sponsored by Big Pharma.

It does not help that a significant number of docs tend to be as obese as their patients; their own advice on health is often ignored.[479] A 2004 national survey in found that 44 percent of doctors are overweight and 6 percent are obese.[480] If doctors worked on their own obesity issues, like doctors who quit smoking in the past to help their patients quit themselves, we would save millions of dollars in health care.[481]

Thankfully, some doctors are now arguing that impaired glucose tolerance, or pre-diabetes, should be considered a disease. This would bring more attention to the IR problem before it becomes a bigger problem: diabetes.[482] Also, insurance companies are starting to investigate the possibility of covering "health coaching" at clinics.[483] Hopefully their efforts will make this indispensable concept take roots.

Nutritionally-Deficient Docs

Metabolic problems are not well addressed by docs who, for the most part, don't receive adequate nutritional education in medical schools. The average doc gets only twenty-four hours on nutrition for the four years in medical school. The little they do get is about calories, servings, and other failed approaches, without the benefit of the new evidence shown in this book.[484] While training in hospitals, docs are exposed to highly questionable food; one-third of hospitals are serving food provided by fast food chains:

"Hospitals may wish to revisit the idea of serving high calorie fast foods in the very place where they also care for the most seriously ill."[485]

"We are giving two different messages by being in the health care profession and promoting health and saying obesity is a huge medical problem . . . and then implicitly encouraging it."[486]

Despite clear evidence that diets high in refined sugars and low in fiber cause sugars to be quickly absorbed, health care workers do not make these reports readily available to their patients.[487] The dogma that high cholesterol is a result of high-fat diets continues to be the mantra in nutritional advice, despite the evidence that a high glycemic index diet is what drives LDL cholesterol elevation.[488] In chapter 26, we will see that it is processed sugar more than saturated fats that drive heart disease; this is why drugs used to treat diabetes also lower cholesterol.[489]

Do You Like Your HMO?

Most insurance companies, for which most docs work, are abandoning coverage for practically all preventive services. The little prevention that is offered tends to be no more than some test to pick up a disease *after* it has started,[490] like a mammogram. Why is prevention so neglected? Insurance companies feel that prevention programs don't return their investments because many patients change insurance coverage; any effort toward prevention would then be accrued by some other insurance company. Poor prevention coverage is likely the reason why only 5 percent of people with diabetes are diagnosed with this condition in a timely manner.[491] Yet, billions of dollars are being spent on drugs and on diabetes's devastating consequences.[492] Given the sweet death epidemic we are having, it is likely to account for most of the doubling of health care costs, which will eat up 20 percent of all money spent in the United States by the end of this decade.[493]

Selling Out?

Early in the 1990s, the AHA started a program to certify foods as "heart-checked." For a fee of thousands of dollars, the AHA allowed certain foods to advertise their "wholesomeness." Several states protested on legal grounds until the program was stopped, only to be re-instituted in 1993—this time to stay. The AHA simply claimed that these arrangements are "certifications, not endorsements."

More than fifty-five companies have 643 "heart smart" products. More than fifty of Kellogg's products have the AHA seal of approval; Frosted Flakes, Cocoa Frosted Flakes, Fruity Marshmallow Krispies, and Pop-Tarts are supposed to be good for you, according to the AHA.

Steps in the Right Direction

Could it be that the AHA is changing? Is it catching on that we have an epidemic of sweet death?

> "The American Heart Association is finally taking aim at our **nation's sweet tooth**, urging consumers to significantly cut back on the amount of sugar they get from such foods as soft drinks, cookies and ice cream. The AHA says most women should limit their sugar intake to 100 calories, or about six teaspoons, a day; for men, the recommendation is 150 calories, or nine teaspoons. The recommendations are likely to prove challenging for many consumers to meet. Just one 12-ounce can of cola has about 130 calories, or eight teaspoons of sugar. Data gathered during a national nutrition survey between 2001 and 2004 suggest that Americans consume on average 355 calories, or more than 22 teaspoons, of sugar a day."[494]

Other than advising patients to cut back or totally eliminate refined sugars from their diet, what else can doctors do? In June 2006, I proposed a program called "Adopt a School" through the Environmental/Public Health Committee I chair at the Utah Medical Association (UMA). Volunteering docs go to a school of their choice to motivate parents, teachers, and students to give up refined sugars. Dr. Catherine Wheeler, a former president of the Utah Medical Association, is now leading the UMA in these efforts.

An HMO in Utah started a new program in 2007 whereby docs are allowed to visit with patients about obesity-related problems twice a month for three months. Heretofore, these types of visits were not covered by HMOs. The doc in charge of prevention for that HMO, who was instrumental in passing this program, was very candid with me. She felt that the reason she was finally successful was that the HMO's bean counters (my words, not hers) were afraid they might have to spend a lot more money on gastric bypass surgeries if that benefit were to be covered for all their patients who demanded it. It doesn't matter why the HMO implemented the program, but that it is finally a reality. Congratulations.

Today, many corporations are beginning to offer wellness training at work simply because they see more productivity out of their employees and they also save small fortunes by lowering health insurance premiums.

Story Time

A patient of mine couldn't control his diabetes; yet, he didn't want to take drugs that his HMO doc recommended. He had a hemoglobin A1c of 8.4 (it is recommended to have this test below 7.0). I put him on a low-glycemic index diet and gave him some of the supplements we will talk about later. His A1c dropped under 7. When my patient told his HMO doc how he had done it, the doc replied, "You shouldn't stay on this diet forever. It may be harmful." This poor patient was forced to go back to the doc covered by his HMO. I hope he stays on the wagon, but it is not likely with that kind of support.

Another patient came to my clinic with a hemoglobin A1c of 9.0. After the same program as the patient above, but with more frequent visits since she had coverage at my clinic, her hemoglobin A1c dropped to 5.6—which is considered normal. She did not use any drugs and she remains "on the wagon."

Chapter 10

Our Children's Bittersweet Lives

The metabolic syndrome is now officially diagnosed in 10 to 20 percent of our children[495] who end up with a higher risk of dying at a young age.[496] Add the fact that one out of three of our children will be diabetic when they grow up and you may understand why our children's generation will be the first one in the history of the world to live less than the preceding generation.[497] This is the main reason why I refer to this problem as "sweet death." I do not feel this is an exaggeration, since the diabetic and obesity issue has been called a pandemic that cost $117 billion in extra health care expenses in the United States in 2000.[498] Depressing, isn't it? It turns out that depression and psychological stress in children are associated with a higher risk of obesity later in life . . .[499] Sweet death will get worse in the United States, unless:

> "In addressing this disturbing trend and preventing its spread, physicians are challenged to look to the broader environment. Successful treatment will require improving the health of individual patients and the larger community (n "ecological model"). For physicians, this means reviving their traditional role as trusted advocates for good health of the public."[500]

Sweet Kids

About one-third of our children are well on their way to becoming diabetics because each year they eat an average of sixty pounds of cakes and cookies, twenty-three gallons of ice cream, seven pounds of potato chips, 365 servings of soda, and 756 doughnuts. No wonder they suffer from poor health, behavior changes, and hyperactivity.[501] Even in kids, electrocardiogram (EKG) changes are more common with this diet.[502]

Doctors now frequently report seeing children and adolescents with high levels of cholesterol, high blood pressure,[503] more heart disease,[504] and adult onset IR. However, the latter is also found in 54 percent of overweight teens and in 17 percent of overweight children.[505] About 1.2 million teens in the United States have been found to have IR.[506]

When children have an abnormal waist/height ratio, they now have a greater risk of developing heart disease[507] because of IR affecting their endothelium, the cell membranes lining their arteries.[508] Sadly, primary care doctors do not identify two-thirds of these obesity-related health problems.[509] Specialty clinics for obese children are popping up, but they are expensive, and not covered by insurance. They also do not appear to be that successful in helping to overcome kids' addiction to sugar. [510]

Children now have positive markers for the metabolic syndrome in their blood, that is, lower adiponectin and higher leptin, which are hormones secreted by fat tissue in their VAT to regulate appetite and metabolism. They also have an elevated CRP;[511] another marker of inflammation, the erythrocyte sedimentation rate (ESR) is also a marker for pre-diabetes and more fat stored in their liver, which is often under-diagnosed.[512] Still, the best marker for future obesity is IR.[513]

Things are getting so bad that Social Services in England have threatened a mother with the loss of her kid's custody because she has allegedly failed to do anything about her eight-year-old son who weighs over 200 pounds. It seems she did not attend scheduled meetings with nurses, dieticians, or government officials who were trying to help her with the problem.[514] Our children are now having trouble fitting into infant car seats;[515] some of them are being offered gastric bypass surgery.[516]

Only when we finally see "Childhood Obesity [as a] Public Health Crisis, [with a] Common Sense Cure"[517] will we begin to address the problem adequately. This article is a reminder that our main goal should be to *prevent* the devastating consequences of metabolic problems in our children. The authors list the problems that our children are seeing because of obesity:

- Psychosocial: Poor self-esteem, depression, and eating disorders.

- Neurological: Pseudotumor cerebri (swollen brain)

- Pulmonary: Sleep apnea, exercise intolerance, asthma

- Gastrointestinal: Gallstones, fatty liver

- Renal: Glomerulosclerosis (scarred filtration apparatus)

- Musculoskeletal: Slipped femur head, Blount's disease, forearm fractures, flat feet

- Cardiovascular: High cholesterol, high blood pressure, coagulation problems, inflammation, endothelial problems and iron-deficiency anemia[518]

- Endocrine: Diabetes, precocious puberty, PCOS, hypogonadism

More dramatically put, obese children who have higher cholesterol have the same "age" in their arteries as adults.[519]

A Cancer Growing in Our Homes, Sweet Homes

No parent can contemplate the awful possibility that one of our children may get cancer. The mere thought sends chills down my spine. It is unimaginable to think of the kind of life my children would have after such a terrible diagnosis. You may feel the same shock I felt when I saw a study on obese children having a quality of life equal to the lives of children with cancer: "The stigmatization directed at obese children by their peers, parents, educators and others is pervasive and often unrelenting".[520]

No wonder they feel as miserable as if they had been diagnosed with cancer. Youngsters who report teasing, rejection, bullying, and other types of abuse because of their weight are two to three times more likely to report suicidal thoughts and suffer from other health issues, such as high blood pressure and eating disorders.

The rest of this chapter is not going to be pretty. Surely we can put up with our own sweet deaths. But watching our children suffer is more than any parent can bear. I suppose we could alleviate their suffering with antipsychotic drug treatments; too bad they cause weight gain, metabolic and cardiovascular adverse effects . . .[521]

Tricked by McD

The relentless ads from fast food joints convince children that McDonald's foods taste better. Even carrots, milk, and apple juice are said to taste better when wrapped in the familiar packaging of the golden arches. Brand "branding" is so powerful that kids

"see a McDonald's label and [they] start salivating . . . [This] is the first study I know of that has shown so simply and clearly that's going on with [marketing to] young children . . . [The kids' perception of taste] was physically altered by the branding."

McDonald's is very aware of this; commenting on the above study, a representative said, "We've always wanted to be part of the solution."[522]

In 2004, the Centers for Disease Control and Prevention (CDC) published the report, "Food Marketing to Children and Youth: Threat or Opportunity." It documents how Big Food intentionally markets junk food to our children. This is a highly profitable practice because children cannot tell the truth in ads. (Come to think of it, many adults cannot either . . .) After reviewing 123 studies on marketing and junk food consumption, the CDC discovered that Big Food hires teams of psychologists and marketers to study the psychology of addiction to purposely hook our children. Big Food knows that kids are a great source of revenue as defenseless consumers.[523]

Children are quite vulnerable to advertisement and peer pressure to eat poorly, particularly in puberty. At this critical time, that is nine to twelve years of age, girls who eat poorly are especially at a higher risk of getting fat.[524] Persuaded by misleading ads, kids spend about $132 billion a year on junk food with their allowances, in addition to their blatant attempts to blackmail their parents into buying them even more garbage. In total, kids controlled a staggering $485 billion in 1999. What do children buy with their allowance? Over half of them buy candy and 39 percent of them get chewing gum. Soft drinks (34 percent), ice cream (33 percent), salty snacks (27 percent), fast food (16 percent), and cookies (18 percent) round up their purchases. Soda alone constitutes 25 percent of the calories consumed by children.[525] In the United States, it is almost impossible to find healthy foods at fast food chains. Nearly every possible combination of children's meals at thirteen restaurants—including Kentucky Fried Chicken (KFC), Taco Bell, Sonic, Jack in the Box and Chick-fil-A—are too high in calories.

A study found 93 percent of 1,474 possible choices at the thirteen chains exceed 430 calories, an amount that is one-third of what the National Institute of Medicine recommends that children ages four through eight should consume in a day.[526] Because of Big Food's "teachings" via commercials, children now know more about "what they are supposed to eat than their parents."

Big Food deliberately plants commercials to persuade children that they need to convince their parents that kids need to make the food choices for the family. Just about every time I go to the grocery store, I spot all-out fights between moms and their addicted children. Kids try very hard to convince their moms to load up the shopping cart with processed sugars. It gives me hope when I see moms put their feet down and refuse to cave in to their kids' demands. "Congress should enact legislation mandating the shift" away from ads enticing children to eat poorly, reports the CDC. Advocacy groups sued Kellogg and Viacom/Nickelodeon over these practices in January 2006. This is a good start, but we are way behind other countries, like Australia. The Aussies ban food ads targeting kids under fourteen years old. Sweden bans cartoons peddling junk food to kids under the age of twelve.[527]

Trix is Not for Kids[528]

When I was in college, I voted for the rabbit to get Trix cereal, too. I proudly wore the button I got in the mail showing a rabbit eating Trix because I practically lived on Trix cereal back then. (No wonder I didn't get any hot dates . . .) I don't know how I got through school eating like that.

Well, Trix cereal is no longer for kids, but Cocoa Puffs cereal is another matter. Big Food has agreed to cut back on TV ads pushing Trix to kids under twelve years of age. However, General Mills will continue to advertise Cocoa Puffs because this cereal has one less gram of sugar per serving than Trix. These measures "will probably amount to a ripple rather than a sea of change in terms of what foods children see pitched on their favorite TV shows." Still, eleven Big Food companies are trotting out these half-baked, caramelized Band-Aids to convince the feds that they don't need government regulation.

Big Food successfully dodged Iowa Senator Tom Harkin's attempt to create a task force to investigate its marketing tactics by announcing these weak changes in its ad campaigns. "The extension will allow for a more thorough examination of new initiatives," said Senator Sam Brown, who was working with Harkin. I hope so. Big Food is now saying that it may turn to healthier food ads and healthier lifestyles if it is not able to reformulate its junk. I am not holding my breath.

Coca-Cola, PepsiCo, McDonald's, the Campbell Soup Company, General Mills, and other companies are also saying they will cut back on radio, print, and Internet advertising. But they are still going to advertise items, like Trix, on "family shows." This loophole is as big as their profits because a significant number of families have children under the age of twelve years of age. According to Nielsen Media Research, *SpongeBob Squarepants* falls in the category of shows that are off-limits to junk food ads. Yet, *American Idol* is a "family show" that qualifies for Big Food to get its sugary mittens on.

Big Food has also agreed to open its marketing plans to the Council of Better Business Bureaus and its Children's Advertising Review Unit in an attempt to show it is socially responsible and wants to help curve our sweet deaths. These are welcome changes, but the $900 million it spends trying to hook kids under the age of twelve will have to be drastically redirected or eliminated for us to believe its newfound social sensitivity. It is very telling that Big Food is talking reform only after it was threatened with regulatory intervention and, in some cases, with the threat of lawsuits. Big Food is unlikely to get many pats on the back because it doesn't come close to implementing the reforms child advocacy groups would prefer to see.

Real changes would involve uniform advertising guidelines to be followed by strict oversight with the authority to enforce violations. "This is great public relations for the companies, but it doesn't go far enough," said Susan Linn, co-founder of Campaign for Commercial-Free Childhood, based in Boston, Mass. "It is going to be impossible to monitor if the companies are actually doing what they say."

Nickelodeon, ABC Family, and Cartoon Network are saying they don't expect to see their ad revenues affected at all. They are probably correct, since Big Food told them "that their ad budgets will not be altered in any meaningful way . . . since [Big Food's] children's ad budget represents only 1 percent of its overall ad budget." I am sure the creative CPAs, lawyers, and marketers will find a way to perpetuate their profitable operations.

For example, PepsiCo has found Gatorade acceptable to advertise to children for sports-related fluid losses, even though Gatorade "only" has 14 grams of sugar, compared to regular Pepsi. PepsiCo is pledging to stop advertising Pepsi to children because it has 28 grams of sugar. It will also stop ads on Cheetos, which have double the amount of fat compared to its baked Cheetos. Quaker Oats' Cap'n Crunch was to be phased out by January 2008, which means that the arcade-style game for children at www.captn-crunch.com may end.

Other Big Food companies are pledging to limit their use of characters like SpongeBob and Scooby-Doo in their ads. Kellogg's said in June 2007 that it will stop advertising Pop-Tarts, Froot Loops, and apple jacks because they have more than 12 grams of sugar, but it will continue to pitch Eggo Waffles, which only have 2 grams.[529] I hope these initiatives bear fruit. But, in my opinion, Big Food will not clean up its act 100 percent until government regulation forces them to do so, much like we saw with the tobacco industry. As noted elsewhere, I believe the Twinkie tax is a good option.

Sweet Schools

Practically every commercial item children are interested in—like toys, books, backpacks, clothing, games, and school supplies—carry Big Food's logos. But a more questionable practice is the direct advertisement it buys on TV channel one—only found in schools. Our kids are practically captive audience in the very places where we would hope they are getting a good education. Big Food invests heavily on mind-numbing commercials on that channel: it pays more than $200,000 for a thirty-second commercial for an annual profit per company of more than $30 million.

This is in addition to the "pouring rights" soda companies buy by paying an average of $30,000 per school, per year, to plant their soda machines in our schools. A legislative audit in Utah discovered that some of the $4 million from the annual sale of pouring rights ends up paying for Costco memberships, cakes, and even a principal's portrait. Legislators discovered that there are no guidelines on how that tainted money is to be spent by schools or what counts as a legitimate school expense.[530]

Many schools are now allowing McDonald's, Burger King, and KFC to open franchises on campus to provide school lunches.[531] Perhaps more puzzling is the ubiquitous practice by teachers to reward students with candy when the latter complete their assignments. In a suburb in Salt Lake City, Utah, they dropped candy from a helicopter after the students finished their reading homework.[532]

Utah schools also have the unfortunate distinction of leading the nation in junk food availability.[533] Interestingly, the same day this report came out, a mother coming to my clinic told me that her daughter's goal to avoid candy at school was ridiculed by her angry teacher who felt the child's decision would cause a disruption in the classroom. It seems that any attempt to correct these problems is met with resistance from not only some parents and some teachers but also from Big Food itself:

"But the intense corporate involvement, along with ex-
emptions that would allow sales of chocolate milk, sports
drinks and diet soda, has caused a rift among food activists
who usually find themselves on the same side of school food
battles. This pits ideas about what children should eat at
school against the political reality of large food corporations
insisting their foods be available to children at all times."[534]

The Center for Science in the Public Interest issued a report
in June 2006 that gave a failing grade to twenty-three states and
a "D" to eight others after evaluating school policies regarding
foods and beverages sold on campus through vending machines,
school stores, and school fundraisers. And who is responsible for
the brainwashing of our children at schools? We are, because we
have repeatedly voted to cut funds for education, leaving poor
teachers and principals so strapped for money that they have no
choice but to strike these "Faustian bargains" with Big Food.

Virtual Couch Potatoes

Our children spend approximately forty hours per week playing video games and watching TV, a figure that is likely to "get
bigger"[535] in the near future, just like their rear ends. Watching TV
not only keeps them from exercising; it also exposes them to even
more advertisements. Their metabolisms get messed up as they
munch on chips, pizzas, sugary cereals, and candy bars.[536] Kids
caught in this virtual reality grow up to be adults who are overweight, unfit, and prone to smoking.[537] A study in Utah showed
that kids watching too much TV (more than two hours a day)
tend to drink more soda, eat junk, and, of course, get fatter. They
estimated that one-seventh of children are consuming too much
soda, defined as more than five soft drinks a week.[538]

Exposure to excessive electromagnetism from our TVs is just
the tip of the iceberg. TV advertisements are full of images promoting refined treats and fast foods.[539] Children between eight
and twelve years of age see an average of twenty-one TV ads promoting junk food each day, or more than 7,600 a year. Not one of
these ads promote fresh fruits and vegetables; only one-fiftieth
advertize healthy foods.[540] As predicted, the ads lead to higher

consumption of bad foods by children and teens[541] who sit, over-dosing on junk food in front of the TV, in a classic and modern version of "bread and circus." Our kids are often found entranced in front of the TV, each day cementing their way to obesity and a sweet death.[542]

Watching TV reduces the time spent in physical activity. If children were to exercise on a daily basis, their chances of developing IR would be much lower.[543] Even though they may remain obese, being fit may trump being fat: there is less IR in obese children who are active.[544]

Kids also get less sleep when they watch too much TV. Kids love staying up watching it, which not only overstimulates their brains with electromagnetism but also cuts into their sleeping time. If a preschooler sleeps less than twelve hours, his or her BMI is likely to be higher.[545] And here is another vicious cycle: the more obese our children are, the more disturbed their sleep becomes.[546]

According to the American Academy of Pediatrics,[547] we should keep our children from watching more than two hours of TV a day. Children under two years of age should not watch any TV at all because it has been linked to brain damage and obesity.[548] If a child already has diabetes, it is harder to control his or her sugar when he or she watches more than two hours of TV a day.[549] Just reducing the amount of time spent watching TV and playing computer games has an important role in preventing sweet death.[550] ADHD and learning difficulties have been show to be more likely to develop when teens watch too much TV.[551]

Some researchers feel that portraying more obese people on TV can help children shed negative stereotypical images about obesity.[552] While overcoming negative stereotypes is a good thing, I can't help but feel a bit uncomfortable about this report. Am I the only one scratching his head on this one? Should we teach our children that their own bulging waistlines are to be accepted as normal?

Video games also contribute to a more sedentary lifestyle.[553] My hometown, Salt Lake City, Utah, where 32 percent of homes have video games, has the dubious distinction of being number one at "thumb-exercising" in the United States.[554] Some docs, myself included, believe that video games are potentially addicting,[555] like anything else, I suppose.

How About *Your* Childhood?

When I was growing up, I would spend every free moment after doing my homework, playing soccer, or swimming at the beach until it got so dark we couldn't see the ball or the bikinis anymore. Today, our children sit in front of their video games and TV practically all day long while physical education classes at school are going the way of the dinosaur.[556] In 1969, 90 percent of kids walked or biked to school. Today, most of them get there by car. Part of it is that we have built our cities and suburbs around the SUV so that kids live further away from their schools. Some kids even feel that walking is "not cool" and exercise is not that important.[557] Between the ages of nine and fifteen, the frequency of exercise falls precipitously.[558]

As a child I walked to school in the snow, uphill both ways; the past looks better in the rearview mirror. Even so, the exploding epidemic of child obesity tells me I am not indulging in "old-gizzard nostalgia" too much.

Story Time

My dad owned a French bistro, full of goodies and Coca-Cola. He advertised in French and Spanish because his bistro was a gathering place for Frogs in Viña del Mar, Chile. He had a huge mural map of Paris that I came to know like the palm of my hand, in which I often had a "mille-feuille" and a Coke. Sugar kicks are nothing new, but the inactivity and the pollution are.

That Parisian map captivated my imagination. I didn't make it to Paris until my medical education and service obligations were done. But, when I got there, I navigated the streets as well as any grumpy Parisian. I went straight to Rue Rodier, having found it on that old map back in my dad's bistro.

Sweet Death Before Birth

Even before we are born, we are exposed to refined sugar. Please, don't get the impression that I am trying to blame our young moms; they already have a lot to deal with. Moms, themselves, are victims of the factors that lead to sweet death. The number of diabetic teens getting pregnant has grown fivefold in the last seven years.[559] This is a significant trend because our children's diet problems begin while in utero. The article, "Pathophysiology of Metabolic Syndrome and its Links to the Perinatal Period,"[560] confirms the fact that children start receiving metabolic signals while in the uterus, which may predispose them to IR when they grow up. An unborn child in the uterus is exposed to environmental clues after the genetic dice has been cast. Practically speaking, moms who eat poorly while pregnant expose their unborn kids to a higher risk of IR and heart problems.[561]

Even fasting glucose considered high-normal in pregnant women increases the risk of neonatal problems. Fasting blood glucose from seventy-five to 105 increases the risk of having a larger baby four to six times while the risk of neonatal hypoglycemia goes up 2.7 times.[562] The latter is a result of higher fetal insulin levels triggered by mom's refined sugar diet.[563] (Insulin has a growth hormone effect.) The best way to screen moms for these pregnancy problems is the two-hour glucose tolerance test.[564]

We could prevent this prenatal sweet environment by encouraging moms to face their sugar addictions for the sake of their unborn children. Despite what is at stake, this is very hard to do because many moms are under the wrong impression that pregnancies give them carte blanche to gain weight by indulging every dietary whim—an attitude supported by our national folklore.

If they decreased their intake of refined sugars and fats and eat more of the right fats, like veggie-based oils and fish, mothers and their unborn children would lower their chances of facing a sweet death later in their lives. When moms eat poorly, they are at risk of developing gestational diabetes, a result of maternal IR. Sadly, the incidence of gestational diabetes is growing rapidly.[565] An increase in mothers' blood pressure before and during pregnancy has been associated with an increase of gestational diabetes.[566] In Utah, the rate of gestational diabetes has doubled from 1.5 percent of pregnant women in 1997 to 3.3 percent in 2006.[567]

Moms who struggle with their weight[568] and their VAT are at higher risk of developing gestational diabetes.[569] A history of a sweet pregnancy increases a mom's risk of developing diabetes and heart problems after she delivers her child,[570] especially if she is genetically susceptible.[571]

Gestational diabetes may be successfully treated with nutrition, lifestyle changes, and medications, like metformin and glyburide.[572] Just as important are the prevention of pregnancy hypertension from vascular disease and the prevention of diabetes in these moms' futures.[573] Unfortunately this problem is often mismanaged.[574]

These moms tend to have larger babies who, even up to eleven years after birth have a twenty times higher risk to develop IR.[575] But being too small at birth is also a problem. These babies also have metabolic problems that may lead to high blood pressure[576] and type 2 diabetes.[577] More ominously, maternal obesity has been shown to increase the risk of preterm deliveries.[578]

Perhaps worse is the effect of a mother's high sugar diet on the developing brain of her baby: more neural tube defects are seen in babies whose moms' are addicted to sugar when they were in utero[579] because this diet lacks B vitamins, glycosacharides, and oils essential for brain development. These same factors seen in obese moms also explain why they bear children with more cardiovascular system and orofacial abnormalities.[580] Fortunately, breastfeeding—which is high in antioxidants, oils, and healthy glycoproteins, such as sialic acid—results in better brain development.[581] The more omega oils moms consume while pregnant, the healthier their birth weights will be.[582] Omega oils are the most critical nutrients for brain development in the fetus.[583]

Unfortunately, most doctors are afraid to incur the wrath of mothers-to-be; docs often avoid telling them that they are packing too much weight through their pregnancies, the very thing these moms *need* to hear the most.[584] Moms could also use more encouragement from docs about safely increasing their activity; they could then lower their risk of gestational diabetes by 72 percent.[585]

Even though nutrigenomics still wins the day, children's genetic make up have some influence on their metabolism. A study in the journal Nature showed that "large, rare chromosomal deletions [are] associated with severe early-onset obesity"[586] The key word is "rare"; rather than missing DNA, kids are more like to be getting too much "KFC".

What Can We Do as Parents?

In a Philadelphia, Penn., middle school, parents felt that doing BMI measurements on their kids was upsetting their body image.[587] In a school district in Denver, Colo., kids were sent home with notes saying they were too obese and that parents needed to do something about it. Parents reacted angrily and the policy of sending notes had to be reconsidered. Only 50 percent of notified parents believed that their kids were really obese.[588]

I agree that we need to be mindful of kids' feelings. Despite official recommendations to check our kids' BMI in schools,[589] I feel this is not a smart way to go about this problem. I much prefer a school-wide program that focuses on all children so that the ones who are a bit overweight are not embarrassed. The program would be based on more physical activity while at school, better school lunches, no vending machines on the premises, and no refined sugar treats to reward their accomplishments. After all, our teachers are already overburdened with duties we, the parents, could do much better at home.

Hopefully, our schools will no longer be part of the problem in the future, but an integral part of the solutions. But the main fields of operation, in my opinion, are our homes, sweet homes. The problem is that our homes are too sweet. As parents, we need to set an example by facing our own sugar addictions if we want our kids to overcome theirs. Family-based weight management programs are more successful, especially when they involve behavioral modification, nutrition education, and more activity. Kids that followed a home-based program had a lower BMI, less fat, and less IR than the kids that just got lectures at school.[590] It is not fair to ask an obese child to change while everyone else at home is munching on Twinkies in front of the TV. If parents are addicted to junk food, their kids will likely follow suit.

Parents could also become more active in Parent-Teacher Association (PTA) organizations to see that the National Institute of Medicine's recommendations for school snacks are implemented. Above all, candy should not be used as rewards for performance and "pouring rights" should be eliminated.

The National Institutes of Health (NIH) is also encouraging more physical activity in schools,[591] such as team sports,[592] because the less fit our kids are, the more IR they have.[593] The Japanese creation, Dance Dance Revolution, a computer program that directs dancing steps on an electronic platform has been implemented in schools in ten states. Children seem to prefer this fun way of physical activity to competitive sports. Competition may have some rather negative and expensive consequences.[594]

Sometimes the metabolic issues are so pronounced that exercise may not help.[595] To maximize the benefits of exercise, the parents of one million children in the United States are paying $40 to $60 an hour to sports clubs' trainers to help their kids shape up.[596] Back in the old days, we had a friend kick our butts to work out harder. Today, I guess we are too busy to go out in the backyard to play with our kids.

The NIH issued a statement in 2002 saying that children should "limit their intake of refined sugars or added sugars to 25 percent of daily calories," which meant that the NIH believed it was okay for our children who were two to three years of age to consume fourteen teaspoonfuls of added sugar each day and seventeen teaspoonfuls for four- and five-year-olds. Fortunately, a study of 5,400 children[597] pointed out that the recommendation of the USDA and the WHO makes more sense: limit added sugar to 6 to 10 percent of calories. The study pointed out that each portion of added sugar keeps children from better foods (vegetables, fruits, etc.), thus decreasing the micronutrients available to them because children have healthier thermostats and will stop eating when they sense they are full with junk. Because of these findings, Cookie Monster, Dora the Explorer, and other heroes have started to tell children that these foods are "sometimes" foods.

Personally, I feel it would be best to advise children to eat sugar only in the company of responsible adults, in controlled situations, and with the mature understanding that treats once in a while are okay. Would you let your kids drink enough alcohol to cover 6 to 10 percent of their daily calories? Sugar is addicting and alcohol is nothing but fermented sugar. Children lack the maturity to handle these toxic foods. You may say that we cannot keep an eye on our children twenty-four hours a day, seven days a week; I agree. This is the same problem we have with alcohol, tobacco, drugs, and sex. So what should we do? We educate them while we still have some influence over them. And our parental example is the best way to teach . . .

About half of the states in the United States are beginning to make efforts to curve this epidemic of obesity and IR. They are targeting soft drinks and junk food sales in schools and demanding that chain restaurants display nutritional information.[598] In chapter 30, we will see why these school- and government-based programs, I am sad to report, are not working.

The Best Thing We May Do as Parents

If you are addicted to sugar, your children are likely to grow up with the same problem. If you think that your "picky eaters" got that behavior out of the blue, think again. For one, their taste buds have grown accustomed to high-sugar foods. There is no way that they will appreciate natural foods that contain less sugar; their palates are ruined.

Secondly, your picky eaters have not only copied your eating habits, but they also have your genes—the same ones that, when left unattended or under the mercy of refined sugars, will surely lead you and them down the path of least resistance. It turns out that there are significant "genetic and environmental influences on children's food neophilia."[599]

What is the best thing you may do to rescue your children from this sweet death? Stop your own addiction and be an example of healthy eating to your little ones.

Story Time

My nine-year-old daughter, Cosette, seldom consumes refined sugars. For example, we ate some almond M&Ms one summer during a car trip to Mesa Verde, Colo., and to the Shakespeare Festival in Cedar City, Utah. I took the time to explain to her that eating M&Ms was okay to keep us (mostly me) awake in the car. Besides, it gets a bit boring driving through the desert. We also have treats like that at baseball games and birthdays.

Time to Think

Here is a curve ball for you: people who eat candy twice a month live longer.[600] Why? Read on.

Mature, integrated, heart-driven people do not have addictions to any substances, ideologies, objects, or people. To eat junk food once in a blue moon is not threatening or tempting to them. Eating something a bit questionable, while enjoying the company of people we love, is more emotionally rewarding than pontificating about good foods in those circumstances. These actualized people are very flexible, which allows them to eat some junk without it becoming addicting — or a federal offense. It is not the candy twice a month that increases longevity, but the person's mature, carefree attitude that allows him or her to enjoy something that might be toxic when ingested too often and in large quantities (as we see some people doing when an addiction is at play).

Salus Populi and Solutions in the Community

In January 2005, the European Union began to crack down on Big Food's marketing and advertising methods. Many school districts in the United States are also opposing its blatant brainwashing of our children. We could follow their example at the federal level.[601] It has been proven that taking soda vending machines out of our schools helps kids lose weight[602] because consumption of one or more of these drinks a day raises the risk of becoming diabetic by 83 percent.[603] Consuming artificially sweetened drinks is no better; these drinks increase cell membrane toxicity, TOILing, and make it harder for the body to know when to stop eating.[604]

While most school programs do not seem to work well, several studies in schools in Berkeley, Calif., and Osceola, Fla., have shown that providing healthier lunches does help students. About 80 percent of their parents end up being positively influenced by their children's change in lifestyle. Of 480 obese students followed by these studies, twenty-three lost unwanted pounds.[605] In order to curve sweet death,

"Schools must focus on increasing children's physical activity and improve their nutrition . . . The selling of candy and sugar drinks must be forbidden. Fast foods loaded with calories and fat must not be available in schools . . . We must put the health and welfare of our children above the financial benefits accrued by selling junk food in school . . . Form the fast food industry to Madison Avenue to Hollywood, the principles of good health—exercise and good nutrition—must be promoted."[606]

Sweet death prevention must start during childhood.[607] Keeping kids from getting fat significantly lowers their risk of having heart disease as adults.[608] But are we really doing what it takes to get the job done? Prevention is clearly the most important, moral, and wise approach.[609] We need to become politically active to fight the tremendous problems facing our children. Working with our schools would be a good start.[610] The AMA has stated that

> We need a "community-based approach to obesity prevention that enlists not only schools, but also businesses, families, restaurants, grocery and convenience stores, and local government."[611]

> "We emphasize intensive lifestyle modification; just handing out a diet sheet doesn't do it . . . They need to see someone on a regular basis for three to four months . . . Large policy changes are needed to have a significant impact on the public health problem of childhood obesity."[612]

Policy changes are good. But what we really need is for *ourselves* to get involved. Our children's futures are at stake.

Part II

E=Mc² and Information/Communication— Main Players in Sweet Death

The last few Nobel Prizes in biology and medicine have been awarded to researchers who are focusing on E&I at the cellular level. Scientists are catching up to the quantum revolution of the early 1900s that showed that E&I are the pillars of everything there is in the universe. Stars, entire galaxies, atoms and their subparticles, Homo sapiens, and every living organism are based on E&I. The same is true of our spiritual and mind/heart issues. According to Integrative Medicine doctors,

> "The current connecting human hearts, love, is identical to the current emerging from the primordial singularity, which gave rise to creation."[613]

Chapter 11

Energy and Information from a Non-physicist

Thanks to quantum physic, a better understanding of E&I is dawning in our society's consciousness. Many books about this concept make the point that, since antiquity, our wisest men and women have known that light, or E&I, are the two flipsides of our existence and the basis of the whole universe. Modern physics has confirmed these concepts that were previously understood through faith, meditation, and/or through the hallucinogenic journeys of shamans.[614]

Albert Einstein understood that energy/light is the very fabric of reality; he was very open to that which is not seen. In fact, he came to "see" these things in dreams. He didn't put "I," for "information," in his famous formula, $E = Mc^2$, but he understood that information is an intrinsic part of "E," or energy. Some feel that "M," for "Matter," also stands for "Memory" because E&I are known to be stored in our bodies, tissues, or matter even outside the brain.[615] In other words, E&I are stored in all fifty to one hundred trillion of our body cells.

Einstein felt that the same principles that govern planets and stars also govern atoms. His main goal was to find a unifying formula for these ideas. He reasoned that organic life, like us and the atoms that make up said matter, must obey the same principles of energy, light, matter, and information that rule the physics of astronomy. His brilliant insights are supported by the fact that DNA, the very blueprint of organic life, emits E&I signals[616] that have been called "biophoton emissions."[617]

The physicist, Erwin Schrödinger, famous for his "cat essays," wrote a lot about how powerful our minds are. He thought that we might be creating the whole universe with the power of our minds.[618] Schrödinger also maintained that life is simply defined as the ability to metabolize or process E&I.[619]

Quantum physic supports those who believe that healing may take place at a distance by the power of intent and by the power of prayer and love, regardless of time and place. Since E&I connect us all, we may all access healing if only we put our egos in their proper subordinate places, below our hearts.

What is Pollution?

It has finally become fashionable to worry about environmental issues, global warming, and pollution. These problems are really E&I issues and the resulting byproducts of energy-making. Even if we believe that global warming is caused by solar changes beyond our control, global warming is still an E&I issue.

The connection between pollution, or free radicals from combustion processes, and our health is very clear. We will see in more detail in chapter 16 how toxicity affects our own use of E&I at the cellular level. Fortunately many doctors are now very concerned about the effect of environmental toxins on our health. [620]

Metaphysics?

Many physicists refuse to link their rigorous scientific work with "new age" thinking[621] and I don't blame them. At times, less rigorous minds adopt a Pollyanna-ish belief that mere wishing, if done sincerely enough, should heal all our suffering, like Rhonda Byrne's book, *The Secret*, maintains. Metaphysicists often use quantum physics principles to explain how this works. As appealing as these beliefs are, they often do not account for the concept that suffering, at times, may be a necessary way to refinement and growth. This is not to say that we may not heal others and ourselves with the power of our intent. But who is to say that

152

all suffering must be eradicated? Do we want to be in a position to tell God, or whatever/whoever one believes in, what is best for us? Are we that in touch with those sources? If you are, I bow before you.

No doubt some of us are able to heal through the power of intent. Perhaps we will all be that powerful in the future. Some believe that in the next few years we may become "Homo luminous" through the transformative E&I stored in our "junk DNA." It turns out that approximately 97 percent of our DNA does not code for any genes. One of the discoverers of DNA, Dr. Francis Crick, felt that DNA was engineered to allow for further development of our species in the future—perhaps as a grand plan originating outside of Earth. He was of the opinion that the chances for DNA to have originated on Earth were as good as that of a Boeing 747 being built after a storm hitting a junkyard.[622]

Reputable scientists are now saying that the E&I stored in our DNA is, indeed, programmed to take us to a higher level of existence when the right time comes.[623] The well-known genius, Ray Kurzweil, entertains these thoughts in his groundbreaking book, *The Singularity is Near*, where he predicts a time "when humans transcend biology."[624] Even Carl Sagan said that Homo sapiens' DNA likely mutated for the better by taking queues from the universe or from spheres outside Earth[625]—an opinion seconded by modern scientists who feel that this evolutionary concept was illustrated in the movie, *2001: A Space Odyssey*.[626]

"In the Beginning, There was Light . . ."

By now, I am sure your wheels are turning; you may have heard your heart whisper that we are all one consciousness: one spirit or one energy. Whether you call this "entity" God or being "at-one-ment" or "implicate order,"[627] you may sense that we are all a part of it, including the Earth and the rest of the universe. Some of you have always known these things, deep within your hearts—your main receiver of E&I. The light of creation from the very beginning shines in our hearts, quickening everything about our body functions, structures, and our very understanding of consciousness.

Let us not fight about the Big Bang Theory or Intelligent Design. Please, slow down a bit and consider that the common denominator to both beliefs is light. There is no need to try to figure out which I favor so that you filter my ideas through your own faith or theories; that would be sad and perhaps a sign that you may need to consider a more integrative approach to life, in general. This cannot happen, unless we operate from our hearts and not our ego-driven brains. Besides, I feel both philosophies are different sides of the same coin. I know this may be offensive to those who believe God created us all without resorting to natural laws. I don't wish to create ill will by stating that I see no problems with a compromise that would have God use these universal laws of E&I to bring about His plans.

Be Lighthearted

Hopefully you are not offended by others' beliefs. Since our hearts are orchestrating the E&I of our bodies and consciousness, it is a good idea to be "lighthearted." In my opinion, becoming "enlightened" is mostly becoming lighthearted. Humor is a sign of humility and of understanding that our brains, logic, and egos are great for survival and self-preservation, but not the final word for seeing things as they really are and for thriving in cooperation and community with our fellowmen. The smaller our egos, the more we love humor, and the more lighthearted we become. When our hearts are placed on the scale against a feather, our lightheartedness may come in handy.

Silly, I know: these are just innocent comments about not taking things too seriously. Silliness comes in handy when we are suffering and when we want to develop intimate relationships.[628] I hope you have at times "laughed your head off" reading this book and that you will consider making a resolution to see the world through lightheartedness and silliness. By the way, "silly" is a derivative of the Greek "selig," which means "blessed." Allan (Bud) Selig, the baseball commissioner, may appreciate this: lots of silliness in Major League Baseball . . .

Holograms = E&I

The whole concept of E&I may be expanded to infinity. If we were to continue to subdivide our body cells, we would get down to the atomic level. After atoms are split asunder, we get down to photons that are nothing but E&I.[629] In fact, our whole bodies are considered by some to be a hologram of E&I.[630] Some scientists think the whole universe is a hologram of E&I,[631] much like you see in the *Matrix* movies.[632]

The whole universe is made up of the same light, or E&I, that "quickens" our bodies, souls, and minds.[633] Whether we call this E&I "God," "Enlightenment," "Nirvana," or anything else for that matter is a decision to be made by each of us, hopefully respecting each others' interpretations of E&I.

The Feathered Serpents

The ancients understood the concept that E&I are at the heart of creation-destruction cycles in the universe as symbolized by the Ouroboros, the snake eating its own tail. In the middle of the circle created by the snake we find a dove, the symbol of communication of information, or "revelation," in the Judeo-Christian tradition. Thoth, the Egyptian God of communication of information, is often represented as holding the Ankh, the key with a closed loop for a handle that represents creation-destruction as well. Thoth is also known as Mercury and Hermes in Roman and Greek mythology, and as Enoch in ancient Palestine.

The caduceous, the symbol of medicine, is represented by a couple of feathered serpents coiling around a staff, very similar to the symbol of Hermes who represents commerce, messengers, integration, healing, and creation-destruction. If you carefully contemplate the "different" meanings of the caduceous, you will see that they are essentially the same thing: representations of E&I. The coiling feathered serpents also represent our DNA, another construct of E&I.[634]

Feathered serpents represented the ancient gods of Mesoamerica, Quetzalcoatl, and Viracocha. Christ spoke of being "wise as a serpent and harmless as a dove." Coincidence? You be the judge. Shiva, the goddess of creation-destruction in India, holds in her four hands all these symbols, too. It is throughout our history; shamans, gurus, prophets, mystics, and avatars—like Christ and Buddha—have alluded to these principles of light, or E&I.

E&I and TOIL

I am hoping that we have already discussed these points enough for you to see that our cells, orchestrated by our hearts,[635] function best when they get the right light (E&I) through good food, good thoughts, good relationships, clean environments, and good detoxification.

Without those optimal conditions, our cells TOIL and disrupt the flow of E&I they need to do their jobs, according to the universal rules of thermodynamics. Cell communication and metabolisms are then disrupted, triggering practically all diseases. Whether we are discussing a heart cell, a brain cell, an intestinal cell—it is all the same. In order to carry out their specific functions, they need E&I to do their job. Even though cells are specialized to do a specific function, they have similar "infrastructure." Whether we are making cars, computers, clothing, or carpets, we need E&I—and somebody to take out the garbage.

Dr. David Deutsch, a renowned physicist, predicted that the day would come when doctors would catch on that human beings also obey the basic principles of thermodynamics, or E&I.[636] To think that humans are outside these basic laws seems incongruous to me; perhaps you will agree after you finish this book. No matter what we are talking about, E&I is the essence of it, even in relationships. Bad E&I from poor communication has poisoned a few of our relationships, don't you agree?

What About the pH?

The potential Hydrogen (pH) of a cell and the extracellular fluids that bathe cells is not just a marker of acidity but of voltage, or E&I. People who emphasize pH as a key to health are quite right. I just wonder if they have considered E&I and all the ramifications discussed above. I also find that emphasizing the pH of every food and obsessing about it is counterproductive. Some people develop a religious zeal about their pH, which may be a bit annoying at a dinner party, especially when they insist on sticking that pH strip under their tongues after each bite. If we were to simply eliminate refined food, especially sugars, our pH would be perfect 99 percent of the time, save for some rare kidney diseases.

Chapter 12

Cell Communication of Energy and Information

As previously mentioned, many of the last ten Nobel Prizes in medicine and biology have turned to cell communication and metabolomics. The cell membranes of each of the fifty to one hundred trillion cells in our bodies are fine-tuned to receive messages of E&I from other cells. Cell membranes need to be healthy and flexible to send and receive these messages. This is possible only when our diets have good amounts of antioxidants, anti-inflammatory micronutrients, minerals, oils, polysaccharides (sugars), and the right amino acids. Then, signals (glycoproteins) of E&I from other cells may hook up to their specific receptors in a lock-and-key fashion. It turns out that the receptors floating on the phospholipids of the cell membrane are also glycoproteins.

Some now believe that this biochemical process of cell communication is really a biophysics process. In other words, biochemical messengers, like insulin and adrenaline, are working through their E&I, or electromagnetic signals. Every biochemical molecule has an electric signature, or E&I.[637]

The phospholipids in cell membranes are arranged much like a sandwich, which allows the membrane to behave like an energy conductor with an insulating layer in between. This structure effectively creates a capacitor of energy much like a regular battery. Since cell membrane receptors and incoming messengers are E&I

158

constructs, one may dilute the E&I of a messenger, like adrenaline, code it as an electronic signal, and e-mail it to the opposite corner of the globe where it may be downloaded and infused into a solution. When said solution is injected into a dog, it makes its heart beat faster,[638] just like mine did when I first read about that study; it has enormous implications . . .

In other words, our cell membranes are E&I receivers, facilitating cell communication of information and metabolism. Cell membranes are also physically connected by "nanotubules," or microscopic filaments made up of connective tissues. Through these nanotubules, cells send each other E&I messages.[639]

Network of E&I

The whole network of cell communication of E&I is called the psycho-neuro-immune-endocrine system.[640] It should have never been divided into its separate components. This network is the reason why everything seems so connected in our body. This network of cell communication of E&I breaks down when our cell membranes become inflexible, rigid and thus unresponsive. Cell membranes lose their ability to function normally through the four mechanisms encapsulated in T.O.I.L.

Our cells' abilities to process E&I is compromised when cells "TOIL"; their communication with one another is not optimal when that is going on. In other words, the network of communication is not healthy. The main reason cells need to communicate is to ensure that adequate E&I is processed or metabolized inside cells.

Our metabolisms generate toxins, or byproducts of energy making, the same as any a combustion engine does while obeying the universal laws of thermodynamics. Toxins created by combustion are also referred to as reactive oxygen species (ROS), oxidants, and free radicals. They must be eliminated or they "jam up" the engine.

Imagine what would happen if someone stuffed your vehicle's muffler with a rag; the process of detoxification would be compromised. Detoxification is like taking out the garbage; it is also known as catabolism. It turns out that ROS (don't confuse these toxins with the ROUS—rodents of unusual size in the movie, *The*

Princess Bride) are responsible for a "long term memory" of high blood glucose stress on arterial walls, even after the glucose levels have been normalized. This just means that even transient indulgence in junk food may have serious oxidative results on our arteries.[641]

Story Time

While I served in Alaska, like you see in the TV series, "Northern Exposure," my kids stayed with me in the summer. I was based in Dillingham, where Sarah Palin's husband, Todd, is from. There wasn't much to do in the late evenings; invariably they would wind up watching their most favorite movie, *The Princess Bride,* over and over again. I was never able to resist sitting along with them; I ended up watching it over a hundred times. I still cannot change channels when I run into it while TV surfing. That wonderful little movie has everything!

Taking Out the Garbage

My main job is to bring home the bread, or "energy." As such, I suppose I am the "lord" of the house. Now, don't have a cow; in old English, "lord" meant "keeper of the bread." Not coincidentally, I am also in charge of taking out the garbage. It is the same in any industry and that is why we have so much pollution on Earth. But to rail against environmental pollution without the understanding that we need E&I to function as a society is, in my opinion, a bit naïve. Some of us, meaning well and having very worthy goals, complain about environmental pollution and try to shut down energy industries while they jet around, drive expensive cars, live in huge mansions in the hills, and use every imaginable electronic gadget. Ironically, some of the gadgets they use to communicate their outstanding resolve to clean up the planet consume enormous amounts of energy.

Our bodies are no different. Each cell, after using up the E&I we ingest in the form of food, needs to get rid of "metabolites," or the garbage produced by the "energy-processing" structures within the cell, the mitochondria. Again, these metabolites are also known as free radicals, oxygen reactive species, and oxidants. Just as we have specialized cells to bring in E&I into every cell (GI tract, lungs, heart, and circulatory system), we have cells that have specialized in getting rid of the garbage produced by all our cells. The "garbage-processing" cells make up the organs that take out the garbage: our intestines, livers, skin, and kidneys.

Since the main engine you are familiar with is in your car, imagine how it would run if you put bad gas in it and, again, stuffed a rag in the exhaust pipe. Some would even point out that thinking unkind thoughts about your jalopy is going to have a negative effect on its performance.[642]

The Sun and E&I

Photosynthesis helps us harness solar light, or E&I, into our bodies by eating good food. No wonder most cultures view eating as a spiritual sacrament. In India, there are reports of gurus taking in solar E&I directly through their eyes, bypassing food altogether. This is great and praise-worthy; but it is fun to eat, too. Imagine procreating without a biological process . . .

It is the same with human societies: they cannot survive without solar E&I. Most wars are triggered by someone wanting someone else's E&I sources. People immigrating from one country to another are "fueled" by their needs for E&I. I don't want to get political on you, but I think you could make some interesting parallels to current political affairs in your country, no matter where you live.

Now, let us look at E&I issues in our bodies and TOILing cell membranes leading to metabolic dysfunction and breakdown of cell communication. The four mechanisms of TOILing will be discussed out of sequence to emphasize the best studied ones first, i.e., inflammation.

(1) Cell Membrane Inflammation

Diabetes is an inflammatory condition.[643] The inflammation of cell membrane receptors and inflammatory messengers trigger TOILing, making the cell membrane develop IR.[644] Even before a diagnosis of diabetes is made we may see that the higher the insulin levels, the higher the markers for inflammation, and vice versa.[645] Simply put, the more sugar we eat, the higher the inflammation in our body.[646]

The metabolic syndrome has also been associated with inflammation.[647]

Increased inflammatory messengers may even predict the risk of future weight gain.[648] In other words, obesity is also an inflammatory condition.[649] The more weight we gain, the more our bodies become inflamed.[650] The more fat tissue one has, the more inflammatory messengers that person releases. This is why weight loss lowers inflammatory markers like CRP with a concomitant reduction of IR.[651] The fact that fat tissues store more toxins creates yet another vicious cycle because environmental toxins increase inflammation and oxidation.

The article, "The Energy Request of Inflammation,"[652] makes the point that inflammatory messengers, like cytokines, play a significant role in our metabolisms. Inflammation itself causes energy to be spent less efficiently; yet another vicious cycle. The same thing happens in any inefficient engine. If it overheats it produces even more "inflammation" making the engine even more inefficient with time. An inflammatory response to pathogens and toxins consumes large amounts of energy in our bodies. Chronic inflammation or overheating of the cell membrane leads to chronic IR.[653]

The immune system at work puts a heavy load on our energy metabolisms. Think of fever: our bodies respond to the inflammation-triggered shortage of energy by allocating energy where it is most needed, the immune system, and by turning down the supply of energy where it is less needed (locomotion, growth, and certain brain functions). To respond quicker, the uptake of glucose into immune system cells does not require insulin.

Infections are inflammatory conditions and inflammation triggers IR; IR triggers inflammation: "acute infections cause IR and even after clinical recovery, some impairment in carbohydrate metabolism persists." Higher white blood cell (WBC) counts are seen in IR.[654] In fact, the highest quartile of WBC had a 50 percent increased risk of diabetes. Aspirin, an anti-inflammatory molecule, reduced glucose by 25 percent, CRP by 15 percent, triglycerides by 50 percent, and insulin clearance by 30 percent.

The paper, "Insulin Resistance (IR) and Chronic Cardiovascular Inflammatory Syndrome,"[655] ties together a lot of related conditions through the mechanism of inflammation. Inflammation causes the lining of arteries to put out messages of distress that lead to coagulation problems, like clots in our legs. This is why obese people have more leg clots.[656] The best known link between IR, inflammation, and cardiovascular function is the subject of many TV commercials these days: disordered lipid metabolism. In other words, IR interferes with the liver's ability to handle cholesterol properly. The reason essential fatty acids have been found to be so helpful with practically all conditions is that they lower TOILing, inflammation, and IR; more about these issues in chapter 26.

(2) Cell Membrane Oxidation

Oxidation is very much like inflammation; it is also involved in diabetes and obesity. Oxidation also raises the inflammatory marker CRP.[657] Cell membrane oxidation leads to IR and to all the complications we see in diabetics.[658] But the cell membrane is not the only thing TOILing: reactive oxygen species found through blood testing also signals oxidative stress in the pancreas, which may lead to insulin secretion problems.[659]

The article, "Is Oxidative Stress the Pathogenic Mechanism Underlying IR, Diabetes, and Cardiovascular Disease? The Common Soil Hypothesis Revisited,"[660] is an excellent review. The "common soil" refers to the cells that make up our tissues. Whether we are dealing with our hearts, kidneys, brains, lungs, bones, etc, these organs constitute a common soil with identical needs for good E&I to live longer, avoid disease, and avoid ending up like the "tin man."[661]

If we are not consuming enough antioxidants in our diets, the products of combustion in our cells (oxidants) and the free radicals we take in from combustion processes in the environment (pollution) scavenge the common soil looking for electrons to satisfy their hunger for completion.[662] In other words, free radicals, oxidants, or reactive oxygen species are a result of energy-making in both our bodies and in the environment.

"Chronic Intake of Potato Chips Increases the Production of Reactive Oxygen Radicals and Increases C-Reactive Protein" is a great article to illustrate the point that bad food will turn you into the tin man.[663]

In the course of producing energy, free radicals donate an electron, but they insist on getting said electron back. Our cell membranes, making up our common terrain, are the most accessible and vulnerable to their predatory behavior. When free radicals scavenge our cell membranes, TOILing begins with dire consequences to our cells' abilities to process E&I and cell communication. And the more we get oxidized, the more fat we accumulate—another vicious cycle.[664]

(3) Cell Membrane and Less Optimal Mitochondrial Function

E&I from the sun are processed in every cell of the body. Specifically, this function takes place in the mitochondria within the cell. Mitochondria are cells themselves; they got into a symbiotic relationship with the bigger cells they live in, our systemic cells. Mitochondrial problems are the "L" in TOILing, which stands for "light" or "love" or "less optimal mitochondrial function." The book, Mitochondrial Medicine,[665] by Salvatore DiMauro, Michio Hirano, and Eric A. Schon summarizes how practically all diseases involve a degree of mitochondrial dysfunction. "Mitohormesis" is the term that describes the control that mitochondrial function exerts on all bodily functions by providing E&I for cells to do their jobs.[666]

Each systemic cell has hundreds of mitochondria cells within. The systemic cells that need the most E&I—the heart, the brain, and muscles in general—have the most mitochondria cells to process that E&I through the Krebs Cycle of phosphorylation. This cycle produces adenosine triphosphate (ATP) as a unit of energy that our cells need to function. Each mitochondria cell produces approximately two million ATP molecules, which vibrate every one ten-thousandth of a second. Multiplying this big number by fifty to one hundred trillion (the number of cells we have in our bodies), gives us a humongous number I am not sure my brain can understand. But my heart manages to orchestrate the E&I that comprise our bodies and consciousness.

This is why intuition wins the day, ahead of intellectualizing and aggrandizing our inflated egos[667] Our old pal Freud, who learned a whole lot of stuff from the woman he and his disaffected sidekick C.J. Jung were in love with, also said that "when confronted with a most difficult decision, it is best to make it from the heart" in the book, *A Most Dangerous Method*, by John Kerr. But I digress . . . or do I?

To cope with less optimal E&I processing, the mitochondria may undergo fusion or fission, creating different arrangements in mitochondria cells found in each systemic cell.[668] The mitochondria need to maximize their ability to eliminate fatty acids, or products of combustion, to optimize their energy-producing function. Failure to do so leads to IR.[669]

The mitochondria are very delicate, but they don't seem to quit working all of a sudden. While they do eventually die (like any other cell), they slowly lose their ability to put out ATP, leading to fatigue and the slow deterioration of function we see in disease and aging.[670] This is particularly true in muscles, especially cardiac muscles and the brain, which need the most E&I. For example, seizures are now felt to be a result of mitochondrial dysfunction due to free radical production and oxidative damage to cellular glycoproteins, lipids, and DNA.[671] The mitochondria's own DNA may also malfunction enough to induce problems in the DNA of the cell itself.[672] Mitochondrial DNA problems are now felt to be "a common cause of chronic morbidity and is more prevalent than has been previously appreciated."[673]

Mitochondrial dysfunction compromises the psycho-neuro-immune-endocrine network of communication of E&I; this leads to obesity and diabetes[674] through IR. This explains why our mitochondrial-dense muscles get infiltrated by fat as we age and become more sedentary;[675] another vicious cycle is at play here because fatty muscles won't work as well. Fatigue ensues, resulting in even less activity. This is another reason why incremental, or gradient, exercise helps fatigue[676] and building up our muscles decreases diabetic tendencies.[677] Practically speaking, it is the signaling of E&I in food that optimizes muscular structure and function.[678]

The process of making energy (ATP phosphorylation) in the mitochondria produces free radicals, or ROS, which are oxidating molecules. They need to be neutralized and eliminated or our "engines will rust."[679] Consequently, mitigating mitochondrial oxidative stress with antioxidants helps reduce IR,[680] whereas diets low in antioxidants, like high sugar diets, increase IR.[681] No wonder that D-ribose, a sugar that acts like an antioxidant, helps mitochondrial production of ATP, or E&I, when taking 5 grams, one to three times a day.[682] Think about healing TOIL of the mitochondrial cell membrane. In subsequent chapters, we will see that the antioxidants alpha lipoic acid and CoQ10 are particularly helpful in mitochondrial function.

The Same Ball of Wax

As you probably have figured out, all four components of TOILing interplay with one another. For example, oxidative/inflammatory damage to the mitochondria in nerve tissues is a key element in diabetes—particularly in neuron dysfunction or neuropathy. This is likely due to a faulty thermostat in the brain.[683] Oxidation of mitochondria is also quite prevalent in neurodegenerative diseases like Alzheimer's and Parkinson's diseases.[684]

Refined diets are low in B complex vitamins like folic acid; this increases oxidation of our DNA and of our cell membranes.[685] Environmental toxins deplete our supply of B complex vitamins and act like free radicals, scavenging cell membranes in our mitochondrial and systemic cell membranes.[686] For example, the more we lack antioxidants—particularly glutathione—the more atherosclerotic lesions we develop on our arterial walls.[687]

Open Sesame

Still, the most insidious problem, at least from this book's perspective, is the IR that mitochondrial dysfunction causes at the cell membrane level.[688]

Each messenger of cell communication requires its own private docking site or receptor. For example, insulin will only attach to insulin receptors, and serotonin to serotonin receptors, much like a key in a specific lock. It turns out that these receptors are really "gates" that require E&I to open and close. In fact, these gates are much like "energy fields"[689] like you see in movies where a shield of energy keeps the matinee idol from momentarily getting out of the aliens' prison. E&I are required to open these gates. The mitochondria provide ATP to fuel this process. If this does not happen efficiently, which is seen as the mitochondria age, we develop IR and resistance to every other cell messenger as well.[690]

Mother Eve's Mitochondrial Genes

Scientists have been able to trace everyone's mitochondrial DNA back to one single woman in prehistoric Africa; she was christened "Eve" because of this. It turns out that the genetics of "mitochondrial defects may play a role in the metabolic syndrome."[691] This article shows that some families have a mutation in their mitochondrial genes: children of type 2 diabetics seem to end up with more IR in muscle cells that show more oxidation in their mitochondria.[692] Even pre-diabetics show a significant decrease in mitochondrial DNA.[693]

Mitochondrial function may be impaired if we lack magnesium, a condition also observed in patients with IR. Some people's genetics are such that they cannot correct low magnesium levels in their cells, unless CoQ10, an antioxidant crucial for mitochondrial function, is supplemented along with magnesium.[694] The antioxidant, CoQ10, has been shown to improve mitochondrial function. Other antioxidants like vitamin C,[695] E, K, lipoic acid, riboflavin, thiamin, niacin, creatine, and carnitine have also been found to help the mitochondria.[696] You may think of supplements for the mitochondria as a "metabolic tune-up."[697]

Optimal mitochondrial function is crucial to avoid developing a sluggish metabolism in our muscles and IR.[698] Then, as noted above, the way we process E&I from solar E&I in food is influenced by genetic tendencies that may be mitigated by the very food we eat.[699] Remember nutrigenomics? Our genes are influenced by our diets, and so is our mitochondrial function.[700] This is yet another vicious cycle if we eat poorly.

What came first: the chicken or the egg? I don't know and neither do I know why the chicken crossed the damn road, but we don't care, as long as we eat lots of vegetables and fruits. The more antioxidants we consume, the better mitochondrial function we have.[701] All the artificial, trans-hydrogenated fats we eat in processed foods alter mitochondria cell membrane function.[702] About 12 percent of mitochondrial function is lost when we eat those plasticized fats.[703]

Communication at the Speed of Light

We have already discussed the view that cell messengers are really working through their energetic, or biophysics, imprints. For example, the E&I contained in the insulin messenger is thought to go into solution in the extracellular fluid bathing all cells.[704] One single molecule of insulin is not as efficient in cell communication as having the E&I of insulin, or its electromagnetic signal, dissolved in the very solution that bathes the receptors on each cell. The experiment that showed that the electromagnetic signal of adrenaline can be e-mailed across the world, downloaded, put in solution, injected into an animal's heart, and have its heart rate go up suggests that this view is correct.[705]

Where the Blubber Hits the Road

The article, "Of the Fit and the Fat: Mitochondrial Abnormalities and Type 2 Diabetes,"[706] reviews the principles of cell membrane dysfunction. It helps us understand why energy-boosting antioxidants like ALA and CoQ10 help decrease IR.[707] Other than the E&I of our thoughts, our spirits, and our hearts, the E&I from our food serves to fuel the mitochondria to "power up" each cell, thereby enabling said cells to carry out whatever their particular function may be. Each cell's DNA determines said function through E&I stored in its genes. At the most basic level, sweet death is due to poor mitochondrial function.[708]

(4) Cell Membrane Toxicity and Glycosylation

Toxicity is a concept generally ignored by most docs who argue that our kidneys, livers, skin, and intestines do a very good job of detoxifying. They feel that we don't need to fuss about detoxification issues very much, unless we are acutely toxic, like having a chemical spill in your neighborhood or some industrial worker, who, after years of battling the alleged offending employer, is told that his disease "is all in his head."

In my opinion, environmental toxins, or free radicals, and the oxidants we make ourselves when we metabolize E&I are serious contributors to cell membrane dysfunction, especially in those of us who have genetic tendencies to detoxify less efficiently. But there is one toxin that is often overlooked, despite its widespread use and abuse. Can you guess what that toxin is? That is right: refined sugars. Most of their damage is due to the fact that they take the place of healthy sugars on the cell membrane.

Environmentalists, as well intended as they are, are concentrating on a few micrograms of toxin exposure, like air pollution, while ignoring the kilograms of refined sugars we eat on a daily basis. They are not wrong. But, as a society, we don't understand the dramatic toxic effects refined sugars have on cell communication, E&I, and how aggressive we need to be to lick our sugar addiction.

Imagine what we could achieve if our sweet deaths also became "an inconvenient truth" and got the same type of coverage environmental pollution is now getting.

Putting it All Together

Once we understand these simple concepts of E&I, TOILing, and poor cell communication, we may see that *all* diseases have the same common roots. Instead of focusing on classifying disease into neat diagnoses, we may then work on the roots of the problem—not the symptoms of each disease—through a pharmaceutical approach. The latter boggles down in minutia and focuses on one pharmaceutical product for each symptom; of course, that is where the money is . . .

No doubt the "one disease/symptom, one drug" approach has helped a lot of people so far by focusing on diagnosing the "leaves" instead of the roots. However, it is my opinion that the science to move beyond this paradigm is here to stay and will eventually win the day.[709]

Chapter 13

Glycobiology: The Sweet Spot

"Glycosylation" is the process of adding Mother Nature's sugars to our proteins so that they are built correctly and function better. This is how we normally make "glycoproteins" the messengers of cell communication and the receptors on cell membranes.[710] The article, "Carbohydrates and Glycobiology: Cinderella's Coach is Ready," tells us that we have known about this for a long time. But it wasn't until recently that we have understood how important glycosylation is in cell communication of E&I. The science that specializes in these concepts is glycobiology.[711] If you want to read more about glycobiology, pick up Dr. Emil I. Mondoa and Mindy Kitei's book, *Sugars That Heal.*[712]

Caramelizing Our Bodies, Like Candy Apples

Genes do not do anything for you unless they are copied from your DNA or transcribed into glucoproteins that carry out genetic messages to other cells, resulting in specific functions and structures in the human body. After all the enthusiasm for gene research, we are discovering that proteomics, or the study of gene function through glycoproteins coded from our DNA, is more important. But even before the dust settled after this dramatic shift of emphasis, glycomics entered the picture, revealing that the function and structure of glycoproteins are dramatically affected by the sugars that are attached to them. This process has been called the "Amadori reaction," the "Maillard reaction," "caramelization," and the "browning of proteins."

Have you noticed that foods cooked at higher temperature tend to taste sweeter?[713] And have you noticed that your shirts are stiffer after dry cleaner staff members used a little starch (a type of sugar) to get them clean? These are some of the day-to-day applications of "caramelization." The problem is that caramelized foods tend to become addicting. They also lose about 50 percent of their nutrients because the high temperatures employed cause more oxidation. In other words, oxidation contributes to poor glycozylation of proteins.[714] This is why it is better to eat our food as raw as possible. If your shirts become stiffer with caramelization, guess what your arteries look like on caramelizing diets?

Again, Mother Nature's sugars modulate the healthy structure and function of proteins. The science of glycobiology has demonstrated that cell membranes TOIL with inflammation, etc., when proteins are glycosylated with refined sugars instead. When this happens, many other problems have been noted—like rejection of transplanted organs, hepatitis, and cancer. The more sugar we eat, the more we affect glycolization of proteins in the liver; this causes the switch that normally shuts off sugar production in the liver to malfunction, adding more sugar into the bloodstream; IR gets worse due to another vicious cycle driven by[715]

> "Harmful inflammatory reactions [that] are often triggered by carbohydrates, as is blood clotting . . . Carbohydrates are central to many processes that are at the core of important diseases, and now that we understand some of those roles, it's not surprising that this has become a hot topic at drug companies."[716]

Sweet Big Pharma

A "hot topic at drug companies . . ." Interesting.

True to our "Homo economicus" nature, a "consortium for functional glycomics" has been founded by Big Pharma to come up with more powerful drugs by attaching good sugars to them.[717] Wouldn't it be better to use glycobiology concepts to convince people to stop eating refined sugars? But there is not much money in this, is there?

Homo economicus has seldom been able to think about the welfare of future generations. Some Native Americans and other Old World cultures don't act on any community issue unless they focused on the impact said decisions would have on their seventh generation. Unfortunately, most people who hold our modern Darwinian capitalism as the best way to do business would consider these enlightened philosophies to be a reflection of lazy and unproductive societies.

More Examples of Glycobiology

(1) There is a rare congenital disorder of glycosylation that affects the GI tract, blood clotting, and neurological problems. When researchers discovered that glycosylation was the common mechanism, they commented that:

> "We have a new perspective on multisystem diseases that we had no way of understanding before. The fact that a simple biochemical defect causes such a wide range of symptoms involving multiple organ systems has been a revelation... Glycobiologists are more confident that a spoonful of sugar will not only make the medicine go down, but replace it with something that works better."[718]

(2) We get more infections when we eat refined sugars. Complex or healthy carbohydrates are essential for the normal function of our immune system. If any cell is attacked it is because the sugars making up the glycoproteins on its surface are not what Mother Nature intended.[719] For example, poor glycolysation of amino acids make infections from the bacteria pseudomonas more virulent.[720]

(3) "Selectins" are carbohydrate-binding proteins that are released by injured cells to attract white blood cells for heal-

ing and fighting potential infections. The manipulation of carbohydrate chains is becoming commonplace to control the immune system.[721]

(4) Digestive enzymes are also glycosylated proteins. Digestive enzymes are powerful anti-inflammatory agents, which is why they lower IR.

(5) Prions are peculiar proteins that replicate or get copied without going through the DNA or RNA process. They may trigger infections like Mad Cow Disease. Prions are unique molecules because of the bad carbohydrates that stick to these proteins. Dr. Stanley Prusiner won the 1997 Nobel Prize in medicine for his work on prions.[722]

(6) The article, "Progressive Glycosylation of Albumin and its Effect on the Binding of Homocysteine May Be a Key Step in the Pathogenesis of Vascular Damage in Diabetes Mellitus,"[723] discusses a hypothesis that makes a whole lot of sense to me because it fits the general concept of TOILing terrain.

Back to "the Planet of the Apes"

The article, "Sugar Separates Humans from Apes,"[724] shows that humans don't have a form of a good sugar called sialic acid in the brain; said sugar allowed the human brain to continue developing well beyond the apes' brain. Could a "devolution" of our brain be triggered by refined sugars in some of us? Don't "go ape" over chocolate cheesecake.

Bloody Example of Glycosylation

Blood types are probably the best known example of glycosylation. Types A and B have an extra sugar molecule on their red blood cell membrane proteins. Type A has acetyl galactose and type B has galactose. Type AB has both sugars; type O has neither. This is why the latter type is more susceptible to the ravages of processed sugar: its butt-naked cell membrane proteins are easily saturated or glycosylated with toxic sugars.

This concept is the basis for the book, *Eat Right For Your Type*, by Dr. Peter J. D'Adamo and Catherine Whitney. There is some merit to this approach. However, the authors studied "in-vitro" (laboratory) reactions in red blood cells when they are exposed to certain foods. This is why I cannot endorse everything the book says. It would be better to study these reactions "in-vivo," or in real people, eating real diets and exposed to real environments. I believe the general idea of the book is still valid. For instance, my practical and personal experience tells me that type O individuals are, indeed, more susceptible to refined sugars, which they should avoid with more vigor, compared to other types. Still, I find the religious zeal with which some people pursue diets according to their blood types a bit counterproductive.

It is simpler to quit refined foods, in general, regardless of the blood type we have. I feel devotees of blood type diets often lose the joy of eating due to their micromanaging. Any diet that is too restrictive is not going to be adhered to for very long. But, again, glycobiology theoretically supports the blood type-diet approach.

The Right Food, the Right Sugars = E&I

Caramelizing proteinsand fats is not only tasty, but it is also vital for cell communication. This process, known as

> "Glycosylation, is the most common form of protein and lipid modification, but its biological significance has long been underestimated. The last decade, however, has witnessed the rapid emergence of the concept of the sugar code of biological information; indeed, monosaccharides represent an alphabet of biological information similar to amino acids and nucleic acids, but with unsurpassed coding capacity."[725]

Consuming processed sugars instead of essential natural sugars is devastating for our cell membranes and glycoproteins; cell communication of E&I will not be optimal if we don't consume the foods or sugars that Mother Nature designed for us to avoid TOILing. These are the natural essential sugars we find in foods: mannose, glucose, xylose, galactose, fucose, N–acetyl glucosamine, N–acetyl galactosamine, and N–acetyl neuraminic acid, or sialic acid.[726]

If we eat a diet based on fruits and vegetables, to the tune of thirteen servings a day, we get these sugars in abundance.[727] Since very few are able to eat like that, these eight sugars may be supplemented with positive results; the sugars reduce TOILing, protein structure, and function by improving glycosylation. The nutritional supplements Glycoessentials (Nature's Sunshine Products) and Ambratose (Mannatec) contain these eight sugars; they are absorbed without being broken down.[728].

Xylitol is often mistakenly thought to be one of these eight essential sugars. It is a natural sweetener, like stevia. These two are the only sweeteners that have been shown to be 100 percent safe. Stevia is an herb that helps insulin secretion.[729] Xylitol, aka "wood or birch sugar," is a polyol sugar or five-carbon sugar alcohol found in birch, raspberries, plums, and corn. It is widely used in a variety of products. These are some of the benefits seen with Xylitol:

- It helps reduce calories and IR.[730]

- In chewing gum, it reduces cavities.[731]

- Appetite suppression[732]

- In cream form, it controls staphyloccocus aureus, an overgrowth on skin, by inhibiting the bug's ability to attach to the glycoproteins of the skin.[733]

- Gingivitis prevention[734]

- Bone strengthening[735]

- Mouthwash for dry mouth[736]

- Reduction of asthma, allergies, and ear/sinus infections[737] (This is why I recommend it for use in sinus irrigation.)

Toxic Sugars

Practically all diseases have a "T," or toxicity component. In my opinion, the most common "T" in TOILing is poor glycosylation due to sweet death. Remember that the four components of TOILing are interacting with one another. This is why poorly-glycosylated proteins act as free radicals, increasing oxidation parameters about fifty times more than those proteins that are not glycosylated.[738]

Chapter 14

An Appeal to Your Vanity:
Age and Glycosylation

The diet we eat is the most important factor on how we age.[739] Some folks may say our genes are more important; perhaps, but the new science of nutrigenomics argues that we may maximize the longevity already coded in our genes through diet. Aging is not as gentle a process when we develop IR from toxic high glycemic diets[740] that trigger excessive insulin secretion. Insulin influences how genes age transcribed[741] and compromises the mitochondria's ability to process energy as it itself ages.[742] Of course, aging, itself, increases IR.[743] Yet another vicious cycle: are you getting dizzy?

In other words, aging is affected by the kinds of sugars we eat. You have heard it say that a cigarette is a like a nail in your coffin. Well, a Twinkie is also a nail in your coffin.

The article, "Diabetes and Advanced Glycosylated End products (AGE),"[744] tells us that poorly-glycosylated proteins alter the structure and function of molecules, increase oxidative stress, and act as inflammatory agents.[745] In other words, the end products of poor glycosylation, or caramelization, speed the onset of death and make disease more likely by increasing TOILing and E&I problems.

When sugars, proteins, and fats are cooked for a long time

at high temperatures, they create more AGE that increase blood vessel damage in diabetics. AGE formation is worsened by high sugar/fat diets and smoking.[746] The bad cholesterol (LDL) becomes more toxic or sticky with inflammation when exposed to AGE products.[747]

The ravages of aging are more pronounced in people with pre-diabetes[748] and diabetes. AGE are responsible for diabetic complications throughout the body; they even disrupt insulin function,[749] molecular formation, enzyme activity, reduce degrading capacity, and alter cell receptors. AGE have been directly implicated with heart disease through the toxic effects that AGE have on the lining of arteries,[750] LDL/bad cholesterol oxidation, eye problems, kidney cell problems, DNA breaks, neuropathy, and Alzheimer's disease. Amyloid formation in the brain, as seen in Alzheimer's disease, has also been linked to AGE formation.[751] Chlorella, a unicellular green algae, may improve Alzheimer's disease by decreasing AGE products.[752]

RAGE Over AGE

"RAGE" is a good word to describe what is going on: the inflamed lining (RAGE) of arteries (endothelium) and the GI tract express receptors for AGE, or RAGE.[753] Our own cells develop receptors for new molecules when they try to make sense of the garbage (AGE) circulating in our bloodstream. This is a reflection of how incredibly malleable, flexible, and adaptable our cells are. They are always trying to make sense of our environment. Cells end up adapting to whatever environment they are exposed to. This is the key concept of nutrigenetics: the foods our ancestors have eaten for thousands of years are best for us. Think of our Japanese friends whose healthy parents quickly become sick when they adapt to the American diet after immigrating to our shores.

This will help you develop a bit of RAGE yourself: Big Food is now placing AGE products in their food to increase the sweet taste. They do so by cooking their products at a high temperature. Big Food knows that very few people like low-heat cooking, which is really not without taste; avoiding high temperature cooking can decrease AGE by 50 percent with a drop of 30 percent in circulating AGE.[754] You may have guessed that Big Food is sweetening its products to maximize profits. But when we see the potential problems that AGE can cause, we have to wonder if Big Food cares about the public's health: Researchers have shown that "RAGE mediated sustained inflammation, coupled with failure or regenerative mechanisms, may lead to irreversible tissue injury."[755]

This is particularly true in the cells lining our arteries, which is why RAGE and AGE molecules affect myocardial energy metabolism and function during episodes of ischemia, or less blood to heart muscle.[756] That RAGE may be used to screen for glycemic control is a pretty good sign that the more RAGE we have, the worse our degree of sweet death.[757]

In my opinion, AGE are being placed in processed food to increase our addiction to refined foods. All the RAGE we develop with AGE-filled processed food and the questionable practices of Big Food are making us age faster.

AGE and Inflammation

The article, "Crosslinking by Advanced Glycation End Products (AGE) Increase the Stiffness of the Collagen Network in Human Articular Cartilage,"[758] tells us that AGE contribute to stiffness not only inside our arteries but throughout our bodies. This is why there is more wrinkling of the skin with high sugar diets.[759] How is that for more motivation? New drugs to neutralize AGE's inflammation are being developed;[760] wouldn't it be better to quit putting AGE in our food?

AGE are also associated with clogging up of arteries in diabetes and renal failure.[761] AGE and poor glycosylation interfere with NOS, the "molecule of the decade."[762] NOS is the system most responsible for inflammation and oxidation in our bodies. This is why antioxidant treatment, like alpha lipoic acid,[763] may reduce the damage created by AGE.[764]

Some people are genetically predisposed to have more problems with inflammation due to NOS polymorphisms in their genes; they are more likely to develop pre-diabetes.[765] Our hormones, in general, not just insulin, are influenced by how our NOS systems work.[766] There is crosstalk between the endocrine

179

system and the NOS system. Remember the psycho-neuro-immune-endocrine network of cell communication. The NOS system also affects our metabolisms by influencing adrenal, thyroid, and insulin function. NOS deficiency behaves much like the metabolic syndrome.

Love Your Gray Hair

Young women tell me that my gray hair makes me look "interesting." Okay, fine, two of my three daughters do.

Aging with grace and dignity to avoid the ravages of chronic illnesses is a worthy goal. However, an escapist approach where death, natural graying, and the gradual loss of function are poorly understood and interpreted as signs of failure seems a bit self-defeating to me. Such an approach robs us of the wisdom that comes from aging and perpetuates the irrational and ubiquitous tendency to devalue seniors while worshipping youth with all its folly and clumsiness.

Living life with constant reminders of our own mortality is quite healthy. We are thus motivated to live life fully—to enjoy the present moment as much as we can. "Carpe diem" (seize the day) is not a hedonistic concept; it is an exhortation to enjoy life as much as we can, provided such enjoyment is coupled with respect for our fellowmen. Then, we may cherish each breath and each sunset with a heart full of gratitude for the gift of life, focusing on the present, instead of obsessing about the past and the future. The latter attitude may keep us from forgiving one another and worrying about problems that never materialize. Living in the present with gray hair and wrinkles has a beauty to it. Don't deprive yourself of aging with wisdom and serenity.

Many cultures understand the wisdom of aging while contemplating their mortality. In our own culture, we celebrate Halloween, which unfortunately has become a time to engorge our children with candy. If you wish to know more about these concepts, read Robert A. F. Thurman's book, *The Tibetan Book of the Dead*.

Chapter 15

Stressed-Out Membranes

Mental, emotional, and spiritual stress may be just as toxic as physical stress is to our cell membranes, especially in the arteries.[767] The more severe our allostatic load (the wear and tear associated with chronic overactivity or suboptimal function of our coping mechanisms), the sicker we get. One of the most serious results of stress is the post-traumatic stress disorder (PTSD). Not surprisingly, it has been documented to increase the risk of metabolic problems.[768]

Stress may impair cell signaling, especially the hormonal messengers that are released to signal TOILing. The most damaging are cortisol, adrenaline, and glucocorticoids from the adrenal glands right above our kidneys. These hormones increase IR. Glucocorticoid genes have been implicated with heart disease, meaning that some of us are more prone to IR and, consequently, heart disease through stress and the adrenal glands.[769]

We Need a Vacation

Overworked people and those lacking sleep are more at risk of developing IR. Lack of sleep mimics the symptoms of diabetes. People who only get four hours of sleep a night have a decrease of 30 percent in insulin secretion. Restoring sleep will normalize the problem, but it takes them 40 percent longer to recover. In fact, chronic loss of sleep may not allow people to recover at all.[770] This can also become a vicious cycle: the more hyperinsulinemia one has, the higher the index of sleep apnea.[771]

This ought to help you get to sleep sooner: people who do not fall asleep within thirty minutes of hitting the pillow have a greater risk of dying prematurely. If you are having trouble falling asleep, read this book when you go to bed. If you still cannot sleep, call me; I have a pair of new shoes you could break in for me as you pace around your bedroom.

Stress causes "glucocorticoid resistance";[772] just like IR, cell membranes TOILing develop resistance to glucocorticoids secreted from the adrenal glands. They are not easily getting inside the cells because of defective cell membrane receptors to glucocorticoids.[773] Not surprisingly, this condition is associated with IR.[774] Why would insulin be the only messenger having trouble getting into cells when its membrane is TOILing?

Resistance to glucocorticoids increases the release of glucocorticoid hormones; they, in turn, increase food intake and the risk of obesity.[775] An overstressed adrenal system will likely cause "growths, or incidentalomas," or benign findings on adrenal gland scans while looking for something else at the time. Adrenal incidentalomas have been associated with early Cushing's syndrome or adrenal failure and IR.[776] No wonder stress reduction helps diabetes and obesity.[777]

Ongoing research is looking into neuropeptide Y, a messenger of cell communication, which has been found to mediate a significant portion of the hypothalamus-adrenal-pituitary (HPA) axis dysfunction when excessive VAT is present. Studies on rats have shown that supplementation with neuropeptide Y keeps rats from suffering the consequences of poor eating and excessive adrenal stress.[778] But don't hold your breath: a practical implementation is way in the distant future. You'd better plan on making some lifestyle changes *now*. Besides, I would wager that the concept of fooling Mother Nature with a chemical is not going to be risk-free. Have we not learned from past experiences?

Early Life

The stress that leads to adrenal problems, and subsequently increases our risk of sweet death, may begin with one's mother's stress during pregnancy. The HPA axis may be thus imprinted in the unborn child so that any stress later in life has more of an impact on how that child's adrenal glands handle it.[779] In other words, early life stress increases our chances of obesity and IR.[780]

Fortunately, a mother's tender loving care (TLC) may counteract the negative effects of her stress on her children. Her loving touches may modulate the expression of the genes regulating hormonal responses to stress.[781] Without mommy's TLC, children have a higher risk of becoming hostile. Their hostility may lead to poor social contacts, thus increasing the risk of developing IR.[782] Their anger inflames their cell membranes (TOIL) and elevates their risk of diabetes.[783]

Unhappy Meals

Food is E&I. It influences how we are built and how we function. Foreign substances like pesticides, food additives, and preservatives end up having an impact on our bodies, too.[784] For example, hyperactivity in children has been associated with chemicals in our food.[785]

Modern agriculture techniques are very stressful to plants and crops, producing stress signals that propagate down the food chain, ultimately influencing our very genes. In other words, our food itself can act as hidden chronic stress signals. The principle of "xenohormesis" states that we may become chronically stressed by non-nutritional signals in our food, like pollutants, in the environment.[786] As you will see below, these signals worsen the "T" of TOIL and thus promote IR and obesity.[787]

This stress on our crops may have also shaped our taste preferences because stress calls for more sugar to "fight or flight." Genetically, we love sugars because we are often stressed out. Our sugar addiction is then a quest for an "unhappy meal" to mitigate the stress.[788] Saturated fats in our diets seem to compromise optimal adrenal function as well.[789]

All of this may sound too far out for you, but when you consider the "Gaia theory"—that Mother Earth is alive and conscious—xenohormesis may make more sense. Even the Holy Book refers to Earth as a living organism.

A Gut Feeling

We cannot "embrace" growth while we try to protect and defend ourselves. To grow, we "open our arms" to new experiences. To protect ourselves, we fold our arms in front of us. This is also true in gut and nutrition issues.

We shift E&I, or blood circulation, from the gut to our "fight or flight" organs when we need to protect ourselves while under stress. By doing so, we deprive our intestines of the ability to adequately process the E&I we need to grow. In other words, we shift invaluable E&I away from our intestinal cells, which causes TOILing of the intestinal lining, and ultimately leaky gut and poor absorption of E&I from our food. Poor food intake then limits our capacity for growth.

Truly, these principles apply "below as they do above . . ."[790]

Story Time

While hosting my radio show, I got a call from a man driving around town. He lamented the fact that he ate very well and exercised regularly, or so he claimed. Yet, he still couldn't lose weight. While talking to me on his cell phone, he got a call on his other cell phone. Remember, he is driving in his car.

"Hello? Oh, yeah . . . Listen, I'll call you back. I'm on the phone talking to a radio station right now. Okay, bye!" [Picking up the cell phone he has me on hold on] "So, Doc, why is it I cannot lose weight?"

Needless to say, we had a discussion on how his overdrive lifestyle increases IR; overwrought adrenal function intensifies cell membrane TOILing.

Stress Management

It is not the stress itself that causes problems with our ability to process E&I; it is how we interpret or handle the stress. Stress is a normal part of life. There will always be spurs under our saddles. Early childhood experiences, even our own inborn temperament, go a long way in programming us to react to stress in different, unique and, at times, dysfunctional ways. This is why it is so critical that we develop self-awareness so that we may be able to heal our ailing heart and diffuse the issues that appear so stressful in our minds.

Superficial issues in our lives easily fool our brains, our logic, and our thinking. "What is important is invisible to the eye. Only with the heart can we see clearly" said the fox to the little prince.[791] Discovering that our egos are not really our true identities is the best way to heal our hearts from any wounds. Forgiving each other and ourselves is the most practical way of living a heart-focused life.

Ultimately, most people under stress cannot lose weight. No wonder that drugs to treat anxiety reduce the neuroendocrine adrenal responses to sugar dysregulation[792] so that people may lose weight. Unfortunately, the addictive nature of these drugs and their side effects may discourage their use.

Licking Sweet Death is not about stress management. Still, chapter 35 is a feeble attempt to address this very important issue. In part IV you will read about nutritional ways to support your adrenal glands; they take quite a beating when you are running around all stressed out. You may remember the time when IR and obesity were heavily advertised as adrenal problems. No doubt, adrenal support is part of the answer.

Chapter 16

Toxic Membranes

We have discussed the "T" in TOILing rather tangentially so far. Now, we will see how toxins in general contribute to the development of practically all diseases, especially those related to the metabolic syndrome. Toxins not only cause cell membrane TOILing, but also jam up cell membrane receptors, disrupting the ability of the real messengers—for instance hormones—to bind to those receptors. Consequently, environmental toxicity issues also worsen IR, diabetes, and obesity,[793] even in normal people.[794]

The most dramatic article I have seen so far on this point is "Persistent Pollutants and the Burden of Diabetes."[795] It documents that Dioxins, polychlorinated biphenyls, dichlorophenyl-dichloroethylene from DDT/DDE, trans-nonachlor, hexachlorobenzene, hexachlorociclohexanes, plus many other chemicals, like phthalates in plastics, are commonly found in humans.[796]

Another study analyzed these persistent organic solvents and fasting plasma glucose concentrations in a random sample of the general population from 1999 to 2002.[797] The prevalence of diabetes was five times higher in groups with higher concentrations of these toxins. The prevalence of diabetes doubled and tripled in the upper quantiles of DDE and other compounds.

The plot "sickens"

Diabetes itself may cause a higher accumulation of persistent organic pollutants because a faulty metabolism inhibits proper detoxification. People with diabetes would be more likely to experience the adverse effects of these pollutants. In other words, obesity does not lead to diabetes if one is not burdened with persistent organic pollutants. Extra fatty padding serves as a vehicle for such chemicals.[798]

A Michigan study corroborated these findings; People with higher PCBs had twice the incidence of diabetes.[799] Dioxins also increase the risk of diabetes.[800] We could therefore conclude that

"The causal role of toxins in diabetes is more likely to be contributory and indirect, i.e., through immunosuppressant, non-genotoxic, perhaps epigenetic mechanisms."[801]

But, the main problem in most diseases is still metabolic and E&I issues secondary to compromised cell communication. The toxins described above, in addition to bad food, and emotional stress, lead to TOILing of our cell membranes; IR, obesity, and diabetes soon follow.[802]

Cell membrane dysfunction leading to diabetes also leads to many other problems, such as resistance to other cell messengers, like neurotransmitters, hormones, and immune messengers. The above toxins have also been associated with cancer, neurologic problems (Parkinson's disease), and many other hormonal problems, especially thyroid and adrenal dysfunction.[803] The concept of toxins messing up our metabolisms and triggering IR is now referred to as "metabolic endotoxemia."[804] In other words, endotoxemia affects the amounts of E&I that are ultimately absorbed into our bodies.[805]

The toxin most talked about at the time of printing was Bisphenol (BPA). It is used in food and beverage containers, especially baby bottles. BPA is found in more than 90 percent of people, just like the other commonly used toxin in plastics: phthalates. The editorial calls for BPA to be labeled a "toxic chemical." In this *Journal of the American Medical Association* (JAMA) study, the oxidative effect of BPA and its tendency to cause IR is documented.

No wonder BPA has been shown to increase the risk of diabetes and heart problems. The article also discusses how these toxins affect the reproductive and neurology systems.[806]

"The Dose Does Not Make the Poison"

Before we get too far into environmental toxins, we need to discuss a little problem that has confused the issue dramatically, especially when we consider that it has been financially beneficial to hide the extent of the problem when it comes to our health and that of the environment.[807] Since the sixteenth century, most people have maintained that "the dose makes the poison," meaning that any substance may be harmful at high doses, even water and oxygen. The FDA has operated under this antiquated dogma since its inception, despite solid evidence that some chemicals may be toxic at very small doses, too.

The "U" curve of toxic exposure is now felt to be a more accurate approximation of what is going on. At very small doses (the beginning of the "U" curve), chemicals may escape detection and detoxification in our bodies so that no initial reaction is seen when exposed. But, in the long run (the end of the "U" curve), said tiny exposures could cause significant damage. The same toxins at a more detectable mid-range level may then be properly eliminated (the bottom of the "U" curve) before damage occurs. This is a common finding for many toxins like

> "endocrine-active chemicals and drugs, for which high doses inhibit (down-regulate) the low response system while initiating a wide array of other adverse effects via different response mechanisms."[808]

Despite these findings most people will still tell you that chemicals in the environment are 100 percent safe in small amounts. You could respond by suggesting they try a drop of water on their forehead over an extended period of time . . .

Let's Not Be "Idiots"

The idiopathic environmental intolerance syndrome (IEI) describes our immune systems overwhelmed by polluted environments; this may lead to practically all diseases because the immune system is involved in all of our body functions. This is one of the reasons why we develop so many inflammatory conditions these days. A new branch of medicine has been created to deal with this concept: immunotoxicology.[809]

"Idiopathic" means, "not knowing the cause" of a problem. Since we now know about TOILing, perhaps we could drop the idiopathic terminology used in many settings. Toxins, by affecting the way cells use E&I, affect the whole network of cell communication. A toxic environment affects our hormones, our immune systems, and our nervous systems. Only an "idiotic" society would soil the very environment that sustains our lives — the very earth we come from. Perhaps we need to keep the "idiopathic" term, after all.

Pollution, again, is an E&I issue. Thankfully, and hopefully not too late, it is now widely accepted that we need to encourage the development of less polluting technologies and stop our "addiction to oil."

Another "idiotic" problem is the environmental oversampling syndrome: people, especially children, are overstimulated by too much noise and visual factors. This may trigger problems with TOILing, especially in the brain.[810] I am of the opinion that bad music and bad entertainment, like some video games and TV shows, not only rot our brains, but our very hearts and souls. The exceptions are *"Weeds"*, *24* and *The Office*, the shows I enjoy, of course.

"What Role Has Nutrition Been Playing in Our Health? The Xenohormesis Connection"

This is the title of an excellent article that puts together many of the concepts discussed so far in this book.[811] The author credits Dr. Anthony J. Yun, Dr. Patrick Y. Lee, and Dr. John D. Doux for coining the term "xenohormesis," or foreign control. These doctors unveiled their cutting-edge ideas in their article, "Are We Eating More Than We Think? Illegitimate Signaling and Xenohormesis as Participants in the Pathogenesis of Obesity."[812] They remind us that the movie *Super Size Me* helped us see that

> "A calorie is not a calorie, meaning that the type of food the calorie is in has E&I beyond its caloric content. The protagonist of the movie, Mr. Spurlock, was becoming 'addicted' and showed 'responses that occur when a person is drugged' [rather] than a result of excess calories alone . . . [He] was eating food that contained substances that negatively altered his cellular signaling systems."

The xenohormesis article mentioned above goes on to say that

> "[The] foreign molecules in food that have been developed over the past five decades may serve as substances that alter cellular signaling and produce a different effect in the body than substances that humans traditionally consumed before the advent of food processing."
>
> "Emerging science recognizes xenohormetic substances as molecules that send signals to receptors on various cells, thereby altering their functions, affecting virtually all physiological processes, including immunity, inflammation, body-fat retention, appetite, blood fat levels, insulin signaling, and cellular division."
>
> "We are witnessing food being redefined as information that alters cellular function..."
>
> "A particular illegitimate cellular signal is chronic stress, which may shift body phenotype to suit a more conservative state that favors storage of energy and obesity...Obese livestock, and unusual fat profiles in farmed fish, meat, eggs may reflect stress phenotypes, a phenomenon known as 'xenohormesis,' and the person consuming these foods assumes the stress phenotype . . . Foods such as diet drinks may generate illegitimate signals by mimicking molecules that the body normally uses for caloric management."
>
> "We have to ask whether an alternative and possibly more successful approach to managing obesity-related dis-

eases than that of calorie restriction alone is to modify the signaling substances in the diet that participate in xeno-hormesis. As has been proposed, this model would suggest that, potentially, the best molecules for managing chronic disease will not come from the discoveries of pharmaceutical chemists, but rather from the 'laboratory' of natural selection in our traditional foods that have been associated with a low incidence of obesity, heart disease, and diabetes."

"[Nutrigenomics] opens the door for the development of an entirely new series of therapeutic agents composed of specified phytochemical concentrates . . . In the case of a person who has been consuming a diet containing illegitimate dietary signals for some time, the question is whether they can consume enough of the necessary substances in their diet to 'turn around' years, if not decades, of faulty cellular signaling. This is where there might be clinical value in specific therapeutic nutritional products that contain concentrates [of legitimate food E&I.]"

Examples of Toxins Affecting E&I

Agent Orange was used during the Vietnam War to exfoliate trees so that soldiers could see the enemy. It has been associated with diabetes[813] because Agent Orange is a form of dioxin that is also pouring out of smokestacks and incinerators throughout the United States. It is also found in pesticides, tampons, and cosmetics.[814] Agent Orange and heavy metals are endocrine disruptors (ED), meaning they mess up our hormonal function. Europeans are much more concerned about ED than Americans are.[815]

Heavy metals like arsenic and mercury are also diabetogenic endocrine disruptors.[816] They are the worst pollution problem in the United States,[817] outside our toxic, refined diets.

A report from Norway suggests a possible link between acidic drinking water and type 1 diabetes. It could be that minerals needed for the cell membrane to function better and for enzyme reactions to take place are depleted in acidic water. Also, the lower pH of acid water interferes with the immune system, allowing more viruses and bacteria to disrupt the sugar regulating pathways of the body. Still, the acidity from refined sugars and soda is a much larger contributor.[818] Speaking of water, arsenic found therein at higher concentrations than recommended has been linked to diabetes.[819]

Tobacco worsens IR[820] and increases the risk of type 2 diabetes.[821] This is why tobacco has been linked to the metabolic syndrome.[822] With passive smoking and polluted air, we are all exposed even though we may not smoke. Sadly, there are still doctors who smoke. They tend to have more diabetes than doctors who choose not to smoke.[823] Mothers who smoke bear children with higher chances of developing diabetes.[824]

And here is another vicious cycle: diabetics are more susceptible to developing problems from air pollution[825] and air pollution increases the risk of cardiac problems in diabetics.[826] Not surprisingly, diabetes and smoking increase the risk of rheumatoid arthritis.[827] Traffic pollution also increases the risk of heart attacks;[828] this happens through TOILing of cells in the cardiovascular system.

Another environmental problem may well be the excessive use of antibiotics, including their use in farm animals. They may be causing an imbalance of intestinal flora (linked to IR) that may contribute to the epidemic of obesity.[829]

Pesticides are made from leftover nerve gas used during World War I and II. As such, they are very toxic to our brain cells. Recently, we have become more aware that they disrupt the whole network of cell communication, the Psycho-Neuro-Immune-Endocrine system by increasing TOILing.[830]

1950s Commercial

Perhaps you were around to see the first TV commercials on pesticides. I remember the one showing a truck driving through a neighborhood, spraying pesticides. Every family decides to come out at that very moment to have a picnic on their front lawn just as the truck goes by in a cloud of chemicals. Those actors should have gotten an Oscar; it was so obvious they were fighting tears as they smiled and bit into their hamburgers. "Chemicals bring us better lives," the voice-over announced . . .

This book cannot highlight the thousands of chemicals, food additives, drugs, preservatives, cosmetics, etc., that are poisoning our cell membranes. While chemicals have been very helpful in many respects, the chemical industry has not factored in the cost of disease, environmental, and social disruption that its chemicals are causing.

The industry also has the annoying habit of denying, and even hiding, evidence that its products may be harmful (remember tobacco, asbestos, and lead?).[831] Don't the industry executives think about their own children being affected by all of their products? Did you know that there have not been more than a dozen studies looking into how these chemicals interact with one another? If you guess that mixing these chemicals may increase their toxic potential, you are unfortunately correct.[832]

Organic Farming

Organically raised food has 50 percent more antioxidants than food grown with pesticides.[833] Why is that? Think of plants fighting against organisms, pests, and weeds to survive; crops develop more antioxidants in the heat of battle. This, alone, is reason enough to prefer organic foods.

When we add the toxicity to ourselves and future generations, and the harm we bring to our environment that makes future farming less assured, we may be motivated to go out of our way and pay a little more for these foods. This is especially true when raised by local farmers, instead of big corporate farms who are starting to cut corners in the production of organic produce—besides using more oil for production and transportation.[834] There is no question that in the long run, and by factoring in many hidden costs to food grown conventionally, it is cheaper to eat organic produce.[835]

The same goes for genetically modified organisms (GMOs), or crops that have had pesticides inserted into their DNA to resist pests and weeds. Conveniently for Monsanto, this blind insertion of foreign genetic material renders crops sterile so that Joe Farmer has to buy new seeds every year from Monsanto. One has to wonder what else these GMO crops may be doing to us. There is already good evidence that they may raise the risk of gastrointestinal problems, including cancer. Not surprisingly, the European Union has banned GMOs from its shelves.[836]

TRANS-Formed by Toxic Trans-Fats

Do you remember the debate about what was better for you, margarine or butter? In those days, "egg-heads," in their arrogance, thought they could improve on Mother Nature's bounty by creating a safer form of bread spread than butter. They told us their motivation was our health. But the evidence is now clear that the motives may have been more in line with their quarterly financial report, if you know what I mean. These artificial oils, or trans-hydrogenated fats, aka trans-hydrogenated fatty acids (TFAs) have been designed mostly to increase shelf life and make oily products more attractive to consumers by increasing taste and consistency. How many of you hate Adam's® Peanut Butter? It doesn't have trans-fats; you have to stir it real well before eating it.

Margarine was eventually shown to be worse than butter because it increased cell membrane rigidity, or the TOILing that increases the risk of IR.[837] But, butter, being a dairy product, is not that innocent either. The whole debate about margarine or butter reminds me of the commercials about light beer: "Great taste . . . Less filling!"

Essential oils keep their chains of carbons linked together by hydrogen atoms. Changing those chemical bonds makes trans-fats. We now know that this change is very toxic to our cells because it messes with E&I and cell communication issues. These little problems have only recently been openly discussed in the media, despite glaring complaints from many scientists over the years. Why the delay? I think you know the answer to that question.

As a result of the IR they trigger, trans-fats have also been associated with cholesterol problems and breast cancer. If we could eliminate trans-fats from our diets, we could cut heart attacks in half and thus save billions of dollars in medical costs and loss of productivity, not to mention a whole lot of "heartache."[838] If I had a pill that cut heart attacks in half, would you take it?

Many states are regulating trans-fats out of restaurants and processed foods. KFC, McDonald's, and other restaurants claim they do not use them—anymore. Some consumers feel these regulations violate their personal freedoms, arguing that they have the right to eat whatever they want. I agree. But, your right to eat garbage stops when I have to pay for your medical bills through higher insurance premiums and many other hidden costs. As I've mentioned before, I feel a better answer is to heavily tax bad food or eliminate taxes on good food only, so that the consumers of trans-fat and refined sugar foods finance the increase in health care expenditures they cause.

Still, the drive to prohibit and regulate trans-fats in our food supply is welcome, as imperfect as it is. Unfortunately, the labels on boxes are not quite as honest as I would prefer them to be. It turns out that they claim "no trans-fats" per portion, because their small, unrealistic portions do not exceed the minimum allowed quantity of trans-fats. If you eat, for example, two to three portions, the amount of trans-fats you consume becomes significant. Do you ever stop at only a handful of potato chips? Or, do you keep digging until you reach the bottom of the bag? If you tend to eat more than a handful, you will have exceeded the allowed minimum of trans-fats. I think it would be best to avoid them altogether.

As we saw above, the trans-fat problem is magnified when the processed foods that contain them are cooked at high temperature and sprinkled with refined sugars for good measure. Do you think there may be a synergistic effect?

Remember that fat, or adipose tissue, is an excellent store of toxic chemicals; TFAs augment this problem.

I don't want to change the world; I just want to change your oil . . .

Truth in Labels?

TFAs are just an example of how labeling laws are routinely circumvented. Hopefully you remember the scandal over processed fruit products; they were found to contain about half of the fruits they claim on their labels.[839] Would it be a stretch to wonder if other processed food labels are also lying?

A related problem is the use of logos to promote "healthier foods." The FDA met with Big Food representatives, watchdog organizations, and medical experts in the fall of 2007 on how to regulate logos designed to "educate" the consumer about those boxed, canned, and bagged items, since there are so many different, confusing and competing symbols and logos. The traffic light logos used in the United Kingdom and Pepsi's "Smart Spot" illustrate these contradictions. The FDA has stated that "there is little consistency among these systems and it is not clear how they may affect market choice," other than increasing profits for Big Food, that is.

In my opinion, it is better to eat food with no labels whatsoever. For the most part, if it has a label, the item has probably been processed. Labeling problems are likely to become more of an issue as China's exports flood the United States and other countries. If China is not able to control, regulate, and patrol its manufacturing industry, especially in food production, we will see more and more questionable and contaminated foods making us sick. China's reaction, so far, was to execute the director of China's FDA after it was forced to face its food production problems; talk about "overkill."[840]

Hope

Our society is now much more aware of environmental issues affecting our health. Hospitals and clinics are making more efforts to "go green" and doctors are more attuned to clinical studies linking toxins and disease. The University Of Utah School Of Medicine now has an elective for medical students on environmental medicine; I have helped teach a section on nutritional detoxification.

Hospitals are trying to reduce the quantity and toxicity of their chemical waste. The Hospital Association of America recently founded "Hospitals for a Healthy Environment"; it is focusing on issues like disposing of mercury in safer ways, saving hospitals approximately 40 percent on the cost of waste management. It is also using more recyclable materials and is becoming more energy efficient. Green facilities for hospital campuses seem to be 5 percent cheaper to build. Since health care consumes more than 15 percent of the nation's Gross National Product (GNP), any changes in this industry are likely to have a significant impact in our communities.[841]

There is much more work to be done to reduce the "T" in TOILing. However, we can take some comfort in the fact that we have made great progress on environmental issues in our country.

Chapter 17

Energy/Information from the Sun

Health hinges on E&I utilization at the cell level for cells to carry out their assigned function and communicate such function to every other cell in the body. Their marching orders are coded in each cell's DNA, which also needs E&I to do its job. Photosynthesis through plants is the main way to tap into solar E&I to fuel all these functions.

There is another mechanism whereby we can absorb E&I directly from the sun, bypassing plants: vitamin D. It turns out to be more than just a vitamin; it's a pro-hormone that shares nuclear receptors with the thyroid hormone. The fact that the thyroid hormone does practically everything, plus the fact that most cells have receptors for vitamin sunshine, explains this pro-hormone's wide ranges of functions.

We absorb solar radiation into E&I through our skin; vitamin D is activated in our kidneys. When we expose our skin to the sun for twenty minutes each day, we produce about twenty thousand international units (IU) of vitamin D. We could probably produce more vitamin D if we run around naked, but this may create a few social problems. Only 10 percent of vitamin D is obtained through food (mostly from fish). There are 10 to 40 micrograms (mcg) of vitamin D per 100 grams of fish.[842] A typical multivitamin has only 400 IU. Dairy and soymilk have approximately 100

IU; cereals have about 65 IU.

If we choose to supplement vitamin D with pills, D3 is more effective than D2.[843] The majority of diabetics have very low levels of vitamin D; this makes us more obese,[844] which elevates IR and arterial inflammation, especially in the neck carotids.[845] IR and diabetes are seen more frequently in people who have both low vitamin D and low levels of calcium.[846] In other words, the lower your vitamin D3 levels, the higher your risk of developing type 2 diabetes.[847] This is why supplementing vitamin D helps with diabetes, weight loss, and normalizes lipids in the blood.[848] Also, there is a strong relationship between metabolic problems and vitamin D levels in adults.[849] Most dramatically, vitamin D supplementation from 300 to 2,000 IU decreases total mortality rates:[850]

> "The ability to turn back the clock on the basic biology of human aging by a full five years via vitamin D supplementation is particularly impressive in light of the more modest, albeit certainly worthwhile, longevity gains to be had from lifestyle modifications . . . We were wrong on vitamin A. We were wrong on vitamin B. We were wrong on vitamin C. We were wrong on vitamin E. Except for K, there is only one letter left, and that is D."[851]

"Sun Worshippers" and Skin Cancer

Before I dive into this subject, I have to admit that I have a bit of an arrogant attitude toward sun exposure. I am fairly swarthy and I grew up as a beach bum in Viña del Mar, Chile. My European side of the family (French father) called me "negrito" or "blacky," especially in the summer. (They thought I didn't sense their contempt, but I did.) Back in those sun-splashed days, I fell in love with Jodie Foster, the Coppertone little girl whose puppy exposed her swimsuit tan lines.

Well, it turns out that darker people have lower levels of vitamin D.[852] T I need to take 10,000 units of vitamin D3 to get my blood levels in the optimal range. Check your blood levels to determine how many units you need; everyone is different.

Having said all that, you may discount what I am about to tell you because of the controversy brewing around skin cancer and solar exposure. Some docs feel that there are less skin cancers, like melanomas, in people who are more exposed to the sun in the equatorial regions.[853] I agree with them because there is data showing that low levels of antioxidants in the skin allow our cells to TOIL, rendering them vulnerable to the toxic effects of excessive sun exposure. This is why foods with higher antioxidant values, like fruits and vegetables, lower the risk of skin cancer.[854]

The Australian Dermatology Association has adopted the above concepts as its policy; it discourages the excessive use of sun-blocking creams.[855] If you are still going to use sun-blocking creams, try Burt's Bees, which is prepared without toxic chemicals.[856]

Isn't it ironic? We fry in the sun, eating Twinkies, and drink soda or other junk low in antioxidants, but we goop up lots of sunscreen that blocks the absorption of vitamin D. I am not saying we should fry without any sunscreen, but that we should not fear casual exposure to the sun, especially if we are eating lots of foods high in antioxidants. Sun tanning is fraught with problems; vanity is not worth the risk. But I am not qualified to judge vanity in my fellowman because I am also afflicted with that little problem . . .

Where Do You Live?

It is estimated that one billion people worldwide have vitamin D deficiency or insufficiency; 40 to 100 percent of the United States population has this problem.[857] For the most part, this is due to inadequate solar exposure for optimal vitamin D production. For instance, Boston, Mass., is 42 degrees of latitude north, which means Bostonians don't get enough sunlight from November through February. It's worse in Canada; people in Toronto (52 degrees north) don't get enough sunlight from October through March.[858] Living close to the sea somewhat mitigates the effects of latitude on vitamin D levels, presumably because of fish intake.[859]

You might think that living in Hawaii may assure you of plenty of vitamin D. Not so: vitamin D blood levels in Hawaiians and in Wisconsin Cheeseheads (sorry, and they are already mad at me after reading about milk!) are about the same. It is possible to have low vitamin D levels despite abundant sun exposure.[860] It seems that the most important factor is our own native ability to transform solar E&I into vitamin D. In other words, we have different efficiency in the enzymes involved in this process. This is why it is now official to recommend vitamin D supplementation, regardless of sun exposure.[861]

There is also considerable seasonal variability to warrant getting our blood levels of vitamin D3 checked. And since we probably have a little extra fat around our middles, we are likely to need even more vitamin D.[862] Catching rays through a window doesn't trigger vitamin D activation. Sorry. Running around naked inside the house won't help either. Tanning beds do help raise vitamin D levels, but it is not worth it; a study found them to be as deadly as arsenic.[863]

"Are Statins Analogues of Vitamin D?"

This is the title of a somewhat controversial article[864] that discusses the possibility that statin drugs to lower cholesterol may be working by maximizing the function of vitamin D. This may be why there are less heart problems in people who have vitamin D levels in the upper limits of normal[865] and more heart attacks with vitamin D deficiency.[866] I agree with the author, who, in my opinion, may have stepped on Big Pharma's toes because he dared to point out that the cholesterol hypothesis inconsistencies have been conveniently dismissed.

Environmental light also influences the levels of vitamin A, or retinoic acid, which has been associated with better lipid levels by optimizing fat metabolism in the liver.[867]

How Much Vitamin D3 Should We Take?

The RDA of 400 IU is not adequate; it has led to one-half of people running around with levels that are too low.[868] In fact, we should probably take about 2,000 IU per day to get our blood levels of vitamin 1, 25-Dihydroxy-vitamin D3 above 80 ng/mL. The range used to be 20 to 60, but you will soon see that lab slip catch up to these new recommendations. And don't worry about taking too much, as long as you don't exceed 15,000 IU per day. It turns out that we absorb calcium much better at those higher levels.[869] You could always check your blood calcium/phosphorus ratio to make sure you are not taking too much.[870]

Again, a lot rides on how your genetic department handles vitamin D activation. Even pre-pregnancy obesity predicts poor vitamin D levels in neonates, which must not be confused with a genetic issue in the child.[871] IR and even cancer of the colon depend on your individual makeup on vitamin D activation[872] and how well you absorb it. Some people have intestinal resistance in their receptors to vitamin D that leads to poor absorption of the vitamin.[873]

Your chances of winding up in some nursing home are high if your vitamin D levels are below twenty-five. You may avoid that fate if your vitamin D levels are above eighty.[874]

Please, get your vitamin D levels checked. If you are below twenty, your doc may prescribe 50,000 units of vitamin D2 once a week for eight to ten weeks, after which that dose may be taken every other week. I feel it is better to take 5,000 to 10,000 units of over-the-counter vitamin D3 everyday in those cases. If your levels are above twenty, take 2,000 to 5,000 units a day.

Taking Too Much Vitamin D?

"When we give 50,000 units once a week for eight weeks, it usually gets the blood level of vitamin D3 to the desired level of greater than 30 ng/mL. People think that's too much vitamin D to take and it will cause vitamin D toxicity, but it's not. I joke with my colleagues when I give my presentation that what is remarkable to me is what physicians seem to remember more from their medical school days than anything else is 'don't ever make your patient vitamin D intoxicated.' They've never seen vitamin D intoxication. They don't know what 50,000 intoxication is, but they know that 50,000 is going to cause [it]. Fifty thousand IU taken once a week a week for eight weeks then every other week is safe. When you go outside in the sun one time in a bathing suit, your body makes 20,000 units . . . Vitamin D intoxication is typically not seen until blood levels are above 150 to 200 ng/mL."[875]

Vitamin Sunshine and Your Bones

Minerals, like calcium, are critical for bone health. If we don't absorb them from the intestines, we are likely to develop bone thinning. Vitamin D is critical for this function: adequate levels increase intestinal absorption of calcium by 45 to 65 percent. Without vitamin D, only 10 percent of calcium and 60 percent of phosphorus are absorbed. A study of 3,270 elderly French women given 1,200 milligrams of calcium and 800 IU of vitamin D3 daily for three years showed a 43 percent reduction in hip fractures and 32 percent in non-vertebral fractures.[876] Drugs for osteoporosis don't do as well; yet, they are "the standard of care" for the treatment of bone thinning problems, despite their significant side effects. One has to wonder why vitamin D, minerals, and optimizing intestinal function are not getting much attention in the treatment of bone thinning . . . In my opinion, the economics of health and disease rule the day. In the end, it is all "show business": break a leg . . .

Vitamin D also helps prevent hip fractures by reducing the risk of falls by 72 percent in the elderly.[877] Presumably, the mechanism of action is improving muscle strength, thereby increasing stability on one's feet.[878]

Not surprisingly, oxidation has been implicated in bone thinning.[879] Again, it is useful to think of our bones TOILing to understand the basic problem bone density issues.

Lack of Sunshine Makes You SAD (and Mad)

It is common knowledge that light makes us feel better. I saw this firsthand when I did my *Northern Exposure* stint in Alaska while paying back my National Health Service obligation. After a divorce, I felt tons better when I splurged by leaving lights on dim in every room of my Quonset house.

Not so long ago, many docs wound up in the slammer for treating their depressed patients with cod liver oil; it is high in vitamin D and omega oils—both indispensable for brain function. I wonder if anyone has apologized to those pioneering, intuitive docs because we now know that vitamin D and omega oils do help with depression[880] and the so-called seasonal affective disorder (SAD). Giving 50,000 IU every two weeks through the winter virtually cures this problem in many people.[881] Vitamin D deficiency has also been linked to schizophrenia, Parkinsonism, and Alzheimer's disease.[882]

"Maintaining vitamin D sufficiency in utero and during early life, to satisfy the vitamin D receptor transcriptional activity in the brain, may be important for brain development as well as for maintenance of mental function later in life."[883]

Story Time

I had to indenture myself to the Feds to pay for medical school by serving one of the thirteen Eskimo Corporations that practically own Alaska. I loved it up there. My friends often joked that I was much like Dr. Fleischmann in the show, *Northern Exposure;* prior to going up to Alaska I also lived in Flushing, NY, and I shared his ethnic looks, grumpiness, ugliness, and his vertical handicap. Anyway, while I was in Alaska I saw a significant number of SAD people. Most of them treated the problem with occasional trips to Hawaii, cross-country skiing, and lots of VCR movies washed down with a few brewskies. Some of them followed our advice to use special lamps to increase their vitamin D levels. Amazingly, I didn't think to check them back in those days: maybe I didn't because I was really SAD myself . . .

The Standard American Diet, another phrase that could use the SAD acronym, surely contributes to the depression seen in Eskimos. The common problem with fire water is also contributing; in my opinion, their culture is subtly and sometimes not so subtly put down as not being as good as the plastic culture we export everywhere.

Vitamin D and Autoimmune Diseases

The risk of getting multiple sclerosis (MS) is much higher when our vitamin D levels are lower.[884] Supplementing vitamin D decreases that risk by 40 percent.[885] In other words, the further North we live, the higher the risk of MS.[886] Maintaining our blood vitamin D levels above seventy-five significantly reduces our risk of MS; if one still gets this disease at those higher levels of vitamin D it doesn't seem to be as severe.[887]

Diabetes is really an autoimmune disease; it is more likely to develop when our vitamin D levels are in or below the old-range of normal.[888] Vitamin D deficiency increases the risk of diabetes by 200 percent. A study of 10,366 children getting 2,000 IU of vitamin D showed a reduction in the risk of developing type 1 diabetes by 80 percent. The risk of IR and metabolic syndrome was also decreased.[889] Arthritis is also an autoimmune disease that is less likely to afflict us when we supplement vitamin D.[890] Keeping our vitamin D levels in the 105-160 range makes autoimmune diseases less common.[891] Anyone having musculoskeletal pain should be checked for low vitamin D levels; this "should be standard practice."[892] When 5,000 to 10,000 IU of vitamin D3 was given to patients with chronic back pain, they all showed clinical improvement.[893]

Vitamin D also improves the function of B and T cells; they are a vital component of our immune system in our circulation. When these cells have optimal levels of vitamin D available, t infections like the flu,[894] the common cold,[895] and tuberculosis are less virulent when we are exposed. By increasing vitamin D levels from under twenty to levels close to thirty ng/mL, a study showed that African-American patients were able to overcome tuberculosis.[896]

Why does vitamin D do so many things? I am hoping you already know the answer to that: E&I. Once we understand how vital E&I is for our cells to carry out their metabolic functions, we can easily see why vitamin D does so many things.[897]

Cancer's "Lighter" Side?

Adequate levels of vitamin D reduce the chances of cancer by 60 percent in older women.[898] Because of many reports, I feel that this anticancer effect is not limited to just older women, but to every one of us. For example, we already know that vitamin D deficiency increases the risk of gastric lymphomas;[899] supplementing it lowers the risk of prostate cancer,[900] and the risk of colon, breast, and ovarian cancer is reduced in half with 1,000 IU of vitamin D per day.[901]

Chapter 18

Laboratory

T he fact that X-rays and ultrasound machines are starting to have problems penetrating all the blubber we carry around should be a sign that we are struggling with our metabolisms. Superman may not be able to see through our clothing anymore; that's probably a good thing for him . . .

The Best Check for Metabolic Issues: Your Beer Belly

A picture paints a thousand words: a quick look at your beer belly advertises your increased risk of developing metabolic problems. If you are trying to impersonate a tree by putting rings around your waist each year, your body is telling you the food you are eating is not good for you. Your waistline is the most practical way to assess IR. Any man with a waist over forty inches, or a woman with a waist over thirty-five inches, is now considered pre-diabetic.[902] As noted above, we do well to keep our waist sizes below one-half of our heights. For instance, if you are six foot tall, or seventy two inches, your waist size should be below thirty six inches.

Our waists, which are a reflection of our VATs, or the fat that we accumulate around the middle, becomes an endocrine tissue whose output of hormones really messes up our thermostats in

206

our brains.[903] This is why the belly is considered by many as the best and most practical way to see how we are handling our metabolisms.[904]

Checking our children's waists is a good idea, especially when they are fairly inactive. Of course, the measurements are relative to their stature.[905] It has been shown that their truncal fat mass affects their metabolic profiles and their HPA axis activity.[906]

The Most Common Tests to Check Our Metabolism

Docs still need to do some bloodletting to quantify one's degree of metabolic dysfunction. Testing will likely corroborate the warning signals your body is already sending you through your belly. The tests can identify patients at risk of developing diabetes ten to fifteen years before they are diagnosed. Unfortunately, there is significant "clinical inertia" when it comes to warning patients about the results of their fight with IR.[907]

The urine glucose test shows the severity of diabetes. Glucose spilling into the urine means that a person has had diabetes for a while and it is not in control; this is not a good test to pick up early tendencies. If this is how you were diagnosed with diabetes, valuable time was wasted; the early signs of IR could have been reversed. In the old days, docs were called "piss prophets" because they would taste their patients' urine to guess how much longer they would live. If the urine were real sweet, the patient would soon die a sweet death. I wonder how they tested for indigestion back then . . .

The fasting glucose in the blood is a better way to pick up early diabetic tendencies. It was considered to be "normal" if a person had a level under 110. This number has been lowered to one hundred. Still, a level over ninety-one indicates a higher risk of developing IR and diabetes,[908] especially when combined with triglyceride levels over 150. There is a higher risk of developing diabetes and/or cardiovascular disease in the upper levels of normal fasting glucose.[909]

If the fasting glucose is over 126 one is already diabetic. Levels of 101 to 126 are called pre-diabetes, or impaired fasting glucose; this is likely to progress to outright diabetes within three years.[910]

Soon, most cell phones will follow the example of the Health-Pia cell phone that will have a built-in glucose meter; it will be easier to monitor one's blood glucose.[911] If you are not diabetic, don't be shy; ask your friends with a glucometer to let you check your fasting blood glucose.

How "Caramelized" Are You?

Remember the Amadori effect or the caramelization of proteins? This means that sugar sticks to proteins in a process called glycosylation, a normal process happening naturally in our cells, but to a smaller degree than what is seen when eating processed sugars. The glycosylated hemoglobin, or Glyco HbA1c, is a test to measure how much sugar is seeping from the bloodstream into the inside of red blood cells where sugar ends up sticking to hemoglobin, a protein.

Normally, no more than 5.5 percent of our hemoglobin is glycosylated, or caramelized. From 5.5 to 6 percent, you may have a degree of IR and an associated higher mortality rate.[912] A glycosylated hemoglobin level above 6 percent is a sign of impending diabetes.[913] The higher the Glyco HbA1c, the more complications we see in diabetics.[914] Also, Glyco HbA1c naturally goes up as we age.[915]

In fact, a glycosylated hemoglobin as low as 5.3 percent peripheral arteries begins to show some damage.[916] Approximately 0.8 percent of people develop diabetes each year with levels below 5.5 percent, a level now erroneously considered to be "normal." From 5.5 to 6 percent, about 2.5 percent of people become diabetics and if they are obese the risk goes up to 4.1 percent each year.[917] This means that caramelization is a continuum: you want to keep the glyco HbA1c number as low as possible.[918] Glycolysation of hemoglobin goes up with age,[919] perhaps because we become "sweeter."

Since our red blood cells only last about three months, this test is checked that often in diabetics to monitor their degree of control. The glycosylated hemoglobin is considered to be an average of the blood glucose levels for the last three months; this is why some feel that it would be cheaper to ignore the glycosylation test and just go with an average of blood sugar levels over that period of time.[920] But most docs think that the glycosylated hemoglobin test is more accurate and it also picks up other caramelized proteins, besides hemoglobin. This is why this test is now considered to be the best way to screen for diabetic tendencies.[921]

Still, a combination of the fasting glucose and the glycosylated hemoglobin is considered by some doctors the most practical blood tests to look for a diagnosis of IR. I would add that these tests could be used to pick up much earlier IR tendencies in order to reverse metabolic issues. Perhaps these easy tests vindicate those docs who have felt that the glucose challenge, 2hGTT, is too complicated.[922]

The Two-Hour Glucose Tolerance Test (2hGTT)

The 2hGTT consists of giving the patient a standard glucose meal after which sugar levels are drawn several times, ending with the two-hour draw. The 2hGTT is three-and-a half times more sensitive than the previous tests discussed[923] and it is better than the BMI in identifying IR.[924] The American Diabetes Association now recommends that the 2hGTT be done routinely to assess patients' risk of developing diabetes; this is sure to tax busy doctors who may not be too thrilled to deal with preventive issues. We need to change this mindset.[925]

The 2hGTT will identify 16 percent of people with pre-diabetes a whole lot earlier in the process of decompensating the metabolism.[926] Hyperinsulinemia may also be measured by this test; doing so is arguably the best predictor for heart disease, even in non-diabetic patients.[927]

Even people with high normal 2hGTT seem to have a degree of IR, which predisposes them to type 2 diabetes.[928] Fully 97 percent of children go on to develop type 1 diabetes when they have an abnormal 2hGTT six months prior to a diagnosis of diabetes.[929]

The 2hGTT could be even more informative if they measured glucose beyond 180 minutes and at ten-minute intervals after they load you up with a nasty and standardized sugar drink.[930] Using alternative ways to run the 2hGTT may be more effective in predicting diabetes development.[931] For instance, in my practice we measure the 2hGTT before and after a meal at IHOP (pancakes). We feel that loading up with pancakes and syrup is more realistic and more reflective of most Americans' lifestyles. I tell my patients I am testing them like that "to smoke them out of the bushes."

I don't recall any of them refusing this test. Yet, most docs believe that patients are not going to be inconvenienced with the 2hGTT. This is why this test is underused. This is why most doctors still use only the fasting glucose that misses a lot of information.[932] I find that taking the time to explain these issues to my patients makes all the difference. Besides, they like the "reprieve" at IHOP.

Make Sure They Check Insulin Levels

When you are scheduled for a 2hGTT, insist that your doctor also checks your "insulin levels."[933] Think about it. Do normal sugar levels completely rule out the possibility that you have IR? No, unless you know how much insulin you needed to pump out to keep the levels of sugar normal. So, the more insulin one puts out, the more IR one has.[934] In fact, checking insulin levels gives us an indication of our potential life expectancy.[935]

The National Asthma Education and Prevention Program also recommends that a ratio of glucose-to-insulin be measured.[936] It proposes that the fasting glucose/insulin ratio should be above 4.5. Insulin levels fasting and at the two-hour mark are more sensitive in picking up IR.[937] The two-hour glucose/insulin ratio is turning out to be a better predictor of cardiovascular problems than imaging tests of the heart like the invasive angiogram.[938] This ratio is also felt to be the best predictor of future risk of type 2 diabetes.[939]

Cholesterol Levels May Reveal IR Tendency

Some researchers feel that the best tests to evaluate our metabolisms are insulin levels and the triglyceride/HDL ratio. The latter ratio should be below four. Looking at your cholesterol levels is probably the most practical lab for assessing IR because most people get their lipids checked routinely. Anyone with a triglyceride level over 130 should be suspected to have the metabolic syndrome.[940] The term "hypertriglyceridemic waist" has been proposed as a way to screen for heart disease. It consists of triglycerids over 130, plus the waist measurement covered above.[941] We will discuss these issues in more detail in chapter 26.

If your triglyceride level is 170 mg?dl and your HDL (good cholesterol) is 40 mg/dl, your ratio of 4.25 is above 4; this points to IR. As you will see below, the cholesterol metabolism is impaired in the liver by higher levels of insulin.

More Testing (I Hope You Have Insurance)

Another test that is getting significant attention in the journals is the intima-media thickness (IMT) to assess the health of the endothelium, or lining of the arteries. The IMT is an ultrasound of the endothelium of the carotid arteries. It is inexpensive, noninvasive, and reliable. The worse the glucose status, the more thickening of the endothelium is documented.[942] The metabolic syndrome makes the carotid lining thicker due to TOILing.[943]

The IMT also tells you your biologic age, compared to your chronologic age. For instance, I took an IMT test when I was fifty years old, chronologically. The IMT estimated that my biologic age, or my wear-and-tear age, was forty-three at the time. This is a great test is you want to fudge about your age, provided you are taking care of yourself.

Testing thyroid and adrenal functions is also helpful because these hormones are related to insulin function; they are altered in the metabolic syndrome. Low normal thyroid function increases the risk of metabolic syndrome.[944] The best way to assess adrenal function is an insulin challenge because it also checks the function of the HPA axis from the brain to the adrenal glands.[945] A rise in morning salivary cortisol signals metabolic problems.[946]

Menstrual problems and ovarian dysfunction are not only symptoms of sex hormonal dysfunction, but of IR as well.[947] We will discuss this concept in more detail in chapter 20. Then there is the quantitative insulin sensitivity check index (QUICKI) test; it measures the two-hour insulin and glucose and non-esterified fatty acids.[948] Sorry, but the QUICKI test has nothing to do with rushed sexual activity . . .

More Testing if You Have Money to Throw Away

The following are tests that researchers use. They are not practical nor necessary your doctors' offices: Fructosamine,

BIGTT test or Beta Cell Impaired Glucose Tolerance Test, Adipocytokines, Lipid peroxides, apolipropotein B/apolipoprotein A-1, an elevated ALT, C-Reactive Protein, Sex hormone-binding globulin, Glycated albumin, HOMA test, or Homeostasis Model Assessment-Insulin Resistance. Ferritin and Transferring, Uric acid elevation, Proinsulin, etc.

Your Savings Account

According to the Academy of Family Practitioners "Many clinicians see diabetes as a simple yes or no issue, which is inconsistent with the current knowledge about progression from normal glucose to diabetes."[949]

This is the principle of organ reserve. Each organ slowly and relentlessly loses its ability to do its job as we age. Tests are mostly designed to pick up a problem way after the first signs of decay have appeared. This is why so many people are told they are okay when their tests are normal, yet they don't feel so good. Using the better tests outlined here, especially the 2hGTT, may pick up a decrease in organ reserve before the organs are diagnosed to be diseased. In other words, we could diagnose IR much earlier, before it becomes diabetes. IR is reversible if you overcome your sugar addiction. If you don't, make sure you budget enough money to buy bigger pants each year.

Early testing may warn you of impending metabolic problems. Pre-diabetes, or impaired glucose tolerance, IGT; it should not be taken lightly, instead

"Impaired glucose tolerance (IGT) should be treated as a disease entity itself, worthy of clinical screening and treatment. Studies have shown that individuals can move in and out of IGT, suggesting that there are potentially reversible components of IGT that could be addressed before its progression to frank diabetes. The most opportune time to intervene is at the beginning of this process, when complications are fewer and less advanced and when patients are younger and possibly more amenable to lifestyle modifications."[950]

Part III

Metabolic Syndrome and All Diseases

We are finally ready to see how practically all diseases, particularly the most dramatic consequence of sweet death—cardiac problems[951]—are metabolic issues. To address this concept, we now have yet another medical journal for people to ignore on their coffee tables, the *Journal Metabolic Syndrome and Related Disorders*. Along with many other publications, it addresses diseases by,

> "[Working with metabolic issues] strikes at the root . . . to promote weight reduction and reduce IR. Treating the underlying causes does not rule out the management of individual risk factors, but it will add strength to the control of multiple risk factors."[952]
>
> "Wellness can be achieved through understanding and addressing the elements of metabolic syndrome . . . The understanding of IR will do more to lead us to wellness than anything that has preceded it."[953]

Don't wait to have a full-blown metabolic problem. Pre-diabetes, the beginning of IR, and metabolic issues should be treated aggressively "as if it were diabetes."[954]

Chapter 19

Defining the Energy and
Information Problem in Health

Finally, we are ready to discuss in detail the modern scourge called the metabolic syndrome, which used to be called "syndrome X." I was an intern at the Texas Medical Center in Houston where I worked my fingers down to the bone in 120 hour weeks thanks to the late Dr. Michael DeBakey's pervading philosophy of squeezing every drop of blood from the indentured house staff. DeBakey was a heart surgeon there; he gets credit for being one of the first docs to notice that most of his heart bypass patients for some unknown reason were diabetic. He would ask his fellow endocrinologists in the hallways why so many diabetics seemed to have more heart problems. Nobody knew back then. Soon, the clustering of diabetes, obesity, hypertension, and high cholesterol that DeBakey and other docs across the country had noticed was christened syndrome X.[955]

Since we have discovered why these diseases run together, the proper name is now the metabolic syndrome. However, Houston, we have a . . .

215

Problem with the Definition: Metabolic Syndrome

After reading the introductory material above, I bet you have guessed what is wrong with the definition of the metabolic syndrome: it does not go far enough. I am sure some of you will agree with me in saying that the metabolic syndrome involves practically all diseases like the author of the article, "Hyperinsulinemic Diseases of Civilization: More Than Just Syndrome X,"[956] argues. All-cause mortality is significantly increased in men with the metabolic syndrome, meaning that the combined mortality of the four diseases making up the limited definition of the metabolic syndrome do not account for the marked increase in mortality seen in patients with the syndrome.[957]

Before we study the evidence pointing to metabolic problems, or E&I issues in all diseases, let's briefly review the main facts about the diseases comprising the metabolic syndrome. We have already discussed diabetes and obesity in some detail. High blood pressure and high cholesterol are next.

High Blood Pressure

The endothelium inside our arteries is not wallpaper, but cell membranes that are TOILing. When the endothelium is irritated, it puts out chemical signals that lead to artery spasms, clotting, and stickiness.[958] Remember that the main reasons for the endothelium to be so dysfunctional are our diets high in refined sugar, [959] a toxic environment, and stress that leads to IR.

The main system of inflammation is the NOS; it triggers vasospasms when alarmed.[960] These spasms cause the diameter of our arteries to shrink, thus triggering a rise in blood pressure.[961] Your blood pressure is mostly going up because you are not handling all the refined sugar in your diet very well.[962] So, if you are a bit chunky and your blood pressure is going up, you are probably developing the metabolic syndrome.[963] Even when our blood pressure is within normal range or in the high-normal range, the levels of oxidative stress,[964] the way our kidneys handle protein, and subtle echocardiographic signs may be clues that people with these metabolic issues will develop outright high blood pressure and heart disease in the future.[965]

The article, "Insulin Resistance/Compensatory Hyperinsulinemia, Essential Hypertension and Cardiovascular Disease,"[966] adds a bit of unintended humor; despite their work relating IR with high blood pressure, the authors still vacillate "only 50 percent of hypertensive patients have hyperinsulinemia." I would blame stress, heavy metals, subclinical thyroid disease, and some rare diseases—like kidney and hormonal issues—for most of the remaining 50 percent of causality.

Hyperisulinemia exposes our kidneys to too much insulin; this compromises optimal function in the kidneys' filtration capacity (see below) and its neuro-hormonal regulation of blood pressure. In other words, IR also affects the kidneys, leading to high blood pressure. This is why several anti-hypertensive drugs work on the kidneys.[967] Calcium channel blocker drugs, like nifedipine, have been shown to reduce IR.[968] Beta-blockers, like carvedilol, also reduce IR.[969] This is likely because of their anti-inflammatory effects. Too bad they have so many side effects. However, you must take them if you are not willing to change your diet.

The relationship between IR and high blood pressure is also implied by the fact that pioglitazone, a drug to treat diabetics, can be used in non-diabetics with hypertension to lower their lurking IR.[970] I am convinced that anyone with high blood pressure is a pre-diabetic until proven otherwise (do the 2hGTT). In fact, even a mild elevation of blood pressure above 140 over 90 is associated with a significant risk for diabetes.[971] If you have a family history of high blood pressure you may have the genes for IR.

Below, you will see how to lower blood pressure with nutritional supplements. I don't recommend this path until my patients have shown a commitment to change their diets. I do not wish to become an enabler with supplements; this already happens all-too-often when docs prescribe pharmaceuticals without any discussion on lifestyle changes. Just a modest weight loss substantially lowers blood pressure.[972] I routinely see patients drop their blood pressure 10 to 60 points by facing their refined sugar addictions without any help from any drug.

High Cholesterol

The main problem with cholesterol is not the cholesterol, per se, but the oxidized cholesterol that creates plaque on the arterial walls.[973] Oxidized, or TOILing, cholesterol becomes "sticky"; it readily sticks to our arteries that are also TOILing and "sticky."[974] In other words, the oxidized/inflamed lining of our arteries cannot be properly repaired by sticky cholesterol: what we get in this situation we see an effect much like Velcro.[975] The clot-forming process is then well on its way to arterial congestion.

It's the Bad Sugars, Not Fat

As we discussed earlier, fat was demonized about thirty years ago when our fat went from the frying pan to the fire—the inflammatory fire of refined sugars. Remember our friends digging for olives in their salads? Fortunately, reason is beginning to prevail; we now have very good evidence that our cholesterol is best improved by low-glycemic index diets. Low-fat diets also help, but not as much.[976]

IR, due to cell membrane TOILing, causes a raise in the levels of insulin in our bloodstreams. The excess of insulin compromises our livers' abilities to handle cholesterol optimally. Liver enzymes, like adipose triglyceride lipase, don't work well with higher insulin levels in the liver.[977] This is why pre-diabetes is associated with cholesterol problems.[978] IR has also been implicated in high cholesterol associated with genetic problems found in certain families.[979]

High cholesterol is not just due to oxidized cholesterol, but also to oxidized sugar.[980] LDL also becomes more toxic (or sticky with inflammation) when exposed to AGE products.[981] As I mentioned, I consider anybody with cholesterol issues to be a pre-diabetic until proven otherwise.

Our focus should be on restricting refined foods, not fats in general. Besides, we need healthy, hopefully vegetarian-based fats to have optimal cell membrane function and structure.[982] Sadly, the drugs used to treat high cholesterol may increase IR. Fortunately, adding vitamin A and CoQ10 opposes this effect and potentiates their cholesterol-lowering activity.[983] Why? Think of TOILing.

Call the Cops

Do we need a "cop" to enforce these concepts so that we quit demonizing fat? Yes: COP stands for cholesterol oxidation products.[984] The relationship between oxidized cholesterol and hyperinsulinemia is so strong that now cholesterol oxides are being used as biomarkers for type 1 and type 2 diabetes.[985] Oxidized lipids also increase our chances of developing problems with clots.[986] Fasting and after-meals glycoxidative and lipoxidative stress markers are found to be elevated in people with type 2 diabetes.[987] Simply put, oxidized LDL is associated with the metabolic syndrome, obesity, IR, and high triglycerides.[988]

If everything is working well and we have lots of antioxidants in our diet, like L-carnitine, our liver keeps cholesterol from oxidizing.[989] When the powerful antioxidant glutathione is supplemented in oral form (liposomal) to mice, oxidized cholesterol drops by 17 percent, enough to stimulate HLDL, reduce macrophage cholesterol by 34 percent, and thus reduce the atherosclerotic area on the arterial wall by 30 percent.[990] But, more often than not, our livers are busy fighting other battles; toxins in the environment tax liver function and excessive refined sugar in the diet elevates insulin levels in the blood.

This extra insulin ends up everywhere, as previously discussed. When it goes to the liver, it jams up the enzymes designed to keep the cholesterol from oxidizing.[991] People who have high triglycerides are more likely to have a hyperinsulinemic effect on the liver, which is betrayed by the hypertriglyceridemic waist.[992] Incidentally, triglycerides yield more information when checked in the non-fasting state.[993]

Natural Little Dutch Boy

The TOILing of the cells making up our arterial walls leads to shrinking and premature death of said cells, creating gaps between them. I have mentioned "leaky gut" a few times. Now, why would the cells lining our guts be the only tissues leaking when all our cells are TOILing? It follows that our arteries are leaking, too. In fact, many diseases have been shown to be due to "leaking tissues."[994] Again, the main cause of our terrains, or common soil, to be TOILing is sweet death.[995]

Guess who, or what, comes to the rescue to plug up those holes like a little Dutch boy? Our old *friend* cholesterol; I emphasize "friend" because we have demonized cholesterol due of our lack of understanding of basic E&I concepts. An overdeveloped need to make profits on drugs to lower cholesterol has also contributed to cholesterol becoming a dirty word.

As noted above, a diet high in antioxidants would allow our livers to produce non-sticky cholesterol and more of the right kind of cell-building cholesterol, the "good" HDL: our "little Dutch boy." Not surprisingly, HDL has been shown to have anti-inflammatory properties.[996] This is why the Mediterranean diet has been shown to reduce cardiovascular risk; it is high in antioxidants,[997] like choline and betaine, which reduce inflammation,[998] TOILing, and mortality.[999]

Linus Pauling, PhD, and his buddy Matthias Rath, MD, routinely lowered cholesterol with a combination of the antioxidant, vitamin C, and the amino acids, lysine and proline; they are indispensable for building up the collagen that constitutes the walls of arterial cells or the "ground" or "terrain" of our arterial lining. When the liver senses that the holes in the arteries are getting fixed, it no longer sees the need to send out cholesterol to patch up said holes; consequently, serum cholesterol levels go down.

Imagine cholesterol saying, "Thanks! Now I don't have to work so hard anymore!"

Big Pharma Strikes Again

It wasn't until Big Pharma came up with statin drugs by extracting the most active chemicals out of fermented red rice (which had been used for millennia in China to treat heart problems) that cholesterol became the enemy. Once the "cure" was isolated in drug form, the "disease" was invented. Statin drugs, whose TV commercials flood our airwaves, are reaping profits of over 30 percent, virtually transforming the way we view the simple issues of E&I and our diets.

These are fighting words, I know, so here is an article that backs up my opinion: "Selling Sickness: The Pharmaceutical Industry and Disease Mongering."[1000]

"There is a lot of money to be made form telling people they are ill."

"The social construction of illness is being replaced by the corporate construction of illness."

"Some forms of medicalization may be described as disease mongering, extending the boundaries of treatable illness to expand market for new products."

"Alliances of pharmaceuticals, doctors and disease groups use the media and expert witnesses to frame conditions as being widespread and severe."

"Disease mongering can include turning ordinary ailments into medical problems, seeing mild symptoms as serious, treating personal problems as medical problems, seeing risks as diseases and framing prevalence estimates to maximize potential markets."

"Corporate funding information should be replaced by independent information."

There is no doubt that these drugs do lower the incidence of heart disease. But they may do so with significant side effects like liver issues and muscle irritation. They also "hit you below the belt": they lower libido by decreasing testosterone production.[1001]

Interestingly, these drugs do have significant antioxidant activity.[1002] I would not be surprised if this were the main mechanism whereby they improve our lipid profiles and slightly lower the incidence of heart disease.[1003] This may be why statin drugs are being studied to help multiple sclerosis; they reduce the TOILing of arteries in a "leaky brain" that allows toxins to penetrate our brains and cause all kinds of problems.[1004] Statin drugs also lower blood pressure, but they do so in those patients with normal pressure, too.[1005]

Then, again, the real marker for usefulness is whether or not anything we do reduces mortality and morbidity—not mere numbers like cholesterol levels. It turns out that total mortality is not reduced by statins, according to pooled data from eight randomized trials:

221

"Frequency of cardiovascular events, a less encompassing outcome, was reduced by statins. However, the absolute risk reduction of 1.5 percent is small, and means that sixty-seven people have to be treated for five years to prevent one event . . . the benefit is limited to men at risk aged thirty to sixty-nine years . . . [These men, when] presented with this evidence, do not choose to take a statin, especially when informed of the potential benefits of lifestyle modification on cardiovascular risk and overall health."[1006]

Good Fats for Fat Heads

We need to stop demonizing cholesterol. It is a necessary molecule to make hormones, steroids, and to build cell membranes, particularly the lining of neurons, the so-called myelin sheath.[1007] Good fats are also necessary for our DNA to function and to be structured optimally.[1008] Creating the impression that cholesterol is bad for us is unlikely to lead to a thorough understanding of high cholesterol in some people.

Trying to lower cholesterol without addressing the underlying causes can have significant side effects like increasing the risk of dementia.[1009] Why? Because 80 percent of our brains are fat: our brains need cholesterol to be structured and to function properly. Again, cholesterol is not the problem; it is oxidized cholesterol. No wonder that cholesterol-lowering drugs have side effects like depression, nightmares, and other neurologic issues. And get this: they also lower the amount of cholesterol in our cell membranes thereby increasing IR.[1010]

Low cholesterol levels are also associated with increased mortality.[1011] The same applies to HDL or the good cholesterol. It is prudent to raise our HDL through non-pharmaceutical means such as exercise, stopping tobacco and alcohol, losing weight and reducing saturated fat intake. It has been shown that 2.4 grams of niacin, a B vitamin, and fish oil improve our HDL, especially in men with IR.[1012] If a person over seventy years of age has an HDL over forty-five, a statin drug to lower the bad cholesterol will not do any good.[1013]

Oh, by the way, a failed drug (Torcetrapib) to raise HDL "killed more people than it actually saved . . . patients on Torcetrapib were 60 percent more likely to die than those taking Lipitor."[1014]

Expanding the Definition of the Metabolic Syndrome

We are now ready to dissect the full meaning of this far-reaching problem. You will see the evidence that practically all diseases involve metabolic problems. Remember the psycho-neuro-immune-endocrine system of cell communication of E&I as you study the next chapters. Focusing on metabolic issues will help practically all diseases by maximizing function in each cell.[1015] We may help restore health without focusing on the disease so much, which is a negative approach perpetuated by the acute care model. Crisis management doesn't work in chronic care very well. Besides, focusing on metabolic issues is a more positive approach and it does not feed the obsession we seem to have with disease.[1016]

Let's begin exploring how every health problem is an issue of E&I, particularly its most common manifestation: IR, or sweet death.

Chapter 20

Metabolic Syndrome and Hormones

T he article, "Hormones and Recalcitrant Obesity,"[1017] goes for the jugular: "About 10 percent of overweight people on a diet cannot lose weight because their metabolism is malfunctioning."

That is the crux of the matter, isn't it? The main hormonal problem they have is the brain-gut-hormonal axis imbalance that worsens their IR. These imbalances trigger suboptimal thyroid function, even though their blood levels of this hormone may appear normal (see below). Many of them also have adrenal hormone issues that compound IR through poor handling of chronic stress and lack of restorative sleep.[1018] We will now discuss how IR compounds all those hormonal problems: ladies first.

Women and Hormones

Let me shock you by saying that irregular menses, premenstrual syndrome (PMS), its severe presentation, premenstrual dysphoric disorder (PMDD) are markers for a higher risk of diabetes in the future because IR mostly drives them.[1019] No wonder that irregular periods increase the risk of heart disease.[1020] When a woman ovulates, an egg flies out of the ovary "on call" (they take turns each month). This leaves a crater-like hole in the ovary that needs to heal. Technically, the crater becomes a cyst, but it quickly resolves, scarring that area of the ovary. Eventually, the ovary will look like a lunar landscape, full of craters, which is when a woman goes into menopause.

Sometimes the monthly crater doesn't heal very quickly; it continues to fill up with blood, creating the kind of cyst that hurts and can become a surgical emergency 50 percent of the time. Sometimes, several cysts are actively "festering," or not healing properly: this is how ovarian hormonal function starts to go awry. Testosterone,[1021] progesterone, and estrogen levels are then compromised, creating many problems, including PMS. If the IR triggering PMS is severe, women may get . . .

Too Many Cysts

IR is the culprit behind the polycystic ovary syndrome (PCOS) that afflicts 6 percent of women. IR is even more severe in PCOS when patients also have the metabolic syndrome.[1022] Even the daughters of women with PCOS have early metabolic derangements.[1023] The excess of insulin generated by IR causes the ovaries to process sex hormones less optimally. The ovaries also develop a new hormone called insulin-like factor 3 that exacerbates the hormonal imbalances seen in PCOS.[1024] Women in this situation have a preponderance of testosterone that leads to hair growth, infertility, and weight gain.[1025] These changes in hormones are the main cause of neuroendocrine problems like depression, anxiety, cognitive issues, and even swelling in PCOS.[1026] And by now you understand why young women with PCOS have early coronary plaque formation.[1027]

Liver Connection

IR leads to elevated levels of insulin in the blood, upsetting every cell, tissue and organ in our body. The liver is no exception (see "fatty liver" below). Its functions become somewhat impaired (detoxification, anti inflammatory, antioxidating, and blood glucose modulation). Endocrine disrupting toxins in the environment are then sub-optimally eliminated; they increase TOIL in all cells when they accumulate in our tissues. The ovaries are particularly affected so that their sex hormones' output is altered.

Consequently, IR aggravates PCOS due to poor diets and xenoestrogenic toxins poorly eliminated. These toxins are chemicals that have estrogen activity in our cells (plastics, pesticides, heavy metals, dioxin, etc.). PCOS improves if we improve the liver's detox and sugar-regulating function of the liver. This is what N-acetyl-cysteine (NAC) does; it's a key amino acid needed to make glutathione in the liver. Glutathione is the master antioxidant that plays a major role in fixing TOIL. In a study involving thirty-seven women with PCOS, 1.8 grams per day of NAC significantly reduced IR.[1028]

Women and Their "Sweet Hearts"

Once we understand that PCOS involves TOILing and IR,[1029] we can see why other organs, like our hearts and arteries, are also affected. Young women with PCOS may have severe endothelial dysfunction, or TOILing of arterial walls,[1030] resulting in a doubling of the incidence of stiff arteries.[1031]

A diet high in refined sugars lacks B-complex, which results in the toxic metabolite homocysteine going up.[1032] Homocysteine correlates with IR, PCOS, and ethnicity.[1033] Refined diets also tend to have more processed fats like trans-hydrogenated fats. Just 2 percent of TFA in our diet can double the risk of anovulatory infertility.[1034] Remember that elevated homocysteine, TFAs, and toxins have been linked with heart disease, too.

Toxins in the environment also worsen infertility, even in males.[1035] Brothers of women with IR and hormonal problems tend to have metabolic problems, too.[1036] "Sexual Dysfunction in Men and Women with Endocrine Disorders" are common in sweet death.[1037]

PCOS and Pregnancies

About 20 percent of women with PCOS have impaired glucose intolerance, or pre-diabetes.[1038] PCOS and even toxemia of pregnancy signal an early beginning of the metabolic syndrome.[1039] No wonder one can screen for ovarian dysfunction with the

2hGTT.[1040] In fact, the glucose/insulin ratio is the best test for IR in PCOS.[1041] We may also screen for PCOS by watching patients' VATs. As noted above, VAT signals IR and inflammation.[1042]

A female fetus exposed to a mother suffering with PCOS will have a greater risk of developing PCOS after birth. This is not necessarily genetics, but the results of the hormonal environment influencing the fetus's nascent ovaries.[1043] Basically, PCOS increases the levels of androgens, like testosterone in utero, causing fetal programming for PCOS to develop in adult life.[1044]

Other Problems Seen with PCOS

Perhaps the problem most reported by women with IR and ovarian dysfunction is hair growth in places where it is not welcome. (I sympathize with this, since now that my dome is thinning I get lots of hair in my ears, nose, and eyebrows.) This is a result of a relative excess of testosterone, given that ovarian hormones are out of balance.[1045] PCOS is present in most women with another common problem: infertility.[1046] About 15 percent of women are infertile; a significant number of them are obese.[1047] As you will see below, most of these women may conceive if they resolve their underlying IR.

Acne is also a common manifestation of the elevated testosterone in PCOS. Not surprisingly, this type of acne may be managed with the diabetic drug, metformin.[1048] Women with ovarian dysfunction due to IR are at risk of developing the metabolic syndrome and cancer, too.[1049] A discussion on cancer and IR in chapter 24 will clarify this statement, although you may already suspect that our immune systems do not work as efficiently when our metabolisms are subpar. You will see that a lot of our immune systems are tied to detoxification issues in the liver that may not function optimally in women with IR.[1050]

Treating PCOS and PMS/PMDD

Controlling IR is the main way to deal with PCOS. Losing weight should be the main goal of treatment.[1051] Essential fatty acids[1052] and alpha lipoic acid, an antioxidant, help by decreasing cell membrane IR.[1053] D-chiro-inositol helps with ovarian problems by strengthening the proteoglycans, or glycoproteins, making up the cell membrane where the IR problem lies.[1054]

Drugs for PCOS may be helpful, but I feel they are often used without trying very hard to address patients' sweet death issues. Besides, these drugs have side effects. Rosiglitazone/avandia reduces IR by working on the cell membrane receptors of insulin. But it has been shown to increase the risk of heart attacks[1055] and bone thinning.[1056] Its cousin drug, actos/pioglitazone, has also been thought to affect the heart; both of them now carry a black box warning, or an alert of potential problems.

Perhaps their side effects are exaggerated. Perhaps most diabetics end up ahead of the game by taking these drugs. But, I feel these are troublesome and repetitive signs that Big Pharma puts profits ahead of our health. This is enough for me to recommend that my patients try not to use these drugs. I write about them benefiting multiple medical conditions to make the point that metabolic, sweet death problems lurk in every disease known to us.

Another drug, metformin/glucophage, tells the liver not to make too much sugar. Metformin reduces AGE in PCOS[1057] and decreases gestational diabetes in women with PCOS.[1058] Unfortunately, metformin may have side effects like renal problems, gastric and intestinal sensitivities, and a loss of B complex due to the latter.[1059] At least it doesn't increase the toxin, homocysteine.[1060]

As always, stress overworks our adrenal glands; this may worsen IR. This is why licorice has been show to help with PCOS by improving adrenal function.[1061] The regulation of DHEA, an adrenal hormone, appears to be disrupted in women who tend to get PCOS.[1062]

Contraception

Have you ever wondered why the pill makes women gain weight? The pill increases IR; vaginal rings don't do it as much;[1063] and the progesterone shot does it more—especially in teens who are already a bit insulin-resistant.[1064] Why is this going on? Think of TOILing ovaries: "T" for toxicity and E&I hormonal signaling disruption.

Sweet Pregnancies

The risk of women dying during childbirth has increased due to more C-sections being done and moms being more obese or suffering from IR.[1065] Fortunately, this is a rare outcome of IR in pregnancy. But the following problems with sweet pregnancies are not so rare.

Preeclampsia, or toxemia of pregnancy, has been linked to endothelial dysfunction. This is why circulation is poor in preeclamsia, causing swelling of the ankles and even high blood pressure. Think: TOILing and leaky arteries.[1066] By now you know why the endothelium is inflamed. Not surprisingly, preeclampsia carries a 5 percent risk of developing diabetes; an elevated blood sugar is often seen in preeclamptic women.[1067] Preeclampsia has been shown to increase the risk of heart disease through its common denominator, IR.[1068]

Mothers and even their children exposed to preeclampsia are at higher risk of type 2 diabetes.[1069] The growth hormone-like protein, insulin growth factor-1 (IGF-1), whose function is adversely impacted by IR, has also been associated with preeclampsia[1070] and prostate cancer.[1071] CoQ10 is an antioxidant indispensable to keep cell membranes intact and open to insulin traffic. When it is not abundant, IR may develop and the risk of preeclampsia increases.[1072]

Gestational diabetes, or elevated insulin and sugar levels in pregnancy, is a milder form of preeclampsia; it is not surprising that it carries a 17 percent risk of turning into pre-diabetes,[1073] diabetes,[1074] and metabolic syndrome issues in a woman's future.[1075] Approximately 4 percent of pregnancies have a degree of diabetes of which 90 percent are diagnosed as gestational diabetes;[1076] this means that women develop a mild form of diabetes while pregnant. This is much like a chain under stress that breaks where its weak link is. Gestational diabetes is linked to inflammation[1077] and IR,[1078] especially in women who get pregnant when they are overweight or have a bit too much around the middle.[1079]

Gestational diabetes is associated with pregnancy-induced hypertension.[1080] Remember the reason why our blood pressure goes up? IR is irritating the endothelium. A previous history of gestational diabetes increases the risk of atherosclerosis or hardening of the arteries after pregnancy.[1081]

Even higher sugar levels in normal pregnancies increase a mother's risk of diabetes by 30 percent.[1082] Modest elevations in their blood sugar increase their future risk of becoming diabetic.[1083] High-normal levels of sugar in non-diabetic pregnant women increase the risk of having a large baby, a first-time cesarean section, neonatal hyperinsulinism, and neonatal hypoglycemia.[1084]

But it is not just refined sugars in pregnancy; processed saturated fats are also contributing to these metabolic problems.[1085] Carrying too much weight in pregnancy increases the risk of premature deliveries[1086] and the risk of babies being too small or too large at birth. These children tend to develop IR at birth and as adults they are likely to have sweet death issues like diabetes and impaired glucose tolerance, or pre-diabetes.[1087] At birth, very small children may even have high blood pressure.[1088] Adipokines, or hormones from adipose tissue (adiponectin, resistin, etc.), have been shown to contribute to the IR seen in pregnancy.[1089]

What Can a Mother Do?

Simply put, she can overcome her sugar addiction.

Higher fiber consumption from a diet free of refined foods and high in fruits and vegetables decreases IR and lowers the risk of toxemia. Foods higher in fiber are naturally lower in fats and refined sugars. High fiber diets help control the rate of absorption of fats and sugars in the intestines.[1090] Meals high in antioxidants, like flavonoids, also inhibit the transport of glucose from the intestines into the blood.[1091] Remember that flavonoids also decrease inflammatory markers, like the CPR,[1092] so that TOIL is addressed.

Women with complicated pregnancies are advised to have a 2hGTT every year because 30 percent of them will develop diabetes.[1093] They would have better pregnancies if they ate low in the glycemic index and exercised regularly.[1094] Because of these IR problems in pregnancy, new recommendations for weight gain have been issued for pregnant women. The goal is to keep IR at bay.[1095]

A report concluded that the odds of getting pregnant with fertility treatments are boosted by 65 percent with acupuncture.[1096] By now, you probably have a fairly good idea why this is so . . . Acupuncture improves E&I in all cells, including ovarian cells and those working on detox pathways. Remember that toxins increase IR. Also, acupuncture is an energy-based treatment much like yoga; they increase glutathione levels, the most powerful antioxidant to reduce TOILing.[1097]

We will discuss treatment in more detail below.

Sweet Menopause

IR causes women to have a more difficult menopause.[1098] The more sugar they eat, the worse "the change" will be. Excessive refined sugars in the diet trigger a rise in insulin, leading to low sugar in the blood that aggravates hot flashes.[1099] Inversely, after menopause women are more likely to develop the metabolic syndrome.[1100] This seems to be aggravated by the predominance of testosterone as they lose estrogen.[1101]

The more compromised our non-sex hormones are as we approach "the change," the more problems we will have with menopause because the dwindling sex hormones are not backed up by the other hormones. In other words, IR worsens thyroid and adrenal function, resulting in a more symptomatic menopause. The same applies to men as we will see below.

Sweet Thyroid Hormones

One of the most serious consequences of hormonal imbalances in the metabolic syndrome is its impact on thyroid function. Diabetics have double the rate of thyroid dysfunction because excessive sugar interferes with the enzyme that transforms inactive thyroid hormone, T4, into its active form, T3.[1102] There are reports that T3 function is intimately linked to the function of insulin[1103] and that thyroid function, through its relationship with IR, affects how arteries perform as they dilate.[1104]

The thyroid-stimulating hormone (TSH) is secreted from the pituitary in the brain in response to a feedback loop signaling low thyroid hormone production from the thyroid gland in the neck.

A high TSH signals compromised thyroid function. Even "normal high" TSH levels have been linked to the metabolic syndrome and IR.[1105] Elevations in serum TSH, IR, serum cholesterol, and endothelial dysfunction are often seen together with subclinical thyroid dysfunction and the metabolic syndrome.[1106] This is why many docs now feel the TSH should not go above 2.0 in the lab report that presently holds that the TSH is okay below 4.5.[1107] Remember that one of the most important functions of the thyroid hormone is E&I; this is much like insulin, if you like.

Besides, IR itself makes the TSH levels appear artificially lower[1108] so that a borderline high level of TSH is likely even higher or more indicative of compromised thyroid function. This lends credence to rebellious docs like me who feel that the diagnosis of thyroid deficiency is poorly handled in our present health care system. IR compromises the feedback loop between thyroid hormone in the neck and TSH.[1109] This means that the TSH test, long worshipped as infallible by most docs, may not be that reliable in many cases, particularly in those who have IR.[1110]

Consider the fact that heart attacks are two-and-a-half times more likely in women with high-normal TSH, meaning a low-normal functioning thyroid.[1111] This illustrates how the TSH, which is the gold standard for monitoring thyroid function in the United States may not be sensitive enough. Another example is the eyes of diabetics. No retinal damage is seen in patients with diabetes when they are taking thyroid hormone replacement. To me, this means that diabetes is also associated with other endocrine abnormalities.

High glucose/insulin levels in the brain also affect the hormone that influences the pituitary release of TSH, the thyroid-releasing hormone (TRH); TRH is also affected by sweet death, compounding the dysfunction of the feedback loop between TSH and the thyroid gland.

Thyroid levels are lower in the metabolic syndrome, probably because of cell membrane resistance to thyroid; think of it as yet another cell communication messenger. In the presence of IR, we must assume that there is also thyroid resistance, in addition to IR directly compromising the rate of conversion of T4 to T3.[1112] In other words, there is also thyroid resistance when our cells TOIL. Think about it: if insulin were the only messenger having trouble getting through our cell membranes, this would be discrimination . . .

Toxins in the environment also cause thyroid resistance by several mechanisms, especially by compromising cell membrane flexibility: think of the "T" in TOIL.[1113] Lacking optimal thyroid function due to the adverse effects of xenoestrogens in the environment (toxins that have an estrogen effect on our bodies) also worsens the symptoms associated with menopause.[1114] These toxins trigger oxidation and inflammation in our tissues, leading to dysfunction of messengers of cell communication, like the thyroid hormone. Degradation of T3 by toxins has also been documented.[1115]

As previously stated, thyroid dysfunction is often seen with IR. I feel it is best to think of all our hormones as if they were joined at the hip. Metabolic issues are pretty much hormonal issues, particularly thyroid and insulin, often found to be a bit compromised in practically all diseases. The function of sex hormones is also compromised since resistance problems in their cell membrane receptors are often associated with the metabolic syndrome.[1116]

Thyroid hormone underfunctioning is often associated with adrenal dysfunction. The higher our cortisol levels (a sign of adrenal stress), the higher the TSH is.[1117] All hormonal messages work together.

Sweet Adrenal Hormones

Elevated stress or an inability to cope with it causes our adrenal glands to be so compromised that they may fail to pick up the slack from dwindling sex hormones at the time of menopausal changes. If our adrenal glands were in good shape, the difficulties associated with menopause would be less significant, mostly because there would be less IR. This is why adrenal supplementation (see below), like DHEA, an adrenal hormone over the counter, is helpful in menopause.[1118]

It turns out that DHEA supplementation is a strong up-regulator of adiponectin gene expression in visceral fat in the metabolic syndrome.[1119] Taking 50 milligrams of DHEA if you are a woman with weak adrenals will help lower your cholesterol.[1120] In fact, the lower the levels of DHEA, the more carotid atherosclerosis there is in type 2 diabetics.[1121] This is likely the result of DHEA's stimulation of endothelial proliferation and angiogenesis.[1122]

Glucocorticoid messages of E&I, or hormones from the adrenal glands, hook onto receptors on cell membranes just like any other message. Glucocorticoids, like their name implies, regulate glucose metabolism. The more stressed we are, the more IR we will have. Glucocorticoid receptors multiply under the stress of IR. In other words, the adrenal glands are overworking due to stress, environmental toxins, and toxic attitudes.[1123]

These factors also create problems with the adrenals' mineralocorticoid hormones (which control the levels of minerals in the body) and sex hormone precursors, which have also been implicated in IR. Levels of minerals like magnesium, vanadium, chromium, and even DHEA are the most affected by hyperinsulinemia.[1124] Predictably, a lack of magnesium increases the risk of diabetes; it is an essential component of normal functioning cell membranes.[1125] Too bad processed foods don't have optimal levels of magnesium.

The effect of stress on our adrenal glands explains why so many people have a tough time losing weight, no matter what they do with exercise or their diets.[1126] At times, the dysfunction in their psycho-neuro-immmune-endocrine system of cell communication is so pronounced that patients suffering from early emotional and physical abuse will always have a marked tendency to hyperinsulinemia. Child abuse is arguably the most serious of the many stressors that may compromise our HPA axis. We may think of early life stress as a trigger to inflammation later in life.[1127] Anybody under stress will have a hard time losing weight because of adrenal oversecretion of the hormones, adrenaline and cortisol.[1128] Unfortunately, cortisol's role in diminishing thyroid hormone activation does not help.

No wonder that expressing one's feelings has been linked to less inflammation in our bodies.[1129]

"Metabolic Syndrome and the Endocrine Stress System"

Hyperactivity of the hypothalamus-pituitary-adrenal (HPA) axis has been associated with visceral obesity. This results in disturbance of glucocorticoid action on peripheral tissues. Those with susceptible glococorticoid receptors on the cell membrane suffer the most.

People with HPA dysfunction tend to have more visceral adipose tissue, VAT, higher blood pressure, cholesterol and fasting insulin and glucose. Glucocorticoid receptors are more numerous in visceral fat. The metabolic syndrome shares many features of adrenal dysfunction: VAT, impaired glucose tolerance, high blood pressure and increased leptin secretion from fat cells. Leptin triggers the release of adrenal hormones (aldosterone, cortisol, and DHEA). Thus, leptin links metabolism and stress regulation. Aldosterone and interleukin-6 secreted by fat cells also raise blood pressure. After relentless and insidious stress,

> "Chronic alterations to the stress system play a major role in the metabolic syndrome." This may be so subtle that the hormone system, particularly the adrenal system, may be stressed without this showing up in testing… Lifestyle 'Westernization' involves excessive high caloric diets, insufficient physical activity and, no less important, chronic exposure to stress."[1130]

"Adrenal incidentalomas," or little benign tumors of the adrenal glands, previously thought to be innocent and incidental findings in tests, while looking for something else, may not be so innocent after all. People with these incidentalomas tend to have higher blood pressure. This is why some researchers feel that,

> "Incidental adrenal adenomas may be an unrecognizable cause of metabolic syndrome. This question is not irrelevant, taking in account the high prevalence of unidentified incidentalomas in the population."[1131]

Classical congenital adrenal hyperplasia also looks like metabolic syndrome. These patients have a tendency to develop metabolic problems. Alterations of the central sympathetic nervous system may also be involved in adrenal issues, contributing to high blood pressure.

Home, Bitter Home

No health-oriented book can be written without touching on domestic violence. Far too many women (and there are some men who are also victimized) are stuck in seemingly impossible situations, fearing for their lives and those of their children. Surely, this situation leads to adrenal dysfunction. Please, consider seeking help, if you are so victimized. If you know of someone suffering under the joke of an abusive spouse, give them the phone number to your state's hotline for domestic violence.

Sexual Abuse, the Adrenals, and Metabolic Problems

We already discussed this thorny issue above. I don't mean to twist the knife, but when one-third of our little girls are being sexually abused in our society, we must not spare any effort to correct this horrendous crime.[1132] As we already discussed, these little ones end up with a disturbed HPA axis that predisposes them to many problems, including IR as they grow older. The problem is so insidious that nearly 100 percent of my so-called "train-wreck" patients have been sexually abused as children.

Now, don't get all upset because I call them train-wrecks. They laugh when I say to their face; they understand I am trying to lighten their heart and load. These poor souls come into my clinic rejected by a health care system that has taught them to focus on every little symptom so that they can get a drug for each one of them while never addressing the real underlying issues of sexual abuse, sweet death, or IR.

They are surprised when I don't appear impatient as they read their "toilet paper roll" of a list of symptoms that is all-too-often interrupted by most docs after less than a minute of recounting. The reason I am not easily flustered by all their symptoms is simple: I boil them all down to E&I, TOILing, and sweet death. Then, I show them that we are going to focus on restoring health instead of managing the symptoms of disease.

But, let us get back to sexual abuse. One of the worst things we can do is deny the victims their day in court. Often families opt to brush the whole thing under the carpet in order to save face or avoid further humiliation in their community. I have seen this in my own foster family and in a former girlfriend. The message is loud and clear when the perpetrators are not disciplined or brought to justice: victimized children feel they are not important when their suffering is so easily dismissed.

I am not arguing for vengeance or blind punishment, although it would be better for all involved, including the perpetrator, if these men were castrated. These are my own feelings, so, I ask for your respect in tolerating this admittedly radical approach. Do we really believe that these men will ever be rehabilitated?

Unfortunately, there is no hope of ever putting this issue to rest in the heart of children, unless the issue is faced straight on and dealt with in a mature manner that hopefully leads to forgiveness.

The reluctance to deal with sexual abuse is likely a result of people's puritanical views of sexuality. I believe we must be tolerant of each other's beliefs and religious attitudes about sex as long as they do not involve underage children, abuse, disrespect, violation, or dishonesty. But our beliefs may become a problem when they inhibit an honest and open discussion of the sexual realities confronting our society.

This is why I believe I get an incredibly negative reaction from some people when I bring up sexual abuse in my sweet death lectures. Again, here is another unsolicited personal feeling of mine that may generate a bit of hate mail: if you find this discussion offensive, I implore you to consider the possibility that you have been sexually abused as a child. It turns out that 90 percent of affected children have no recollection of these events because the most common coping mechanism in childhood is denial and memory lapses.

So that you may see that I am not speaking from a pedestal, I want you to know that I, too, was sexually abused as a child. After openly examining this episode and forgiving the perpetrator, I can honestly say this part of my life is settled and has no bearing in my present life. I encourage you to seek help if you have been the victim of sexual abuse. It may still be playing a factor on your metabolism and perhaps other issues, such as chronic fatigue and fibromyalgia.[1133]

Politics, Economics, and the Adrenal Glands

If it seems strange that a health book gets a bit political at times, or if you feel that a doc shouldn't get involved in these matters, you may want to skip this section . . .

The article, "Status Syndrome,"[1134] discusses the issues of lack of control, poverty, and disenfranchisement of poor people significantly impacting their health:

> "Low control or lack of autonomy and low social participation are likely to be important contributors [to poor health] . . . Social gradient is associated with dysfunction of the pituitary hypothalamus adrenal axis . . . Stress at work is associated with the metabolic syndrome."

In my opinion, our republican democracy has been hijacked by large groups of people with lots of money, which perpetuates or institutionalizes poverty in our country. Corporatism, or fascism, is the name we must use when a "revolving door" is installed between jobs going to and from big corporations and government. These privileged people are maneuvering both political parties, much like puppets on strings. Please do not buy into the orchestrated attacks each party launches on the other. In my opinion, they are staged to divert your attention from the puppets' master who wants you to "pay no attention to the man behind the curtain."

I am not saying that money is the problem, but the way it is used when it is the vehicle of greed and oppression of those less fortunate. In my opinion, "noblesse oblige": if we are privileged and wealthy, we have a moral obligation to help the less fortunate without dismissing them as deserving of their lesser fortunes.

Our health care system is not immune to these political and economic issues in our country's affairs. The health insurance companies, Big Food, and Big Pharma are involved in this game, largely looking out for their own interests, rather than the public's interest. You may want to read Maggie Mahar's book, *Money-Driven Medicine*, and the article by Robert Sapolsky, titled, "Poverty and Health."[1135]

The idea that poor people have worse health than affluent

people is due to lack of access to health care and poor nutrition being outdated; poor people have worse health because they are angry over their disenfranchisement from the riches our country now largely reserves for the more affluent citizens. These issues nag at them, increasing the risk of adrenal gland dysfunction, which, as you know contributes to metabolic disorders.

A Bookworm's Brain Droppings

Our world literature is full of examples of human suffering. My personal favorite is *Les Miserables* by Victor Hugo. What is yours? I also recommend Pablo Neruda, Gabriel Garcia Marquez, Nelson DeMille, Tom Robbins, Carl Hiassen, and the classics. Does it seem strange to find literature in a book on health? Perhaps the Columbia Medical School program designed to teach literature to medical doctors will spread to the rest of our country's schools. At Columbia, they feel literature teaches young doctors empathy and reflection, as noted in the article, "Narrative Medicine: A Model for Empathy, Reflection, Profession, and Trust."[1136]

Despite the intense pressure to read medical stuff in medical school, I would leave textbooks at school so that at home I could read Shakespeare, Dostoyevsky, Tolstoy, Moliere, de Beauvoir, Asimov, H. Miller, etc. Some of you will say that I shouldn't have done that, judging by my roguish attitude. But I graduated in the middle of my class without overdoing the memorizing that is required for success in medical school. I assure you that "thinking skills" are not emphasized as much as memorizing skills in our docs' education. Are you surprised?

At home, I was never able to study in my basement office where I fashioned a desk with a door sitting atop two barrels. Instead, I would wind up reading in my kids' playroom where I felt close to them, despite the noise. They grew up seeing their dad studying all the time and hearing how important it is to get an education in our modern society.

The best way to overcome negative social issues is education. As far back as I have looked in my genealogy, I am the only member of my family who graduated from a university. As an immigrant to this country when I was in junior high school, I have experienced some of the all-too-common stresses of foreign-born Americans. But my education has been the greatest equalizer and, consequently, my stress levels have been reduced to a very manageable level.

The bottom line is that I took an oath to help alleviate my patients' suffering; implementing said oath has taken me in the direction of E&I in food and prevention, in general.

The AMA's Stand

Despite the politics, I choose to work with the AMA in Utah because we recognize that,

"The responsibilities of the physician extend not only to the individual but also to society and demand his cooperation and participation in activities, which have as their objective the improvement of the health and welfare of the individual and the community . . . As good citizens it is the duty of physicians to be ever vigilant for the welfare of the community."

Other Hormones

IR significantly affects prolactin from the pituitary gland. This is the hormone that women secrete to breastfeed. When men produce it in higher amounts, it is often a sign of pituitary malfunction. Other hormones, like ghrelin and sex hormones (androgens), are also affected by IR—especially in women with PCOS.[1137] Ghrelin is a hormone produced by the stomach to talk to the brain about thermostat issues. Ghrelin will likely be used as a drug to decrease appetite in the future.[1138] Another hormone, obestatin, has also been found to come out of the stomach to signal a decrease in appetite. It may also be used to help people lose weight.

What About Men?

Testosterone is converted to estrogen to become functional (the enzyme, aromatase, is in charge of doing this). Consequently, men have many estrogen issues, too. This is an example of "the queen being the power behind the king." If you play chess, you know what I mean. We need to keep this vital survival principle in mind . . .

Of course, testosterone does have function before it is converted to estrogen. It makes men smell really bad, fight, and watch too much sports on TV while we scratch places on our bodies that ought to be left alone. It's also responsible for us getting a lot of hair where we don't necessarily want it. Sometimes, testosterone makes us rush too much blood away from our brain, precipitating very peculiar situations. (I will leave it at that.)

IR increases when men go through andropause, the guys' equivalent of menopause.[1139] In fact, lower testosterone levels increase the levels of caramelized proteins, like the test glycosylated hemoglobin A1c demonstrates.[1140] Some men may be too proud to admit that their testosterone levels are going south. I hope that men reading this get their testosterone levels checked. At least, do it for the Mrs.[1141]

Losing Muscles

One of the main problems in aging men and women is the loss of muscle mass (sarcopenia) and the concomitant increase in fat—conditions seen regularly with low testosterone levels. The loss of muscle is not necessarily because of getting old or from a deficiency in protein synthesis, but an increase in IR that accelerates muscle protein degradation.[1142] In fact, older men make more muscle than younger men.[1143] The real problem is sweet death: the more IR we have, and this is worse in diabetics, the more muscle mass we lose.[1144] Also, protein glycosylation defects may result in muscle diseases.[1145]

To make matters worse, low testosterone makes men in their forties and fifties put on more fat tissue on, which worsens IR, inflames our arterial lining, and piles up rings on our trunks.[1146] Yet another vicious cycle; this one is really not fun, since it makes it harder to keep our women interested . . .

Hitting Below the Belt

Here is the worst vicious cycle in the testosterone department: IR lowers testosterone and low testosterone worsens IR, especially when our cells are TOILing with inflammation.[1147] That inflammation is part of this problem is not surprising; sex hormone-binding globulin (SHBG) is produced in the liver; it may be inflamed with elevated insulin. This makes SHBG go up and thus binds more testosterone, making it less available inside the cell.[1148] Approximately 92 percent of men with low testosterone have IR and 65 percent have the metabolic syndrome.[1149]

Men get an inflamed endothelium when they lack testosterone and estrogen. This is why castration for prostate cancer increases the risk of cardiac death in men by 2.5 percent in five years.[1150] (I don't recommend this as a form of contraception . . .)

Since the lining of our arteries is inflamed in every artery, IR and low testosterone also affect the ones facilitating an erection. See below; I mean, see the *section* below . . .

Sweet Limpness

Erectile dysfunction (ED) is an early sign of endothelial inflammation.[1151] Just as the TOILing arteries of the penis are going into spasms that restrict blood flow to trigger an erection, your arteries throughout your body are TOILing. Why would the arteries of the penis be the only ones to suffer? I know you think you are special and gifted in that area, but . . .

Glycosylated hemoglobin A1C levels going up are correlated with more inflammation in our arteries. This takes place by compromising the NOS system of inflammation in the arteries where the amino acid L-arginine is critical to avoid arterial spasms. A dysfunctional NOS system leads to more clot formation, abnormal cardiovascular reflexes, and changes in temperature perception, which explains ED.[1152] ED has also been linked to a lack of B vitamins; this raises the levels of the inflammatory molecule homocysteine.[1153] Diets high in refined foods don't have adequate amounts of B vitamins, or arginine.

In 1998, the research on NOS and arginine won the Nobel Prize in Medicine. It led to the creation of Viagra®. Not that I am complaining; but the role of arginine in ED is seldom discussed when Viagra is prescribed. There is good evidence that arginine—especially when combined with the antioxidant, pycnogenol,[1154] and the herb, Korean ginseng (all of which lower IR)—can work just as well as Viagra:

> "Korean red ginseng (panax ginseng), 900 milligrams three times day works as well as sildenafil/Viagra to achieve and maintain an erection sufficient for intercourse, even in a population with severe erectile dysfunction. It is a reasonable, non-prescription treatment, especially for men with reservations about taking Viagra. A 500-milligram capsule of panax ginseng costs about six cents compared with $10 for a tablet of Viagra."[1155]

Your dates just got cheaper . . . Since arginine dilates blood vessels, it also lowers blood pressure, especially when combined with another amino acid, N-acetyl-cysteine.[1156]

In other words, obesity, IR and hyperinsulinemia are linked to ED;[1157] these factors have also been associated with alopecia.[1158] Of course, if you are bald and have too many rings around the middle you may not get too many chances to need Viagra. Sorry, I couldn't resist; I know that being bald is a sensitive issue.

Is it worth it to indulge on Twinkies only to have trouble with ED? Can you imagine what would happen if Twinkies carried a warning like this? *Warning: The surgeon general has decreed that consumption of Twinkies leads to erectile dysfunction.*

Do you want to have a good sex life? Quit the sweets. Eating bonbons as a seduction move is not likely to work very well in the long run, my friend.[1159] Let's be blunt: if you cannot lay off the Lays® Potato Chips, they may be all the lays you get.

Please don't write me a letter; lighten up.

Supplementing Testosterone

Supplementing testosterone and its adrenal precursor, DHEA has been shown to reduce IR.[1160] Normal levels of testosterone in men are associated with lower risks of developing IR.[1161] DHEA has also been shown to reduce abdominal fat in adults[1162] and increase our metabolic rates, especially when combined with green tea,[1163] which improves our metabolism by decreasing IR.[1164] This is why green tea helps to reduce abdominal fat.[1165]

Testosterone increases insulin sensitivity in peripheral tissues, but it decreases it in the liver. This may be why there are contrasting studies on the effects of testosterone supplementation,[1166] especially when it comes to women, who may have a higher risk of diabetes when they supplement this hormone.[1167] Some docs feel that:

" . . . Testosterone use to treat metabolic syndrome may also lead to the prevention of urological complications commonly associated with these chronic states, such as neurologic bladder and erectile dysfunction Physicians must be mindful to evaluate hypogonadism in all men diagnosed with metabolic syndrome as well as metabolic syndrome in all men diagnosed with hypogonadism."[1168]

Prostate Cancer with Testosterone Treatment?

If testosterone supplementation is recommended, it is advisable to keep an eye on the prostate specific antigen (PSA), a protein that goes up with prostate cancer. PSA is also secreted in women, particularly those who are more hirsute and have polycystic ovarian syndrome. In other words, hyperinsulinemia affects both androgenic and estrogenic functions.[1169] If your PSA is going up, more testing is required, including a biopsy and a very intimate exam with a finger. So, always choose a doc with a thinner finger. In my clinic, I keep an oversized "Utah Jazz #1" foam finger, just for kicks . . .

In my opinion, the fear of prostate cancer from testosterone supplementation has been exaggerated, resulting in many men being kept from therapy that would literally change their lives. Besides, restoring low levels of testosterone to normal would theoretically only "normalize" the risk of prostate cancer—not increase it. Also, remember that prostate cancer is linked to IR,[1170] which means that our own native testosterone is not likely to become a problem unless our immune systems are compromised by problems, like IR. In the chapter on cancer, you will see why there is more cancer in people with metabolic problems.[1171]

Xenoestrogenic toxins in the environment that act like estrogen fuel prostate cancer, like breast cancer.[1172] Milk is often contaminated with these toxins:

> "High milk consumption has consistently not been associated with lower risk of fractures in large prospective studies, whereas increased risks of advanced or fatal prostate cancer have been observed in many studies."[1173]

When patients are told about the potential risks of testosterone replacement, most of them still choose to take the hormone anyway. Men realize that the potential gain in their relationships with the feminine element (or other men) is worth the risk. Several male patients, however, have told me they would rather "die with their boots on."

Testosterone supplementation is also neglected in females. Other than a higher risk of growing facial hair and an irresistible urge to watch sports on TV while burping and scratching too much, testosterone replacement is very safe and it should be part of the standard package of estrogen replacement in most women. Adding testosterone does not increase the risk of cancer. In fact, it may lower it.[1174] Get your levels of testosterone checked if your partner keeps complaining that you'd rather watch *The Jay Leno Show* at night instead of you-know-what.

Sweet Growth Hormone

Insulin growth factor-1 (IGF-1) is a protein from the liver that functions much like growth hormone. It needs to be over 152 in the blood. Below 152, the risk of developing IR increases.[1175] By optimizing the blood levels of IGF-1, we may reduce inflammation, oxidation,[1176] and decrease the progression of plaque formation.[1177]

A lack of sulfur (cruciferous vegetables, garlic, onions, and eggs) in our diets can influence the healthy genetic expression of the IGF-1 gene.[1178] By increasing the intake of sulfur-containing foods, decreasing refined sugar, and supplementing IGF-1 in people who have a deficiency of IFG-1, we may reduce the risk of developing the metabolic syndrome.

Your Beer Belly: Beyond Cosmetics

Fat cells in the "spare tire" around our waistlines secrete hormones and neuronal signals. These fat cells' messengers are called adipokines; they include leptin (which signals the brain to control appetite), tumor growth factor alpha, angiotensinogen (a hormone controlling blood pressure in the kidneys), adiponectin, and resistin. These hormones lead to higher clotting risks, the metabolic syndrome,[1179] IR, and an inability to lose weight.[1180] Remember VAT?[1181]

Here is another vicious cycle: the bigger the beer belly, the more disrupted our metabolism is, since these hormones increase IR, and the more IR, the bigger the belly and the higher the risk of heart disease.[1182] In other words, VAT increases TOILing, specifically inflammation and oxidation,[1183] which accelerates clogging of our arteries, thus compromising transport of E&I.[1184] Hopefully we will soon reach a "better understanding of multi-organ crosstalk in the pathogenesis of diet-induced obesity."[1185] Translation: just like we talked about above, calories are not the main issue. Our disturbed thermostats are. It turns out that we may be obese, but avoid becoming diabetic, if our belly hormones are well balanced.[1186]

Chapter 21

Metabolic Syndrome and the Genito-Urinary System

E levated insulin levels in the bloodstream (a result of IR) reach every corner of our bodies, including our kidneys. After all, our kidneys are blood vessels that have specialized in filtrating toxins out of circulation. The more TOILing there is in the lining of our arteries (endothelium), the more kidney filtration declines.[1187] Remember how devastating IR is to the lining cells of our arteries. Diabetes, itself, is terribly hard on the kidneys. A significant number of diabetics end up with kidney problems. Diabetics with kidney problems do much better on a low-glycemic index diet.[1188]

Even before blood pressure goes up and tests for IR are positive, the kidneys can show a decrease in function with high sugar diets that further increase insulin levels.[1189] Within five years of developing signs of the metabolic syndrome, we may have chronic kidney disease.[1190] Obesity, a cousin of IR, decreases kidney function even as early as childhood.[1191]

HFCS, one of the biggest causes of obesity, seems to be particularly damaging to our kidneys.[1192] Our high sugar diets are a common factor by the time our blood pressure levels go up, a symptom of our kidneys definitely having circulatory problems.[1193]

Kidney damage is common by the time we become diabetic; docs are very vigilant about kidney function when they screen patients every three months, much like the "piss prophets" of old. Most diabetics have kidneys that don't function 100 percent, even when their kidney blood tests appear to be normal. It turns out that diabetics with more rings around their trunks have a higher risk of kidney damage. For each four extra inches around the middle, the risk of protein spilling out in the urine—a sign of kidneys being affected by diabetes—goes up 34 percent.[1194] In other words, VAT increases the risk of renal disease in diabetics.[1195] Chronic renal problems are often seen in people with the metabolic syndrome.[1196]

In outright renal failure, obesity and subpar muscle mass (sarcopenia) increase inflammation and increase mortality.[1197] If we end up having hemodialysis, IR worsens the risk of vascular injury.[1198]

Gout and Fat Kings

Have you wondered why a fat king sitting with a swollen toe elevated on a pillow often portrays gout? When the normal filtrating function of the kidneys is impaired by the hyperinsulinemia triggered by IR, uric acid (a product of protein metabolism) builds up in the bloodstream. What may happen next is that uric acid crystals may precipitate out of solution.[1199] These uric acid crystals may lodge in our joints, particularly in our feet and hands. In other words, Gout is an IR condition:

> "This shows that firmly held views on diet need revisiting. There is much work to be done before prescribing allopurinol, a drug that cuts down on the formation of uric acid."[1200]

Not surprisingly, uric acid elevation is a risk for cardiac problems and high blood pressure: IR is the common denominator. High insulin levels are found in 95 percent of people with gout. Gout sufferers have three times a higher risk of the metabolic syndrome.[1201] Given that gout is associated with obesity and body fat,[1202] it is no wonder that the incidence of gout is climbing at alarming rates.[1203]

People with gout have impaired endothelial vasodilatation and more clotting.[1204] Even by itself, uric acid is an inflammatory agent associated with cardiovascular and renal disease.[1205] Now you can see why high uric acid is associated with higher mortality,[1206] particularly in middle-aged men.[1207]

Even children and adolescents are now showing higher levels of uric acid when they have the metabolic syndrome.[1208] This means that we will soon see our children developing gout. A study showed that teens with high blood pressure and high cholesterol reduced their blood pressure by taking allopurinol, a drug used to get rid of uric acid in the kidneys.[1209] Hmmm . . . I wonder if they thought to help them by reducing IR through dietary changes.

The Gouty Merry-Go-Round

Most docs tell their gout patients to eat less protein to cut down on protein metabolism because that is where uric acid comes from. What do people eat when they cut down on proteins? They turn to sugars and refined carbohydrates that perpetuate the gout problem. No wonder gout sufferers are condemned to stay on pain medication and allopurinol at great risk of significant side effects. Would it not be easier to treat the underlying condition, hyperinsulinemia and IR? In doing so, the kidneys could filter out uric acid more efficiently.

Making matters worse, most of the drugs used to treat the metabolic syndrome also elevate uric acid.[1210] Are you tired of "vicious cycles"? We keep chasing our tails, don't we?

Don't Be Like Sisyphus

If you don't get what you are about to read, you and Sisyphus will be rolling that old stone up the hill for the rest of your lives. When the kidneys are exposed to hyperinsulinemia and IR, they form kidney stones; the kidneys' filtration function is universally impaired.[1211]

Anybody with kidney stones would do well to be screened for IR. While you are waiting for the doc to send you the labora-

249

tory results, relax and have a cup of coffee; it has been shown to lower uric acid levels by reducing IR.[1212]

Rushing Around to Pee

Have you seen those commercials showing people rushing around looking for a toilet to emergently pee? Some are very funny, like the one with the middle-aged guys boating; can't the one who has to go so badly just whip it out and pee overboard? Now, don't pretend to be shocked. I bet you have done it yourself . . .

Big Pharma is trying to sell you a drug to stop the signals of bladder-lining TOILing, or irritation, without addressing the reason why you have that "going problem" in the first place.

It turns out that IR also affects the rest of the urinary system; interstitial cystitis or bladder irritation causes frequent and urgent urination. The mechanism is simple: the cells lining the bladder are TOILing. Bladder irritation has also been linked to a lack of protective glycosaminoglycans (healthy sugars in good diets) on the bladder lining. Thusly, irritants, like bad foods, food additives, and toxins being eliminated in the urine, irritate the lining of the bladder that is already too sensitive and inflamed. This triggers muscle spasms because the bladder is wrapped in a layer of muscle. This is the *real* reason why you have to rush around to pee, particularly when you first walk through the door at home.[1213]

TOILing and IR also explain urinary incontinence.[1214] Of course, incontinency is often seen after childbirth because of excessive stretching of the pelvic musculature. Even so, IR worsens this problem.

Do you want to take a pill to stop these symptoms, or would you prefer to fix the TOILing of your bladder lining? Stop your SAD diet and supplement the amino acid L-arginine; it reduces the tendency to spasms in the bladder.[1215] Antioxidants like MSM sulfur[1216] and capsaicin (in red peppers) also help.[1217]

The Canary in the Mine

Xenoestrogens in the environment are more likely to affect our prostates when they TOIL; then they grow larger. This is why we have to get up to pee so much at night. The problem is called benign prostatic hypertrophy (BPH). In other words, an enlarged prostate is a canary in the mine signaling that we are lacking anti-oxidants.[1218] Not surprisingly, BPH is worse in diabetics.[1219]

When we have beer bellies, or too much VAT, the fat therein acts like an endocrine organ producing too much aromatase, the enzyme that turns testosterone into estrogen. The more VAT we have, the more estrogen men are exposed to. The more estrogen, the more prostate problems we may have. Still hung up on the rather cumbersome BMI? I feel that the

> "The waist circumference is a home run in terms of prediction . . . The results even surprised us . . . The waist circumference may be a more accurate predictor of metabolic problems than the BMI . . . Belly fat is almost a separate organ . . . a new gland . . . By altering our metabolism, perhaps you fuel prostate growth."[1220]

A large VAT also increases the risk of having an elevated PSA, prostate volume, and ejaculatory and erectile dysfunction.[1221] If you want to shoot blanks, keep eating those Twinkies.

Researchers noticed that these metabolic problems from a large VAT that cause urinary issues also lead to more hypertension and diabetes. Not surprisingly, they found that those patients had higher glucose levels, more IR, and more cholesterol problems. They are now proposing that urinary problems be incorporated into the mainstream definition of the metabolic syndrome.

Drugs for the Kidneys and Their Metabolism

ACE inhibitor drugs work on the kidneys (ramipril, quinapril, etc.) to lower IR and blood pressure.[1222] These drugs focus on the kidneys' hormonal systems, much like the herbs hawthorn[1223] and hibiscus sabdariffa do. The latter, works better than the drugs above, to lower high blood pressure with no side effects.[1224] A new drug, pyridoxamine (K-13), improves renal function; interestingly, it does so by counteracting TOILing, or the oxidating and inflammatory effect of AGE products.[1225]

251

Chapter 22

Metabolic Syndrome and the Immune System

We briefly discussed the immune system under the concept of glycosylation because the immune system is nothing more than glycoproteins. In other words, the immune system's "messengers" cannot function properly if they get stuck with the wrong sugars. The article, "Complex Carbohydrates are Essential in the Correct Functioning of the Immune System,"[1226] explains that the more refined sugars you eat, the more compromised your defenses will be.

Sweet death causes our immune systems to work overtime. For example, our infection-fighting white blood cells, like CD4 and CD8, and total lymphocytes go up when our BMIs are too high.[1227] Two cans of Coca-Cola can depress your white blood cell function by 92 percent for as long as five hours.[1228] Now you know why you keep getting colds and your sinuses are stuffed up to the rafters.

Stress and the Immune System

World literature is full of examples of characters getting pneumonia or tuberculosis after some emotional catastrophe, like a failed love affair, occurs. Back then, the connection between stress and the immune system was not clouded by over-intellectualizing or micromanaging the simplicity of the human condition. I will never forget the doc who crucified me at a lecture when I said that stress down-regulates the immune system . . .

The adrenal glands are overworked with stress because of the HPA axis connection. The resulting hormonal imbalance ends up increasing the risk of IR and compromising the immune system. To make matters worse, this relationship is bidirectional, meaning that an inflamed immune system also affects the HPA axis and the adrenal glands.[1229] In other words, systemic inflammation—like we see in obesity—activates the HPA axis, resulting in cortisol going up and the thyroid hormone being less active,[1230] both of which worsen IR.

Immune System and Our Metabolism

The article, "The Intricate Interface Between the Immune System and Metabolism,"[1231] tells us that food intake regulates our metabolism and the immune system. In other words, bad food triggers inflammation through dysregulation of the immune system. Cytokines, hormones, neuropeptides, and transcription factors are messengers of cell communication in the psycho-neuro-endocrine-immune system that governs both our metabolisms and our immune systems.

Our metabolisms generate byproducts, or free radicals/oxidants, the same way the environmental toxins produced by any engine work in our industries. Our immune systems are also in charge of eliminating these free radicals. This is why this system would be better named the immune-toxicology system. As you already know, our detox pathways are most represented in the intestines and the liver. This is why even small amounts of toxins in our food and environment may significantly compromise our immune systems. This is again the "hormesis" word at play.[1232] And where do we process food and toxins?

Our Intestines: The Forgotten Immune System

Despite Dr. Elie Metchnikoff's Nobel Prize winning research in 1908, the concept that most of the immune system is in the intestines had been relegated to "alternative medicine," until recently.[1233] Many researchers are resurrecting Metchnikoff's work, showing that we have a symbiotic relationship with the good microorganisms we have in the intestines:

> "What if we discover that our entire evolution is a side effect of the requirements of the microbes in our guts? Maybe those organisms needed to modify their hosts to be more efficient in finding certain foods for them. If so, it's about time we turned the tables. From now on, by gosh, they work for us."[1234]

Amazingly, 10 percent of our body weight is due to bacteria living in our intestines. Since these guys outnumber our body cells ten-to-one, most of the genes we pack around belong to them, not us. What a humbling proposition, one that may help us not be so arrogant and concede that this is not the *Planet of the Apes,* nor the Planet of Humans, but, as the article suggests, "The Planet of Bacteria."[1235]

Metchnikoff talked about the close relationship between our intestines and our immune systems from the time we were amebas (if you don't believe in evolution, just bear with me). Back then, amebas had only two things to worry about: eat or be eaten. Come to think of it, this attitude still prevails in the business world. The close relationship between eating and the immune system, or our way of defending ourselves from being eaten, is regaining its proper place in modern health care.

Besides, when do we get E&I? Our intestines: eating poorly, particularly foods high in refined sugars, will alter the delicate balance of friendly intestinal flora, the very foundation of the immune system in the intestines.[1236] Remember that good bacteria in the intestines keep bad organisms out and help us digest and metabolize food better. Also think about how we prepare milk, bread, yogurt, and cheese: we add friendly bacteria.

We were taught that most of the immune system is circulating in the blood in the form of white blood cells, antibodies, immunoglobulins, etc. While these molecules are very important, they take their marching orders from the intestinal immune system where they learn what is "self" and what is not. There is an "internal conversation between tissues and the cells of the immune system;

we may regain a renewed sense of the self that we have lost."[1237]

There is a "seductive talk" is going on between the tissues of the GI tract and our friendly bacteria in order to put up a fight against invading organisms. The authors of the article, "Host-Pathogen Interactions: The Seduction of Molecular Cross Talk"[1238] state that

> "We are currently witnessing a transition period between the now classical concept of 'cellular microbiology' and the new concept of 'tissular microbiology.'"

Think about it: if you are going to defend yourself against an invader, would you not place most of your defenses at the site they attack the most? Most bugs try to get us through the foods we eat besides our airways and skin. No wonder these tissues are imbued with antibiotic-like chemicals to defend us.[1239] The old concept of the "terrain" as an important factor in infection is being revived.[1240] But, most people may still consider our genetic tendencies as the most important factor on how our terrains behave. Again, remember "nutrigenomics," which also contributes to gut health.[1241] Still, the debate over which is more important—nurture or nature—will never end.[1242]

Think of the circulating immune system as cops on the highways. We need them there, but most crimes are nevertheless committed in the neighborhoods, bars, stadiums, etc. In other words, most "crimes" are committed in the "tissues," not the blood. Tissues are a bunch of specialized cells that need to have E&I and good membranes to communicate to do their specialized jobs and keep the immune system humming.

About one-fifth of us have what we call irritable bowel syndrome (IBS). If you're not one of these lucky people, have you ever wondered what the heck is irritating them? It seems obvious; yet, you only get pills to bring down the inflammation while nothing is done to treat the imbalance of intestinal flora created by all the garbage we eat and the excessive use of chlorinated water and antibiotics. It turns out that IBS has been linked to auto-immunes diseases and depression.[1243] You may easily figure out the immune angle, but depression? In chapter 25, we will study the brain-gut connection a bit more.

Vaccines

Let's open Pandora's box, take out a can of worms, and toss it into a hornets' nest, shall we?

Some of you hate vaccines; but, as much as we may not like them, they seem to be the lesser of two evils. Our immune systems are compromised by pollution, living in close proximity with our fellowmen, and eating poorly. No wonder we get so many infections. But to say that we don't need vaccines or that they are harmless are extreme positions that ignore the complexity of the issues involved.

I have taken a middle-of-the road approach, which, no doubt doesn't make anyone happy. Then, again, I warned you: I am a synthesizer, not a fighter. Yet, I believe that the millions of dollars in sales at stake are clouding the issue.

The studies on vaccines and neurologic problems are controversial. They seem to be interpreted differently, according to what one believes beforehand and who paid for them. Are vaccines truly implicated in autism, ADD, and other problems? I don't know. But it is clear that mercury is; it has been used in vaccines as a preservative. Despite reports that this is no longer the case, there are persistent rumors that some vaccines still contain mercury.

Vaccines probably interfere with the glycosylation process of the immune system, thus increasing autoimmune disorders. Approximately 3 percent of immunized children develop autoimmune problems: they have more antibodies to thyroid, gonads, and a positive rheumatoid factor. Maybe this is why 15 percent of people have antibodies to the thyroid gland.[1244] Of course, toxins in the environment have a lot to do with this problem, too.

With a natural infection, the adrenal glands have three days to prevent autoimmunity by producing glucocorticoids, which are the adrenal hormones in charge of regulating sugar. With vaccines, the adrenals don't have time to react. Live rubella, coxsackie B, and mumps vaccines may then increase the risk of diabetes.[1245]

I believe we are vaccinating our children too soon, too fast, and with too much all at once. Their immune systems are not very mature when they are right out of the hospital. Those who believe this way of vaccinating is harmless do not seem to have a reason why our children are having so many problems with their psycho-neuro-endocrine-immune systems. The negative studies that have shown no association between vaccines and these problems are creating a false sense of security in our docs. I believe these studies are not asking the right questions, so the answers leave a lot to be desired.

Since I don't have great answers either, I have chosen a more cautious approach to vaccination until we know more about this issue. I immunized my little girl one vaccine at a time when she turned twelve months of age. I also kept her out of daycare centers. Is this the best way to go about vaccinating our children? I don't know. Until we do, let us be cautious and more tolerant of our divergent points of view.

Interestingly, many health practitioners have the same misguivings about H1N1 vaccination.[1246] Health workers In the State of New York reversed a policy that tried to make H1N1 vaccination for them in the fall of 2009.[1247] And in Texas, half of doctors oppose vaccination for Human Papilloma virus.[1248] As 2009 dwindles, it has become clearer that H1N1 was not as big a concern as it was "marketed" at the beginning of the flu season. Could it be that the whole thing was driven, at least in part, by Big Pharma's profit machine?[1249]

By the way; why was the public not made more aware that half of the fatalities seen with H1N1 were obese? Would you have wanted to know that the obese have a six times greater risk of doing poorly when infected with H1N1?[1250] IR, sweet death compromises our immune system.

Chapter 23

Metabolic Syndrome and Cancer

"When cells turn against the body (cancer), their cell surface carbohydrate profile is altered."[1251] Translation: cell membranes are TOILing, or toxic from refined sugars, trans-hydrogenated fats, excessive animal proteins, toxic, and emotional environments so that our immune systems are unable to protect us from mutating cells that become cancerous. Plainly put, refined sugar[1252] and obesity increase the risk of cancer[1253] and the higher mortality associated with it.[1254] PET scanning for tumors is based on the principle that tumors have a different metabolic rate of sugar.

Dr. Otto Warburg won the 1931 Nobel Prize for his work on metabolism and cancer. He determined that "obesity and carbohydrate excess predisposes people to cancer . . . [This is why] caloric restriction has been shown to lower 60 percent for cancers." His brilliant insight was rehashed in the clever British article "Cancer's Sweet Tooth: the Janus effect of glucose metabolism in tumorigenesis."[1255] Dr. Warburg went on to say that:

> "The prime cause of cancer is the replacement of the respiration of oxygen in normal body cells by a fermentation of sugar. All normal body cells meet their energy needs by respiration of oxygen, whereas cancer cells meet their energy

needs in great part by fermentation. All normal body cells are thus obligate aerobes, whereas cancer cells are partial anaerobes . . . Oxygen is dethroned in the cancer cells and replaced by an energy-yielding reaction of the lowest living forms, a fermentation of sugar."[1256]

TOILing With Cancer

Knowing about E&I and TOIL issues predicts that tumors harbor defective mitochondria. Early tumors seem to use up more ATP (mitochondrial function), but advanced tumors do not. In fact, two recent papers have squarely zeroed in on E&I as a way to deal with cancer: "Tumor Biology: How Signaling Processes Translate to Therapy" talks about cellular communication of information. "Metabolic Targeting As an Anticancer Strategy: Dawn of a New Era?" talks about the mitochondria and our metabolism.[1257]

Cancer is an oxidating and inflammatory condition.[1258] By now you know what is causing the TOILing. With the excess of refined sugar in our diets comes an excess of insulin in our bloodstreams, or hyperinsulinemia; this has been linked to prostate,[1259] pancreatic, colon,[1260] endometrial or uterine cancer,[1261] and bladder cancer.[1262]

The 2009 Nobel Prize in medicine was awarded for research on telomeres—the region of repetitive DNA at the end of a chromosome—which protect the ends of chromosomes from destruction. It turns out that antioxidants protect these telomeres from TOILing, thus prolonging life and reducing the risk of cancer.[1263]

Cancer's Sweet Tooth and Obesity

The higher the fasting glucose is, the higher the risk of getting cancer.[1264] An abnormal 2hGTT also increases the risk.[1265] There is more cancer in obese people who are more likely to suffer from IR that inhibits their immune systems.[1266] For example, adiposity and the metabolic syndrome increase the risk of breast cancer.[1267]

Another reason for obesity to be associated with more cancer is the fact that more cancer-triggering toxins are stored in fat. Corn syrup/oil, widespread in processed foods, has tetrahy-

259

drofurandiol; it has xenoestrogenic activity. It has been linked to prostate and breast cancer.[1268]

Obesity also raises levels of IGF-1, which fuels cancer growth like growth hormone does.[1269] A high BMI has been associated with a higher risk of colorectal neoplasia.[1270] This is why being born a "lightweight," like me, has been shown to have a lower risk of breast cancer.[1271] Hyperinsulinemia, IGT, IR, and diabetes are seen more often in survivors of childhood cancers. This is why screening kids' waist/height ratios is suggested.[1272] Since sweet death and its companion the metabolic syndrome are involved in all diseases, not just cancer,[1273] especially when we are obese.[1274]

Eating low glycemic index foods reduces the risk of cancer[1275] and increases longevity. For example, diet and exercise modify breast cancer risks.[1276] PPAR molecules, like omega oils, have an anti-tumor effect: less colon cancer is noted with omega oils.[1277] These PPAR nutrients are reduced in obesity.[1278] There is a 50 percent reduction of pancreatic cancer risk just by walking or hiking one-and-a-half hours per week because these activities reduce obesity and IR.[1279] Exercise lowers the risk of breast cancer significantly.[1280]

Cancer and Metabolism

The Harvard Medical School Division of Nutrition presented a whole symposium on E&I in food, how we process it in our bodies, and how our metabolisms affect cancer tendencies:

> "This symposium and future research will guide the development of effective cancer prevention strategies through nutritional and lifestyle modifications that alleviate metabolic syndrome."[1281]

It The symposium reiterated that the metabolic syndrome and IR have been shown to increase our risk of getting cancer, especially colorectal, prostate, and breast cancer.[1282] Other than TOIL, researchers focused on communication messengers, like leptin, TNF, IGF-1, and adiponectin.[1283] They also looked at epigenetic, or post-translation, effects of IR on the genetic tendencies that may lead to cancer. In other words, IR and the metabolic defects

260

that are triggered by our poor diets modulate the copying of potentially cancerous genes.[1284]

They concluded that nutrition to diminish metabolic problems should be explored in depth to reduce our risk of cancer.[1285]
For instance, reducing animal fat from the diet reduces the risk of
breast cancer[1286] and "prostate cancer prevention [is possible] by
nutritional means to alleviate metabolic syndrome."[1287] They also
recommended supplementing soy and tea together to reduce elevated estrogen levels that drive prostate and breast cancer.[1288]

As discussed above, genes that predispose to cancer may be
turned off by proper nutrition, thereby preventing the development of cancer. The article, "Genome Health Nutrigenomics and
Nutrigenetics: Diagnosis and Nutritional Treatment of Genome
Damage on an Individual Basis," is a good review of this concept.[1289]

"Apoptosis (Cell Death) by Dietary Factors"[1290]

Here is another great article from *Carcinogenesis: Integrative
Cancer Research*; let me step out of the way . . .

> "In spite of substantial progress in the development of
> anticancer therapies, the incidence of cancer is still increas-
> ing worldwide. Recently, chemoprevention by the use of
> naturally occurring dietary substances is considered as a
> practical approach to reduce the ever-increasing incidence
> of cancer."

> "By making modifications in the diet, more than two-
> thirds of human cancers could be prevented . . . Dietary
> chemopreventive compounds offer great potential in the
> fight against cancer by inhibiting the carcinogenesis process
> through the regulation of cell defensive and cell death ma-
> chineries."

> "Apoptosis, a form of programmed cell death, plays a
> fundamental role in the maintenance of tissues and organ
> systems by providing a controlled cell deletion to balanced
> cell proliferation. The last decade has witnessed an exponen-
> tial increase in the number of studies investigating how dif-
> ferent components of the diet interact at the molecular and

cellular level to determine the fate of a cell. It is now apparent that many dietary chemopreventive agents with promise for human consumption can also preferentially inhibit the growth of tumor cells by targeting one or more signaling intermediates leading to induction of apoptosis."

"The two major pathways that initiate apoptosis are extrinsic (death receptor-mediated), and intrinsic (mitochondrial mediated). Mitogenic and stress responsive pathways are involved in the regulation of apoptotic signaling. Noteworthy is the crosstalk between some of these pathways."

Translation: cell communication of E&I.

Here is a list of nutrients found to work in apoptosis and the foods that they are in:

- ECGC: Green Tea
- Curcumin: Turmeric
- Genistein: Soy
- I3C: Cruciferous
- Sulpharanes: Cruciferous
- Beta Carotenes: Vegetables
- Resveratrol: Grapes
- Isothiocyanates: Cruciferous
- Luteolin: Celery, Green Peppers, Peppermints
- Lycopene: Tomatoes
- Anthocyanins: Pomegranates, Wolfberries, Plankton, Algae
- Delphidin: Pigmented Fruits, Berries
- Lupeol/Sylimarin: Mangoes, Olive Oil, Herbs
- Gingerol: Ginger
- Capsaicin: Red Peppers
- Sulfur: Onions, Garlic

At risk of restating the obvious: avoiding a sweet death could prevent two-thirds of cancers. If I told you that there is a pill that would reduce your risk of cancer by two-thirds, would you buy it?

Fighting Words

The present paradigm of attacking cancer is based on killing the cancer as if it were a bug. This worn-out approach is failing because it does not encourage our "tissular immune systems" to keep the cancer in check. The book, *The War on Cancer: an anatomy of failure, a blueprint for the future,* by Guy B. Faguet, agrees.[1291] Think of tuberculosis: you may have it, but the bug responsible for it has been cocooned by your tissular immune system in a tough, scar-like cyst in your lungs so that it is practically isolated from the rest of the body. Would you want chemotherapy for it? Would you want to cut it out? I say, "Let sleeping dogs lie."

Of course, there are circumstances where we may want every available tool to deal with cancer. It is pretty scary to be told we have it. Yet, this is a personal decision that should be honored by all involved. Unfortunately, many patients are railroaded into futile, expensive, and often harmful courses of chemotherapy, radiation, and surgery in their last few months of life.[1292]

I leave you to ponder why an oncologist at the Huntsman Center for Cancer in Salt Lake City, Utah, refused to read a copy of the article, "Apoptosis (Cell Death) by Dietary Factors." One of my patients with breast cancer in remission took a copy of it to her doc to explain why her breast cancer had totally disappeared. This was to the surprise of the oncologist, who still recommended a protocol of chemotherapy. My patient asked, "Why would I go through that if my cancer is gone?" The doc responded, "That is what we do."

I was not there and I may be guilty of passing on an "anecdotal tale." Still, you be the judge about the doc who would not read a peer-reviewed article about her very line of work. Could it be that her worldview was threatened? In my opinion, this episode illustrates why so many docs still take refuge in the statement that "there is not enough evidence on nutrition and cancer."

Another disturbing book, *The Secret History of the War on Cancer,* by Devra Davis documents very well that the roots of cancer, polluted environments, poor diets, and stress have been de-emphasized in favor of money-making, seldom ineffective, and more aggressive modes of therapy that fight hard to keep "alternative" modes like nutrition from getting traction.[1293]

Chapter 24

Metabolic Syndrome and the Mind/Brain

The most famous Alzheimer's patient, former president Ronald Reagan, had a well-known sweet tooth. Remember his jellybeans on the oval office's desk? It turns out that our brains take quite a beating from sweet death. Chronic TOILing in the brain from too much insulin, IR, obesity,[1294] and metabolic problems[1295] increase our chances of Alzheimer's disease.[1296] "Crazy about sugar" takes on a whole new meaning, doesn't it?

Our aging-brain issues are really best understood by referring to them as "neurometabolic" problems.[1297] Neurodegenerative diseases, like Parkinson's, have also been documented to involve significant alterations in our metabolisms.[1298] At best, high blood sugar contributes to bad moods and cognitive problems[1299] and at worst it increases our chances of dementia, particularly in diabetics.[1300] Diabetes in midlife raises the risk of developing Alzheimer's disease or dementia by 70 percent.[1301]

Type 3 Diabetes?

The connection between IR and Alzheimer's disease is so well documented that the neurometabolic problems stemming from diabetes and its effects on the brain is now referred to as "type 3 diabetes."[1302] Some of our brains will be affected more than others' as we get older.[1303] Do you feel lucky? I wouldn't bet on you dodging Alzheimer's disease if you have a lot of rings around your midriff; a study followed 6,600 patients for twenty-seven years into their midlife. Those with a beer belly had a 35 percent higher risk of getting Alzheimer's disease.[1304]

Alzheimer's patients cannot bind oxidating AGE molecules very well because they have reduced RAGE receptors for them. This causes even more TOILing in the brain.[1305] Hyperinsulinemia is the cause of amyloid plaques in the brain of Alzheimer's patients. These plaques are thought to be due to chronic inflammation in the brain that accelerates brain aging. Type 1 diabetic patients have MRIs that show older brains than one would expect for their chronologic ages.[1306]

Stress and Brain Aging

If we are under too much stress, and we don't handle it very well, our brains age faster and we are more at risk of getting Alzheimer's disease and other neurodegenerative diseases. Higher cortisol levels due to stress and IR increases cognitive dysfunction[1307] and the risk of depression.[1308] The HPA axis dysregulation from stress significantly impairs memory in type 2 diabetes.[1309] Predictably, good insulin signaling suppresses toxicity of amyloid aggregates.[1310] Translation: less amyloid plaques are seen when healing TOILing controls IR.

After a meal high in sugar, even normal people may notice a decrease in cognitive performance right after said meal.[1311] (Don't use this as an excuse not to tip 20 percent.) Have you noticed some brain fog after your banana split? Patients with only IR, not yet full-blown diabetes, show brain changes by positron emission tomography (PET) scanning of the brain years before they are diagnosed to have Alzheimer's disease.[1312] The metabolic syndrome has been linked to white lesions on brain MRIs[1313] and cognitive decline is more pronounced in people with the metabolic syndrome[1314] and diabetes.[1315]

"Leaky Brain"

You are now familiar with "leaky gut." Well, there is "leaky brain," too. Once we understand that a TOILing intestinal lining may lead to mucosal permeability, we may see that the same process may occur anywhere in the body. It turns out that poor glucose processing also makes the brain more "leaky," allowing toxins to enter the brain more easily. The blood-brain barrier (BBB) is weakened by age and IR; they accelerate the rate at which the brain's blood vessels become leaky from cell membrane TOILing.[1316]

It is not surprising that the BBB is impaired in Alzheimer's disease.[1317] Glucose at high levels is toxic to the central nervous system.[1318] Environmental toxins may not get inside the brain to trigger TOILing of neurons, unless the BBB is leaky from TOILing.[1319] In other words, we are all exposed to toxins, like pesticides, but our nutrigenomic factors make it so that each of us is affected differently.

A leaky BBB is more likely when we lower our cholesterol too much. Remember that cell membranes are made up mostly of phospholipids and that cholesterol goes up to stop tissues from leaking. The most important phospholipid in the cell membranes of brain neurons is cerebrosterol.[1320] When we insist on lowering cholesterol too, much (under 150 mg/dl) we mess with cerebrosterol, thereby increasing our chances of Parkinson's disease[1321] and dementia.[1322] This is why we would do well to eat a lot of nuts, so we don't go nuts.[1323] (No, nuts don't make you gain weight.)[1324]

Not surprisingly, a leaky BBB has been linked to high blood pressure,[1325] which, as you now know, is a function of IR. High blood pressure is going to increase brain cell aging and dysfunction. Fixing the TOILing that leads to "leaky brain" helps with practically all neurologic problems. This is why coffee, which is high in antioxidants and thus reduces IR, has been shown to protect the BBB from cholesterol-induced leakage.[1326]

"Is the Brain on Fire?"

Every time I see the title of the article, "Is the Brain on Fire?"[1327] I think of Hitler screaming on the phone, "Is Paris burning?" to the general who disobeyed his orders to blow up Paris, France, as the Nazis withdrew in front of the allied armies. Is your brain burning? It turns out that neurodegenerative diseases like Alzheimer's disease, ALS, MS, and Parkinson's disease are inflammatory problems.[1328] This "neuro-inflammation"[1329] likely comes from our refined foods, stressful lifestyles, and free radicals from the environment. Pesticides are potent neurotoxins that add to the TOILing we see with high sugar diets as the article, "High Glucose Induce[d] Oxidative Stress and Mitochondrial Dysfunction in Neurons," attests.[1330]

This is why drugs designed to treat diabetes, the peroxisome proliferator activator receptor (PPAR) drugs, like avandia/rosiglitazone and actos/pioglitazone, have been shown to help with multiple sclerosis through their anti-diabetic and anti-inflammatory action.[1331] EFAs have been shown to have PPAR activity, too.[1332] Remember that insulin needs receptors on the cell membrane to work. Not surprisingly, these drugs, like EFA, have been shown to be of benefit in practically all conditions.

Your Brain on Insulin

"Insulin acts in the brain to aid memory and thinking."[1333] It seems obvious that insulin would do that because it is the main E&I molecule in our bodies. Insulin dysregulation sets the stage for neurodegenerative diseases, like Alzheimer's disease.[1334] IR, even before advancing to diabetes, increases brain inflammation and beta amyloid plaque formation, the hallmark of Alzheimer's disease. "Treating insulin resistance might improve memory and even avert cognitive decline in people with mild cognitive impairment."[1335] Higher levels of insulin cause hypoglycemia and raise the risk of dementia in the elderly.[1336]

PET scans of the brain have shown marked differences in brain function between insulin resistant patients and normal ones. Even totally normal adults with no IR see a quick improvement of memory by sniffing insulin through the nose.[1337] Hmmm, would you rather just stop eating so many jellybeans?

Another little problem with too much insulin in the brain is that it compromises serotonin function. Serotonin is the happy neurotransmitter that Big Pharma works on to create antidepressant medications. Taking an antidepressant is okay if you are so depressed that you may hurt yourself or others. But there are many other ways to get help if your depression is IR-driven, like taking 600 milligrams of chromium. Chromium reduces IR[1338] and more dramatically so in diabetics with the right genes.[1339] Just keeping blood sugar levels under control reduces our risk of dementia.[1340]

Insulysin, a normal molecule in the brain to break down insulin, is lacking in Alzheimer's disease.[1341] This results in higher levels of insulin in the brain; insulin then becomes an inflammatory agent. Of course, if insulin levels are too low, our brains don't get enough sugar, or E&I. In these cases, intranasal insulin has also been shown to lower the risk of cognitive decline.[1342]

Other kind of messengers, insulin-like growth factors, which act much like growth hormone, have been shown to have a profound effect on the brain, particularly in its development and in maintaining normal central nervous system functions.[1343]

Halloween's Trick (Sweet Death) or Treat (Ritalin)

I feel bad for all those moms who have had their keen observation that refined sugar make their kids hyperactive shot down by health care workers who insist that candy has nothing to do with this problem. After Halloween, teachers can also see the obvious link between candy and ADHD. While some may feel that IR is only theoretically possible to be associated with hyperactivity,[1344] other health workers routinely improve, if not cure ADHD, by avoiding sweet death and supplementing the nutrients that have been absent from their high sugar and processed astronaut food.

But Big Food and the Sugar Association of America are not going to see their cash cow threatened. Routinely, they plant articles in the media that would lead the unsuspecting to believe there is nothing wrong with sugar and no association with ADHD. A laughable study sponsored by General Mills, Coca-Cola, PepsiCo and Royal Crown Cola International gave only five teaspoonfuls of sugar to the control group—spit in the bucket compared to the amounts of sugar our kids eat in a regular day. Obviously, kids didn't react at all.[1345] Better-designed and independent studies consistently show that there is an association between sweet death and ADHD.[1346]

Even "bad moods" have been associated with hypoglycemia, a natural result of high-sugar diets that trigger more insulin production.[1347] This is especially true in children and in me; I get really grumpy waiting in lines at restaurants. Eating too much sugar causes our brains not to function as well after a meal;[1348] this is another excuse I use to get out of doing the dishes afterwards. Refined sugar messes with our brain's cognitive functions and brainwave patterns;[1349] it also triggers emotional distress.[1350]

A study found that a low-glycemic index diet free of food preservatives, colorings, and heavy metals, when supplemented by essential fatty acids, B vitamins, multiple minerals, grapeseed, soy, amino acids, alpha lipoic acid, probiotics, and milk thistle was as helpful as treating these children with Ritalin.[1351] Kids also do better on intellectual tasks in school when they eat well and supplement a protein-rich formula.[1352] By trying this approach before prescribing Ritalin (if parents are willing to fight this battle), 90 percent of children avoid Ritalin in my experience.

Ritalin has been associated with a higher risk of cardiovascular problems[1353] and it has been linked to a three-fold increase in cancer risk through chromosome abnormalities.[1354] While Ritalin may be the only way to help children who are severely afflicted, the fact that 40 percent of them have side effects, 11 percent stop the drug and lose half an inch and two pounds in seventy weeks may mean that we could be less cavalier about prescribing Ritalin at the drop of a witch's hat.[1355]

Many feel that ADHD is not a disease, but a creation of busy teachers and Big Pharma. To continue to medicalize our kids for discipline and attention issues is not a wise approach, in my opinion.

Rumor Has It . . .

The following rumor has not been adequately corroborated: according to Michael Downing, author of the book, *Spring Forward: the annual madness of Daylight Saving Time* (DST), the sugar industry lobbied Congress to delay the implementation of DST the fall of 2007 for one week, so that Halloween would have more daylight time for kids to go out and "trick" more candy out of their neighbors.[1356]

Sweet Brain and Neurodegeneration

Multiple sclerosis is also a brain inflammatory condition; it is not surprising that it shares a genetic susceptibility with diabetes,[1357] which is partly the reason why type 1 diabetics have a risk of multiple sclerosis three times higher.[1358] Multiple sclerosis is also linked to adrenal dysfunction, an important factor in blood sugar dysregulation.[1359] The brain runs on a very narrow or specific level of sugar in the blood. Any variance in how much sugar in the blood supplies the brain can have significant consequences.

Sweet death, or diabetes, has also been associated with Huntington's disease,[1360] Alzheimer's disease, multiple sclerosis, and Parkinson's disease.[1361] Some believe that a higher fruit intake increases the risk of Parkinson's disease;[1362] I feel this is due to the pesticides in fruit. They have been associated with Parkinson's disease.[1363] Remember that pesticides were derived from World War II leftover nerve gas. Isn't it amazing that we have been brainwashed to believe that pesticides could be 100 percent safe?

When combined with too much iron, the pesticide, paraquat, is even more harmful to the brain. Not surprisingly, mice treated with a synthetic antioxidant (EUK-189), had significantly less brain cell death in the area of the brain associated with Parkinson's disease:

> "These findings support the notion that environmental Parkinson's disease factors may act synergistically... and that iron and paraquat may act via common oxidative stress-mediated mechanisms."[1364]

This is another example of TOILing terrain creating E&I issues in the brain terrain.[1365] Oxidation of brain cells by toxins may also be treated with natural antioxidants.[1366] But the money is in creating artificial drugs that mimic natural compounds, like dopamine. After enough time goes by, Big Pharma stops telling us that its drugs are mostly copied from Mother Nature.

Co-creators With Mother Nature

The Chilean doctors, Humberto Maturana and Francisco Varela, won the Nobel Prize in biology for the work they eloquently explain in their book, *The Tree of Knowledge*.[1367] They coined the term "autopoesis" or "making yourself," which is exactly what we do constantly by consuming E&I from our food. In other words, we influence how our bodies and, more importantly, our brains continue to grow and completely replace themselves every month.[1368] Before these two docs showed up, we used to think that the brain stopped evolving and changing when we were teenagers.

The 167th National Meeting of the American Association for the Advancement of Science confirmed their observations. Indeed, our brains keep developing and changing even after the age of forty. The article, "Neurodegeneration: A Failure of Neuroregeneration?" tells us that the brain is in a dynamic state of equilibrium between degeneration and regeneration, just like any other tissue in the body.[1369] By eating well, we assure ourselves of a better new brain tomorrow.[1370] This is an example of the thermodynamic concept of "creation-destruction."

The great doc Linus Pauling, winner of two Nobel Prizes, coined the term "orthomolecular psychiatry," arguing that we may improve and even heal any psychiatric condition by being mindful to the E&I we get from our food.[1371] Mainstream psychiatrists rejected his opinions back in the 1970s, when we didn't have very much information on metabolic, E&I, and nutritional issues. The fact that psychiatry was, at the time, desperately trying to prove itself to be a "hard science" by relying on scientific pharmaceuticals didn't help Pauling's research see the light of day.

The introduction of Nazi-developed antidepressants and sedatives helped the present view that nutrition is not viable mode of treatment in mental illness.[1372] It is easy to see why nutrition has not been a particularly profitable endeavor in health care. In my opinion, revisiting the work of Pauling, Maturana, and Varela with a view to do the best and most cost-effective thing for people is likely to reverse these mistaken notions. Neuroscientists give us more food for thought:

"Understanding the molecular basis of the effects of food on cognition will help us to determine how best to manipulate diet in order to increase the resistance to neurons to insults and promote mental fitness."[1373]

Sweet Brain and Other Diseases

A modified or healthier Atkin's Diet helps children with seizures as much as the Ketogenic Diet does. The latter diet is high in fats, which produce more energy for the brain and the raw material to make more brain cells because 80 percent of the brain is fat.[1374] Low sugar in the blood can impair driving and a poor balance of sugar in the brain compromises overall performance in normal people.[1375]

Migraines are worse on high-sugar diets[1376] and in the obese.[1377] I hope it is not surprising to you to read that weight gain in people who suffer from migraines may raise the risk of cardiovascular problems.[1378] The metabolic syndrome increases the risk of depression, bipolar disorder, and schizophrenia. About 80 percent of patients with depression and bipolar disorder have at least one metabolic syndrome marker and 50 percent of them have a VAT (beer belly) a little too big.[1379] And it works the other way around, too: depression increases our abdominal girth.[1380] Even pre-diabetes (impaired 2hGTT) and the metabolic syndrome haves been associated with depression.[1381]

Higher cortisol levels, which produce more glucose, have also been associated with depression.[1382] Refined carbohydrates have been reported to interfere with the messenger or neurotransmitter serotonin,[1383] 95 percent of which is found in the GI tract. Refined sugars block the absorption of B-complex from the intestines that are needed for the enzymes that convert amino acids into neurotransmitters, an imbalance of which leads to depression.

It gets worse: neurotransmitters are glycoproteins.[1384] Imagine the quality of neurotransmitters people have when they eat excessive refined sugars. IR inhibits the conversion of the amino acid l-tryptophan to 5HTP and then serotonin.[1385] When we struggle controlling glucose levels in our bloodstreams, a problem often seen in pre-diabetics and diabetics, we have a tendency to develop more depression.[1386] Not surprisingly, tryptophan is lacking in obese patients.[1387] And it works the other way around, too: glutamate and GABA are neurotransmitters that have been found to have receptors for insulin secretion in the pancreas.[1388]

Diabetics and patients with the metabolic syndrome are well known for having more strokes and poor cognitive function as a result of compromised blood flow to the brain.[1389] From 1999 to 2004, strokes tripled in middle-aged women; they had two extra inches around their waists.[1390] Women who had signs of circulation problems revealed in their mammograms also tended to have higher sugar levels in their blood, more somnolence and, not surprisingly, more strokes.[1391]

Hyperinsulinemic patients also have more neurological problems everywhere (feet, stomach, intestines, eyes, etc.) due to poor blood flow to the nerves wiring those areas. Even non-diabetics with recent transient ischemic attacks or pre-strokes and strokes are found to have more IR after the fact:[1392] most of them have an impaired two-hour GTT.[1393]

Schizophrenia has also been linked to poor nutrition. After the Chinese famine of 1959 to1961, the rate of schizophrenia doubled.[1394] In other words, a starved brain is going to suffer from poor communication of E&I due to TOILing. Some feel that there is an impairment of neuronal glucose uptake in these patients' brains.[1395] Idiopathic neuropathy or unexplained numbness or motor dysfunction in the legs may be the first indication of pre-diabetes.[1396] Tourette's syndrome, the disease where people feel compelled to yell and curse at inappropriate times, is associated with metabolic problems, or glucose utilization in the brain.[1397]

Sweet Death May Land You in Prison

Daily candy consumption in childhood increases the likelihood of violent behavior in adulthood.[1398] In susceptible people it may even lead to criminal activity: sixty nine % of children who eat candy daily wind up in prison, compared to forty two % control group by age 34.[1399] Pre-diabetes, or abnormal 2hGTT, is more common in violent offenders[1400] who may be engaged in extreme "trick or treating.", which is similar to children hooked on refined sugars.[1401] In fact, the worse the diet, the worse the nature of the crime.[1402]

273

Some prison systems have shown that there is a drop in antisocial behavior in juvenile inmates when they take away the soda machines in their dorms for three months. A study reported a 45 percent decrease in disciplinary actions, 82 percent drop in assaults, 77 percent less thefts, and 65 percent less "horseplay" when soda was withheld.[1403] (Some people are so addicted to sugar that they may wind up in jail themselves if they were kept from their liquid candy fix.)

In several New York State correctional schools, an increase in fruits, vegetables, and whole grains increased performance by 16 percent and the number of children thought to be disabled dropped from 125,000 to 74,000.[1404] Their IQs, conduct, brain function and personality improved.[1405] A National Health Institute study showed that eating more salmon in jail reduced the rate of homicides.

Have you been wondering why these simple changes are not widely implemented in our penal system? Could it be that those in charge do not want to see their spending budgets reduced, which would certainly occur if their inmates were to shape up by addressing their sweet deaths?[1406]

Other "Sweet Hormones" and the Brain

IGF-1, the hormone that works much like growth hormone, is also involved in clearing the amyloid plaques that increase neuronal TOILing and lead to Alzheimer's disease. TNF alpha, an inflammatory molecule, hinders this process: amyloid plaques are then more likely to form in the TOILing brain. The brain also secretes IGF-1 and insulin; these hormones also have metabolic, neurotrophic, neuromodulatory, neuroprotective, neurogenesis, and neuroendocrine functions. "IGF [is a] promising therapeutic target for the treatment of neurodegenerative disorders."[1407] IGF-1 has also been shown to improve glucose tolerance.[1408]

Our rushed lifestyles cause our adrenal glands to work overtime. They produce mostly adrenaline and cortisol, two hormones that increase sugar production and aggravate IR.[1409] When stressed, most people end up sleep-deprived, which also worsens IR.[1410] Sleep breathing problems, like sleep apnea (a brain problem aggravated by central obesity), has been associated with IR.[1411]

Chronic loss of sleep may not allow people to recover from IR.[1412] You already know about this vicious cycle: the more hyperinsulinemia one has, the worse sleep apnea gets.[1413] Surprisingly, sleep deprivation helps in depression, if the patient has higher brain glucose levels and metabolism.[1414]

Even marital stress can aggravate the metabolic syndrome through adrenal strain.[1415] "Honey, you are going to make me diabetic!"

DHEA, an adrenal hormone, affects the hippocampus; it is involved in learning, memory, and cognitive function.[1416] DHEA replacement reduces the damage caused by the dysfunction of the HPA axis. Not surprisingly, low levels of DHEA correlate with high levels of amyloid plaques.[1417]

"Maybe?"

At a 2002 international symposium on Alzheimer's disease in Stockholm, Sweden, experts timidly ventured that, "We are beginning to realize that what is good for the heart may be good for the brain." They listed the typical factors that lead to heart disease as being similar to the factors that lead to Alzheimer's disease. Maybe? Understanding TOILing and E&I issues would remove such tepid declaration.

Atherosclerosis, or hardening of the arteries, makes the problem worse because the brain needs optimal circulation to get adequate E&I.[1418] The Mediterranean diet, often associated with lower rates of cardiac disease also lowers the risk of Alzheimer's.[1419] With time, "experts" will admit that all diseases are E&I concepts.

TOILing of the brain is caused mostly by our metabolic problems. Our brain cells are deprived of E&I or glucose, problems often seen early in the course of Alzheimer's disease. How else could we explain the fact that an elevated uric acid, a consequence of IR working on the kidneys, is associated with suboptimal circulation to the brain of older patients?[1420] Without good E&I the brain turns to alternative sources of energy (we should do the same in the United States) like ketones that are produced from fat metabolism. A new drug that mimics a ketone, AC-1202 ketasyn, has been found to improve learning, memory, and cognition in Alzheimer's disease patients, especially those who have the APOEε4 gene. Nutrigenomic principles give us:

> "Further evidence of the link between Alzheimer's disease and glucose metabolism . . . AC-1202 might provide a new approach to treating other neurodegenerative disorders characterized by neuronal hypometabolism."[1421]

"Neuronal hypometabolism," I like that. But I am not sure about the emphasis on a pharmaceutical approach that has significant side effects in lieu of facing our sweet deaths. Maybe we need to be patient with our experts. It turns out that AC-1202 works by increasing the levels of beta hydroxybutyrate, a natural molecule our probiotics or friendly intestinal flora produce when they are healthy.[1422] In the next chapter we will discuss the link between the gut and the brain, exemplified by the research leading to AC-1202.

"Diet and Lifestyle Interventions Lower Risk of Dementia"[1423]

A diet high in fruits and vegetables, folic acid, moderate alcohol consumption, adequate social and mental activity, and exercise are the cornerstone of prevention. This was determined by a study on separated twins; genetics plays a minor role.[1424]

A vicious cycle: more dementia leads to more social isolation and vise versa.

Factors increasing risk of dementia: strokes (six-fold), periodontal disease (four-fold), and low education. More inflammation at an early age contributes to brain inflammation. The main causes of early inflammation are periodontal decay, and poor nutrition. Both are associated with refined diets and a lack of vitamin D. The latter is likely due to people not being active outside, where they would get more sunlight. Strokes are linked to cardiovascular issues. So, poor circulation, also from poor diets, is a major factor in dementia.

Polyphenols are antioxidants that are found in fruits and vegetables. Drinking vegetable or fruit juice three times a week reduces the risk of dementia by 75 percent.

Folic acid lowers homocysteine, a toxic that goes up with a lack of this nutrient. Diets high in refined breads and pasta lack folic acid. A decrease of homocysteine of 26 percent (when given folic acid) reduced the risk of Alzheimer's disease.

Chapter 25

Metabolic Syndrome and the Second Brain: The Intestinal Tract

The importance of the gut and its effect on our bodies is underscored by the fact that most hormones come from the intestines. We have already discussed the influence of hormones on our brain thermostats. Prepare to develop a renewed understanding and appreciation for our lowly intestines: simply put, our metabolisms depend on our intestinal functions and the foods we eat on a regular basis.[1425]

In my opinion, it is in the gut where most physics concepts, especially thermodynamics, are applied in a practical way to our bodies. This is why I find the acronym, GUT, for "grand unified theory," somewhat ironic. GUT stands for the physicists' holy grail: finding an integrative approach to everything in the universe.[1426] In my opinion, the GUT in health is in the gut and the E&I in the food it metabolizes.

The Second Brain

If you are old like me, you may remember being stunned by the opening scene of the 1969 movie, *2001: A Space Odyssey.* Watching the moon, earth, and sun rise to the tune of "Thus Spake Zarathustra" left me breathless.

278

We didn't make it back to the moon in 2001 but we did gain considerable understanding on the amazing brain-gut connection. The Brits must have been equally taken by Stanley Kubrick, judging by the name they gave their brain-gut symposium, "The 2001 Brain Gut Odyssey."[1427] It recognized what many have known for centuries: most neurotransmitters, which are glycoproteins, are found in the intestines.[1428] The Brits are not alone. Entire symposiums are being dedicated to the topic of "the second brain," a term coined by Dr. Michael Gershon in his book, *The Second Brain: A Groundbreaking New Understanding of Nervous Disorders of the Stomach and Intestine.*[1429] Even more recent and less technical is the report from a symposium in Paris called, "The Intelligent Intestine."[1430]

Earlier, we talked about hormones from the intestines talking to the brain to regulate our metabolisms. The messenger in vogue at the time of printing was GLP-1, or glucagon-like peptide-1, which messes up our metabolisms by abnormally signaling our brains after ingesting bad foods, like ice cream.[1431] GLP-1 triggers IR after high-fat meals and reduces the amount of energy spent in metabolizing said toxic food.[1432] Try this on for size: I have never seen a person with brain/mind problems, such as depression, who did not have intestinal problems to go along.

Sadly, the vital role of the intestines as the organs through which we get E&I from the sun is often ignored. For instance, a lot of people with a diagnosis of depression are told that their intestinal symptoms are "all in their heads." They may well be in some of them, but not all. If a relationship goes only one way (brain to gut), then it would be the only example in physics where that happens because the whole universe is built on bidirectional relationships. In other words, the gut influences the brain, too.

Many diseases seem to have a connection to intestinal function as the article, "IBS, Depression, and Autoimmune Diseases,"[1433] describes. The fact that selective serotonin reuptake inhibitors (SSRI) agents to treat depression (prozac, zoloft, etc.) have been found to have significant anti-fungal activity[1434] should make you think a bit. Take a few moments to absorb the impact of this statement.

We know it is normal to have some yeast species in the intestines, but when we eat Twinkies all day long we overfeed this bug. It turns out that yeast loves refined sugars. Excessive candida overgrowth in the intestines blocks thiaminase, the essential enzyme for neurotransmitter synthesis, through the thiamine pathway and thus compromises the synthesis of serotonin. Refined sugars also have a direct toxic effect on our metabolisms, in addition to selecting out toxic organisms, like yeast, in the intestines. Fungal overgrowth in the intestines has also been shown to interfere with the intestines' immune system.[1435]

Could it be that the SSRI's anti-depressant action may in part be due to their antifungal action? The fact that 95 percent of serotonin is found in the intestines may keep you scratching you head a little longer.[1436]

And how about this: tryptan drugs, like Imitrex, are serotonin agents used to treat migraines. Not surprisingly, migraine sufferers often have some degree of depression.[1437] The brain-gut connection explains why people with migraines often have intestinal problems, too. Understanding this concept has helped many of my patients get rid of their migraines and depression by improving their brain-gut connection when they optimize E&I intake and metabolism.

Prozac and Our Metabolism

Antidepressants and antipsychotic drugs have been shown to mess up our thermostats in the brain and thereby increase the risk of IR and diabetes.[1438] The drugs used to treat schizophrenia and other serious psychiatric conditions are notorious for causing weight gain through IR.[1439]

If you are depressed about your weight, don't even think to take antidepressants: they have been linked to weight gain and a 40 percent increase risk of the metabolic syndrome. More than two thousand patients were studied between 2005 and 2006. Their waist circumferences, lipids, and fasting glucose levels were followed. Those treated with antidepressants also had a 120 percent increase in cholesterol problems.[1440]

Getting on Your Vagus Nerve

The vagus nerve is thought to be a cranial nerve, meaning that it comes out of your head to talk to the gut, mainly the stomach. It is not surprising that the vagus nerve is also involved in controlling E&I issues and our levels of sugar in the blood.[1441] What may be surprising to you is the fact that the vagus nerve, when dissected to look at its fibers or the tails of the neurons that make up the nerve itself, reveals that one-third of these neurons go from the head to the stomach, and . . . you guessed it, two-thirds go from the stomach to the head. Who is controlling whom?

This reminds me of Lao Tzu's, *Tao Te Ching:*

> "The river is mightier than the stream, because it is below
>   the stream.
> The ocean is mightier than the river, because it is below the
>   river.
> So is the woman mightier than the man, because she is below
>   him."

Relax: Lao Tzu is talking about the feminine and masculine in us all.

Refined foods, especially fats, get on your vagus nerve, leading to more inflammation.[1442]

The Psycho-Neuro-Endocrine-Immune System

The neurologic system works hand-in-hand with our hormones. In fact, many feel that hormones and neurotransmitters share many functions. Above, we saw that the intestinal hormone insulin acts like a neurotransmitter in the brain.

The hormone, ghrelin, is made in the stomach to signal hunger to the brain; it triggers a release of growth hormone in the pituitary gland of the brain. Ghrelin also helps with the digestion of foods, including sugar. [1443] Stomach bypass surgeries often fail to keep the weight off for many reasons. One of them might be that this invasive approach is disrupting the connection between the stomach and the brain and ghrelin's function. Ghrelin circulates at levels inversely proportional to the size of body fat. Ingested nutrients acutely suppress ghrelin levels; so do other hormones, like insulin and leptin. The latter is produced by fat cells. Any derangement in the amount of these hormones is likely to impair one's ability to regulate appetite and fat storage.[1444]

IGF-1 is a liver protein that has much the same function as growth hormone. IGF-1 has been found to be associated with IR when its levels drop below 152.[1445] IGF-1 dysfunction has also been associated with Crohn's disease, metabolic bone disease, and muscle wasting.[1446] Two other hormones in the GI tract have also been shown to work with the brain to regulate hunger and appetite: intestinal hormone PPY3-36 and cholecystokinin. These "gut peptides [are critical] in the regulation of food intake and energy homeostasis."[1447]

Inflamed Intestines Alter Cell Communication

Dr. Elie Metchnikoff won the 1908 Nobel Prize in Medicine by showing that 60 percent of the immune system is in the intestines.[1448] The ramifications of this profound fact are far reaching.

Wheat, processed foods, trans-fats, preservatives, colorants, environmental toxins, antibiotics, drugs, chlorinated water, etc., trigger various degrees of immune reactions like inflammatory changes in the intestines that spill out into our bodies. This bad E&I also messes up our metabolisms in our guts by disturbing several organs' functions, like our livers and pancreases, and by altering the delicate balance of friendly and not-so-friendly microflora in the intestines.

Yeast is not the only bug to take advantage of these changes in the gut. Other toxic organisms are also playing: viruses, parasites, and mutating bacteria. These bad guys take advantage of the weakened friendly bacteria, or probiotics.[1449] As you saw in a previous chapter, these friendly organisms have a lot to say about how we metabolize and handle food.[1450] There are more than five hundred species of these good guys; they are responsible for 10 percent of our body weight. Due to the hostile environment we often create inside our intestines, even what we consider benign bacteria may turn on us and become harmful. A good example is the bacteria, klebsiella.[1451]

I had an interesting discussion with doctors at the Cleveland

Clinic; they refused to believe that klebsiella could be the reason one of my patients was having rheumatologic problems. The article, "The Gut in Ankylosing Spondylitis and Other Arthropathies: Inflammation Beneath the Surface,"[1452] exposing "turncoat" klebsiella didn't seem to mean anything to them. I guess our minds seem to be conditioned to think, "either/or." Once a bug is thought to be benign, it is hard to believe it can go bad. I guess they didn't see the movie, *Spider-Man 3*. (In chapter 27, we will talk about the concept of arthritic problems and their association with intestinal inflammation.)

There is "a thin line between gut-friendly and pathogen."[1453] Still, many docs do not believe that an overgrowth of mutating intestinal bacteria, viruses, parasites, and yeast could turn into a problem. For instance, most docs attribute yeast growth in stool cultures to "contamination" of the stool sample. Other docs go as far as to say that "there are no parasites in America."

I wonder where they think the worms that eat our bodies in a closed casket come from when we kick the bucket?

More on Wheat Allergies

Celiac disease in the gut, an extreme expression of gluten intolerance, is twenty times more likely to be associated with diabetes.[1454] Eliminating gluten from the diet for six months improves insulin sensitivity in many patients.[1455] In fact, we now recommend that all type 1 diabetics be screened for celiac disease.[1456] Approximately 12 percent of type 1 diabetic children already have celiac disease;[1457] it's imperative to screen these children for it—an intervention commonly ignored.[1458] This explains why wheat allergies are under-diagnosed.[1459] Some genetically-susceptible people, the ones carrying the HLA-DQB1 gene, seem to have more intestinal problems with gluten.[1460]

Wheat intolerance is another example of the interconnection of cell messengers working through the psycho-neuro-endocrine-immune system network: diabetes and wheat intolerance are signs of a disrupted immune system. This is why wheat may cause depression, headaches, schizophrenia, Tourette's, bipolar disorder, and many other neurologic problems. Wheat allergy is also directly harmful to the brain, especially the white matter.

"Wheat sensitivity can be primarily and sometimes exclusively a neurological disease."[1461]

The Bible tells you to eat wheat. The problem is that we have refined this God-given grain too much and our intestines are already beat up pretty good by our refined diets and are very sensitive to further insults, especially when we eat wheat day in and out. Remember that process food is wheat-based.

Nothing New Under the Sun

Most gastroenterologists tell my patients that colitis, like IBS, Crohn's disease, and ulcerative colitis have nothing to do with their diets. This is why I had to smile when I saw the article, "Novel Pathophysiological Concepts of Inflammatory Bowel Disease."[1462] And what was so novel? The very concepts that Metchnikoff advanced to earn him the Nobel Prize in medicine in 1908: the interaction of the food we eat with our microbiota in the intestines determines the amount of inflammation therein. The fact that patients with Crohn's disease seem to have altered glycoproteins lining their intestinal walls would strengthen this concept.[1463]

The TOILing of the cell membranes lining the intestines, which is aggravated by an imbalance of intestinal organisms,[1464] causes an increase in permeability of the lining of the intestines, a condition often referred as "leaky gut." The inflammation brewing therein may then spill out to every corner of the body. Not surprisingly, this "increased intestinal permeability precedes clinical onset of type 1 diabetes"[1465] because leaky gut is a cause and consequence of poor E&I processing and TOILing. And here is another vicious cycle: IR worsens with intestinal inflammation.[1466]

Sisyphus Stoning You, Again

Another poorly understood IR problem is gallbladder stones.[1467] Most people with this problem have their gallbladders taken out without any mention of why they ended up forming stones in the first place. In fact, most of them continue to have abdominal problems, even after the gallbladder is gone. This is because nothing was done for the underlying problem: IR.

Hyperinsulinemia causes liver cells to be exposed to higher levels of insulin that impairs their function. These patients' livers start making thicker bile that will end up precipitating out of solution and form stones inside the gallbladder.[1468] This is why cholelithiasis, the medical name for stones in the gallbladder, has been associated with higher triglyceride levels—the lipid that goes up with IR.[1469] Have you wondered why most people with gallbladder problems tend to be obese women in their forties who have had several children? We are taught in medical school that gallbladder stones are seen in fat fertile females over forty—not very sensitive, I know, but don't shoot the messenger . . .

The idea that gallbladder stones are caused by excessive fat in the diet is wrong. In fact, eating more nuts and more protein reduces the risk of gallbladder stones.[1470] It is true that eating fat triggers contractions of the inflamed gallbladder, already carrying irritating stones within. But the stones themselves were formed over the years by refined sugar, not fat. It is understandable but wrong to think that fat created the stones because people hurt more when they eat fat.

Unfortunately, this misunderstanding causes them to avoid fat and eat more sugar to satisfy their hunger. Since the gallbladder is now gone, bile is dripping out of the liver without anywhere to sit in storage, waiting to squirt out when a meal comes down the plumbing. The end result is that these poor people cannot digest fats properly; this is complicated by the fact that stones are (in some patients) still being formed, but now only inside the liver. Can you now see why lots of patients continue to feel discomfort after the surgery to take the gall bladder out?

To make problems worse, the thicker (and sicker bile) triggered by IR causes constipation and irritation in the bowels,[1471] which causes our metabolisms/digestion of E&I in the intestines to be further compromised. More TOILing and more IR will follow.

A diet low in the glycemic index is the answer: "fruit and vegetable consumption [reduce the] risk of cholecystectomy in women."[1472]

Chunky Liver

This is not the name of a canned soup . . .

Having established that the liver is a bit soaked in too much sugar and insulin, you may see why people with the metabolic syndrome tend to suffer from "Fatty Liver."[1473] The article, "Fatty Liver a Novel Component of the Metabolic Syndrome,"[1474] goes into more detail. About seventy million people in the United States have Fatty Liver and 25 percent of them have a severe form of this problem.[1475] Sadly, Fatty Liver is now seen in about 50 percent of children over the age of five who are obese and in 10 percent of all children: "Experts predict those who have [Fatty Liver] as a kid may need a transplant by their thirties and forties."[1476] A transplant? What a dire consequence of our thoughtless facilitation of the food politics in our society that led to their sweet death . . .

If you were startled by this report on liver transplants for kids like I was, you and I may be republicans; apparently people who startle easily tend to be republicans, according to the journal, *Science* . . .[1477]

Blood tests may pick up Fatty Liver, but I would rather get an ultrasound of the liver.[1478] Still, ultrasounds, normal blood tests, and gross appearance of the liver do not rule out obesity-related liver disease.[1479] It is best to simply assume that Fatty Liver is present when we are dealing with metabolic problems.

Worst of all, Fatty Liver is the reason behind most liver damage in the United States. Number two is over-the-counter Tylenol. Alcohol is the third largest cause of liver problems.[1480] Yet, many docs still believe that we can't have oxidative stress in the liver without alcohol. Why? I don't know. You would have to ask them. It turns out that TOILing, or oxidation that leads to IR, is the main problem with Fatty Liver.[1481] The liver itself also develops IR when we succumb to systemic IR.[1482] There are other causes for Fatty Liver, such as infections and chemicals that act synergistically with metabolic issues.[1483]

Since Fatty Liver is a function of IR[1484] and inflammation,[1485] it also leads to hypertension,[1486] cardiovascular diseases, type 2 diabetes,[1487] strokes, and peripheral arterial disease. Of course, Fatty Liver is associated with more VAT,[1488] but it seems like Fatty

Liver, itself, is a more powerful predictor of metabolic problems than VAT.[1489] IR compromises our immune systems, making viral infections of the liver more likely. These infections worsen Fatty Liver and increase the risk of scarring of liver tissues with chronic infections, like chronic hepatitis C. As you may have predicted, chronic hepatitis worsens IR.[1490] Hepatic activation of inflammatory markers leads to more liver and systemic cells IR.[1491] This vicious cycle is more pronounced in those with a genetic tendency.[1492]

Sadly, many people are told that their Fatty Livers, when found on an incidental ultrasound, means nothing and that there is nothing that can be done about it. This is not true. We must control our sweet deaths and eat diets that don't trigger IR.[1493] This is why controlling IR with a drug like pioglytazone improves Fatty Liver.[1494] Hopefully you would ask for a low-glycemic diet before trying a potentially problematic drug that might hurt your liver. If you protect your liver from the effects of any drug with the detoxifying amino acid N-Acetyl-Cysteine, NAC, it will also help the liver lose its fatty deposits.[1495] In general, vitamin B complex and betaine help reduce TOILing in a Fatty Liver.[1496] Exercise also helps.[1497]

Chapter 26

Metabolic Syndrome and the Heart

L et's shed some "sunshine" on this rapidly changing field; the fact that the super antioxidant vitamin D is critical for heart health[1498] points to heart problems coming from the oxidation and inflammation[1499] (TOILing) seen in IR,[1500] particularly in the obese[1501] and in diabetics who have higher AGE products.[1502] Higher than normal insulin levels have a significant impact on our cardiovascular systems[1503] and our peripheral arteries, in particular,[1504] by triggering TOILing through an up-regulated immune system.[1505] In fact, a 1 percent elevation of GlycoHb increases the risk of cardiac disease by 11 percent.[1506]

Researchers are focusing on this simple concept to help us with cardiometabolic issues and several other chronic health problems. They can get pretty fancy with the biochemistry (i.e., selective kinase response modulators, and phosphoinositol-3-kinase), but I assure you it all boils down to cell communication of E&I. The article, "Type 2 Diabetes and Heart Disease: All Roads Lead to Insulin Signaling," goes into more detail on IR and hyperinsulinemia being the main mechanisms of heart disease.[1507]

Many docs now refer to the whole sticky mess of heart disease as "cardiometabolic syndrome."[1508] There is now a Cardiometabolic E-Journal Club dedicated to E&I and TOILing issues. Understanding the metabolic syndrome leads to better management of heart disease,[1509] earlier predictions of future diabetes,[1510] and a decrease in all-cause mortality,[1511] especially in those who have had bypass surgery.[1512]

Our waist circumferences are a very practical way to predict future risk of heart disease because VAT predicts coronary artery calcification.[1513] The American Diabetes Association, the Obesity Society, and the American Society for Nutrition have teamed up to raise awareness on these issues. They feel that more studies are needed to pin down the exact waist measurements that signal future sweet death.[1514] I am not sure why they don't like the already widely publicized measurements that consistently show IR when men have a waist circumference over forty inches and women have one over thirty-five inches.

What Your Parents Didn't Know

I always ask patients if they have a family history of diabetes. Often, they say no while acknowledging that Uncle Bob had a heart attack in his forties. Too bad we didn't know back then that Uncle Bob was probably at least a pre-diabetic. In all likelihood, he worried a lot about fats in his diet, but felt okay about eating a lot of sugary desserts.

It turns out that about 90 percent of people with heart problems have pre-diabetes, diabetes, and/or metabolic syndrome problems,[1515] especially the elderly.[1516] This relationship is perhaps the most practical breakthrough in medicine in many years. Now we know that the spasms and clogging of the arteries that lead to lack of blood to the heart begin with IR.[1517] By the time a person winds up in the hospital with a heart attack, that person does worse the higher his or her average blood sugars are.[1518]

Excessive sugar and insulin in the bloodstream irritate or inflame/oxidize the lining of the arteries, which puts out glycoprotein messengers, like ICAM and VCAM,[1519] that make the endothelium or lining cell membranes of the arteries become stickier. Stress also increases ICAM messengers; this means that stress increases cardiovascular disease.[1520] TOILing endothelium is noted even in teens when they are overweight.[1521]

TOILing sets in—oxidative and inflammatory stress,[1522]—leading to spasms of the muscles wrapping the arteries, endothelial stickiness, clotting, and eventually the formation of a clot. In other words, the arterial terrain becomes fertile ground for life-threatening decrease in blood flow as the article, "Diabetes and Cardiovascular Disease and Common Soil Hypothesis," tells us.[1523] The more oxidized the terrain is, the more heart disease we will have.[1524]

Heart disease is an inflammatory condition best addressed by the article, "Attacking the Metabolic Syndrome to Reduce Atherosclerotic Risk."[1525] Heart disease is arguably the scariest form of sweet death and metabolic problems.[1526] By eating diets high in antioxidants, we may decrease the TOILing of the lining of our arteries[1527] and of our hearts[1528] to improve not only their function but their structure, too.

We have already discussed the role of fats; nowadays, they are emphasized a bit too much at the expense of refined sugars. Also, salt intake takes some attention away from our sweet tooth without understanding that the excess of salt in our diets merely compounds the toxic effect of metabolic issues in the kidneys.[1529]

And so it is that anyone of us with a family history of heart disease is likely to be at risk of developing IR, diabetes, and obesity *if* you don't follow the simple principles of nutrigenetics.

Still Genetics

Those of us with the genotype APOE 2 and 3 seem to have less genetic tendencies to developing a poor lipid profile than those of us with the APOE 4 genotype.[1530] The latter is also associated with a higher risk of developing neurodegenerative brain diseases, like Alzheimer's disease. Also, heart disease is more likely in patients with poor glycemic control in their blood when they have the gene variant 9p21.[1531]

As you continue to read about these types of findings, keep firmly in mind the lessons learned from nutrigenetics and nutrigenomics.

Don't Wait for the Clot to Form

Heart disease is brewing years before the clots form.
There is a continuous relationship between sugar and en-

dothelium inflammation in everyone, not just in diabetic patients: the more sugar we eat, the more dysfunctional the arterial lining becomes.[1532] The obese have subclinical or not-yet-noticeable heart disease.[1533]

Heart disease begins when we start to have problems metabolizing sugar, causing a hyperinsulinemic condition.[1534] This means that even pre-diabetics have an increase risk for heart disease.[1535] Insulin is directly toxic to the endothelium; it triggers atheromas or abnormal growths on the endothelium.[1536] Once we have a heart attack, the race is on. Our tendency to pre-diabetes and diabetes escalates.[1537]

Don't wait for the clot to form: make sure you are screened with some of the metabolic tests noted in the laboratory chapter. Therein we also discussed the IMT test that can detect endothelial inflammation caused by the metabolic syndrome very early.[1538]

The Lining of Our Arteries is Not Wallpaper

The circulatory system is critical for transportation of E&I to optimize the structuring and functioning of our cells, fuel waste disposal, and cell communication. If there is poor circulation, our whole bodies will be affected. This is a critical concept to understand. Our freeway system in the United States was created over fifty years ago; it is often credited for the massive explosion of economic growth in our country during and directly after World War II.[1539] Communication of E&I in our bodies is also heavily dependent on our "highways" of transit.

Excessive sugar in the bloodstream and its accompanying rise in insulin (IR) cause inflammation of the lining of all organs, particularly the lining of arteries or endothelium.[1540] This is exactly what is also going on in peripheral arterial disease (PAD),[1541] which is a fancy name for poor circulation to your limbs.

Endothelial Medicine,[1542] a book by William C. Aird, refers to this concept as "an entity unto itself." It recognizes that the health of cell membranes lining not only our arteries, but practically all tissues and organs, is a critical common denominator to almost all diseases. Older docs referred to this concept as "the terrain." Unfortunately, the authors do not go into nutrition, stress, or environmental toxicity (TOIL) issues as the cause of endothelial problems. Rather, they focus on pharmaceutical products (nitrates, steroids, statins) and gadgets (stents) to address the symptoms of TOIL.

The article, "Endothelium as an Endocrine Organ,"[1543] clarifies these concepts quite well. The endothelium is participating in this massive orchestra of communication of E&I to keep our metabolisms going. Diabetes and obesity are associated with endothelial dysfunction[1544] that leads to heart disease, strokes, blindness, nerve impairment (particularly in the lower extremities), gallbladder stones, kidney stones, high cholesterol, hypertension, ovarian dysfunction, reproductive problems, pre-eclampsia, depression, thyroid dysfunction, arthritis, asthma, allergies, difficult menopause, Alzheimer's disease, Parkinson's diseases, cancer, etc.

These complications are some of the reasons why it is so sad to now find obese children with endothelial dysfunction.[1545] A study found that obese children have the arteries of a forty-five-year-old person.[1546] Even patients with IR may have signs of early endothelial dysfunction.[1547] Endothelial dysfunction begins with our poor diets.[1548] How may we then repair our TOILing endothelium? Clean up the environment, handle stress better, and eat a low-glycemic index diet with judicious supplementation of micronutrients, like antioxidants to control oxidative stress.[1549] If necessary, drugs like Metformin[1550] reduce heart failure morbidity and mortality.[1551]

The bottom line: the more we control IR, the better the health of our arterial walls.[1552] This is why diets high in antioxidants reduce the risk of heart disease.[1553]

SOS From Our NOS

The research into the cell messenger, nitric oxide synthase (NOS), won the Nobel Prize in medicine in 1998 and the honor of being dubbed the "molecule of the decade." NOS is the cornerstone of the system of cell communication that governs our TOILing at the cellular level, particularly in those cells lining our arteries—the endothelium.

The Nobel academy got a "charge" awarding the three docs who made the "dynamite" discovery of NOS. As you know, Alfred Nobel himself made his fortune with dynamite. The "nitric" in NOS is a pretty good clue because it is the main ingredient in TNT. It turns out that we had known for quite a while that dynamite workers would get horrendous headaches when exposed to nitric products. Some smart doc figured that this was happening because of arterial dilatation in the brain. This serendipitous discovery led to the famous little pills people put under the tongue when they are having chest pain from restriction of blood flow to the heart, aka angina. Nitroglycerin has been a very good old drug for the relief of cardiac circulatory issues.

Viagra and its Humble Origins

The NOS research was also used to come up with sildenafil/ Viagra. When the NOS system works optimally, our arteries dilate effectively, especially where we may need it in certain situations. So what may cause the NOS to perform less efficiently, thus triggering erectile dysfunction (ED)? Below we will review in more detail that ED is a function of IR.

One of the best-kept secrets about NOS is the amino acid L-arginine. It's one of the main steps in the healthy functioning of NOS.[1554] Making sure that we get enough L-arginine in our diets, which we cannot do unless we eat a wholesome diet of lean meats, flavonoids (like quercetin and green tea),[1555] and plenty of fiber to make sure that L-arginine is well absorbed from intestines,[1556] helps our arteries become are less likely to go into spasms when we are TOILing.[1557] (This is sometimes the case in patients with heart disease.)[1558] NOS blockade reduces adiposity and IR,[1559] conditions that may be reversed by supplementing L-arginine,[1560] thereby improving the treatment of the metabolic syndrome.[1561]

Now, why do you think Pfizer came up with Viagra instead of telling us about our relative lack of L-arginine contributing to ED? I am not complaining; everybody seems to be pretty happy with Viagra. But I am merely pointing out how Big Pharma loves to treat the symptoms instead of the underlying problems.

Story Time

While on-call one night, a kid trying to beef up his weightlifting program passed out after taking L-arginine. It is often used by body-builders to increase blood flow to their muscles to make them bigger; too bad it also lowers blood pressure. He called me at 4:00 a.m. to tell me this . . .

Please, don't take L-arginine unless you are seeing an integrative doc.

Making New Blood Vessels

Creation/destruction, the forces that sustain our entire universe have nit spared our bodies. They are always getting "remodeled" to keep them from TOILing and leaking. We complain about road maintenance in the summer, right? Well, our arteries are always being remodeled or maintained, too, *if* we eat right.

The article, "Angiogenesis in Health and Disease,"[1562] links practically all diseases to a dysregulation of angiogenesis, the making of new arteries. Without proper transportation, without highways, E&I don't get to where they need to: our cells. Angiogenic factors, or messengers, put out to make new cells amplify the inflammatory process by recruiting white cells and affecting their function. Hemostasis (equilibrium) and angiogenesis are closely linked. Ultimately, IR and hyperglycemia are strong contributors to endothelial inflammation, which is related to dysregulated angiogenesis, especially in the severely obese.[1563]

According to the above article, these are the problems we may see when we don't make new arteries very well: malignancy, ischemia (lack of blood), inflammation, infections, immune disorders, neurodegeneration, hypertension, brain ischemia, respiratory distress, osteoporosis, cancer, obesity, psoriasis, warts, dermatitis, Kaposi's sarcoma, diabetic retinopathy, primary pulmonary hypertension, asthma, nasal polyps, Crohn's disease, ulcerative colitis, periodontal disease, ascites (free fluid in abdominal cavity from liver problems), endometriosis, uterine bleeding, ovarian cysts, arthritis, synovitis, osteomyelitis, Alzheimer's disease, ALS, strokes, atherosclerosis, hypertension, diabetes, ulcers, hair loss, menorrhagia, pulmonary fibrosis, emphysema, nephropathy, and bone fracture healing.

It'd be better to say *all* diseases are associated with poor blood vessel formation. If you are like me, you will only remember "hair loss" from that list . . .

Drugs or Stents? How About Neither?

A stent is a little hollow tube inserted inside a clogged up coronary artery to restore blood flow to the heart muscle to treat chest pain (angina) and/or a heart attack. Restricted blood flow to the heart muscle deprives those cells of oxygen and E&I to carry out their functions. As much as stents seem to quickly restore blood flow—after years of using these expensive devices at such a critical time—an article came out saying that rosuvastatin/Crestor®, used to lower cholesterol, is just as effective at unclogging our coronaries as stents are.[1564] Interesting . . .

It turns out that the company making rosuvastatin financed the study; we have to wonder how valid the results are because pharmaceutical companies have been shown to look out mostly for shareholders interests, not the health of the people.[1565] We also have to question the evidence for rosuvastatin and the stent because 80 percent of what modern medicine has to offer has little, if any evidence, according to a surgeon-turned-mathematician/statistician.[1566] In fact, cholesterol-lowering drugs bite the dust on a regular basis after better evidence is finally released. Often, their negative pre-marketing studies are not made public until troublesome side effects become obvious a few years after their launch in the market.

The last example of this little problem before this printing is Vytorin, a combination of ezetimibe/simvastatin. This drug sold well because it did lower cholesterol, but nagging questions remained about its ability to really prevent heart attacks or arterial clogging, the real endpoints. In other words, it doesn't matter that a drug lowers cholesterol if people keep having heart attacks and strokes. The ENHANCE study reached this conclusion in 2006, but the drug companies did not release their results, despite pressure from the FDA to do so at the time. After several warning letters, the results were published in February 2008. They claimed that it took them longer than estimated to review the results of forty thousand ultrasounds of the carotids.

> "These are companies that do trials all the time, and it's hard to accept the fact that they said the analysis was more complicated than they expected, which resulted in the delay."[1567]

The drug companies even tried to change the endpoints after the study was concluded: at the outset, they checked 3 points on the carotid artery for plaque formation, which they wanted to reduce to only 1 carotid point. The companies stated that they had an "unnamed advisory panel" recommend that the endpoints be changed, a group that excluded the trial's primary investigator, Dr. John J. P. Kastelein from the Netherlands.[1568]

Despite all these concerns, the American Heart Association and the American College of Cardiology urge cautious interpretation of these results, stating that no conclusion may be drawn from a single study. Fair enough, but both a panel of cardiologists and the *New England Journal of Medicine* editor have stated that Vytorin and ezetimibe should not be used but in more extreme cases.[1569]

Let's see what results larger studies bring when they conclude in 2012. What are you betting on? That a European Society of Cardiology study, now in its fourth year, is showing no reduction in "major cardiovascular events" with ezetimibe[1570] may be an indication that it would be prudent to bet against this drug.

Let's Chew the Fat Some More

Many doctors are beginning to question the whole cholesterol hypothesis, according to the article, "Cholesterol Veers Off Script,"[1571] because of the Vytorin problem, joining many other doctors who never quite bought into it from the beginning.[1572] You should consider joining us, too.

It is estimated that 80 percent of heart disease could be avoided if we simply ate better.[1573] Avoiding saturated fats and refined sugars reduces IR[1574] and even unclogs our arteries with a good diet. Dr. Dean Ornish's advice to eat that way has proven to be true, even in patients who were told they would not survive without bypass surgery, stents, or heavy-duty drugs.[1575] Even after a heart attack, we do better the lower our blood sugar levels are.[1576]

Interestingly, drugs used to treat cholesterol, like rosuvastatin, seem to work even in patients with normal serum lipids. A study showed that the incidence of strokes, heart attacks, and other circulatory problems decreased significantly with statin drugs because they have an anti-inflammatory action and not necessarily because they lowered cholesterol.[1577] Could it be why statin drugs improve the treatment of pneumonia, an inflammatory problem?[1578] In fact, any drug used to treat heart disease or clogging of the arteries seems to have anti-inflammatory and antioxidant properties.[1579] For instance, new drugs for angina (pFOX inhibitors) like ranolazine inhibit the oxidation of fatty acids and reduce glycosylated hemoglobin.[1580] In my opinion these are TOILing issues.

Story Time

If you are a staunch republican, skip this section.

Did you know that former president Bill Clinton was told he needed a heart bypass to survive his fast food fix? He refused the heart bypass because he didn't want to become a republican.

I warned you; don't complain.

Since almost every other commercial we see on TV is about a cholesterol-lowering drug, I need to keep bringing up my take on this sticky subject for equal time: lots of articles, like, "Fatty Acid, Dyslipidemia and Insulin Resistance,"[1581] are consistently ignored by mainstream medicine because the "standard of care" dictates that you quickly get a drug to lower your cholesterol, despite clear recommendations by the American Heart Association that "therapeutic lifestyle changes" (TLC) be used first. TLC, like low-tech diet and exercise advice, are supposed to be implemented for six months prior to prescribing cholesterol-lowering drugs.[1582]

But some doctors have told me they feel patients don't respond to TLC talks. This is very likely true. I wonder if the docs' body language and sometimes outright casual discussions on lifestyle changes have anything to do with their patients' alleged unresponsiveness. Cavalier advice like "eat a balanced diet" thrown out in passing only convey to the patient the lack of importance diet and exercise has in the eyes of the doc. It is not unusual for highly educated docs to feel that nutrition is below their academic prowess.

We must address patients' sugar and trans-fats addictions in order to lower cholesterol. As you already know, cholesterol is not a problem unless the liver does not keep cholesterol from getting oxidized, which happens when our liver cells are overwhelmed by excessive insulin in the bloodstream, a result of IR.[1583] The hallmark of IR affecting the liver's processing of fats is an elevation of triglycerides; when they go over 442 milligrams/deciliters, the risk of heart disease is significantly elevated.[1584] In fact, if triglycerides steadily go up over five years, the risk of diabetes increases.[1585]

Demonizing cholesterol is not the answer.

Good Fats

Fats, in general, were demonized to market cholesterol-lowering drugs without any attempt to single out saturated and trans-hydrogenated fats. These bad fats are, indeed, problematic; they up-regulate the immune system, leading to TOILing in the liver, and a subsequent elevation of cholesterol.[1586] Unfortunately, the "bad fat" axe also fell on omega oils, monounsaturated fats, and polyunsaturated fatty acids (PUFA). These good fats have been repeatedly shown to reduce atherosclerosis and heart disease by about 19 percent.[1587]

In fact, raising the levels of essential fatty acids would have eight times the impact of distributing automated external defibrillating machines in public places and two times the effect of implanting cardioverter defibrillators in patients.[1588] No wonder the American Heart Association recommends that all heart patients supplement omega oils.[1589]

Remember that omega oils lower IR. They also stabilize plaque after it has formed[1590] and improve heart rhythm.[1591] Omega oils also lower cholesterol.[1592] If one decides to still take drugs to lower cholesterol, omega oils potentiate their effects.[1593] Even if we still eat high-fat diets, omega oils reduce the stiffness of our arteries seen immediately after such meals.[1594]

It turns out eggs, occasionally vilified as bad food for cholesterol, increase the HDL—the good cholesterol—*if* people get off refined sugar diets that increase the real problem behind lipid problems, IR.[1595] The same may be said about avocados, olives, nuts, veggie fats (in general), and fish.

New Fats

Docs are always finding new types of cholesterol molecules to demonize and each new finding is supposed to be the best indicator that one is at higher risk for heart disease. The latest candidates for this fleeting honor are the apolipoproteins. By looking at the ratio of apoB/apoA-1, one gets an indication of how serious the cardiometabolic and IR problems are.[1596] Unfortunately, there is already evidence that these new fats are no better than the cheaper "meat-and-potatoes" total cholesterol levels.[1597]

Still, I find the research on apolipoproteins interesting because an elevated apoB/apoA-1 ratio signals significant IR and a higher risk of heart disease in the future.[1598] This is very helpful because we often see elderly people with high cholesterol; yet, they have never had a stroke or a heart attack. Clearly, the problem is not the elevated cholesterol, but the underlying IR and E&I problems of cardiometabolism. The fact that apoB and the apoA-1 are processed in the liver and in the intestines is also very appealing to me: remember Fatty Liver and probiotics?

Blaming Bugs

Have you heard that heart disease may be due to a bacterial or viral infection? As appealing as it is to blame others for our own problems, this theory has been put to rest: a review of nine studies enrolling more than eleven thousand patients showed no improvement in heart disease with the use of antibiotics.[1599] It seems that the main problem is TOILing, or inflammation of the arterial lining, without any signs of infection.[1600] Once inflammation sets in, the lining of the arteries becomes sticky: bugs love to dive into it. Chlamydia, H. pylori, and cytomegalovirus seem to be associated with hardening of the arteries only after the CRP is elevated.[1601]

In other words, the metabolic syndrome increases the risk of arterial inflammation that leads to atherosclerosis and major heart problems more than the bugs that may be found floating around in the bloodstream.[1602] When bacteria and viruses are found frolicking in the endothelium, it is because they are taking advantage of an optimal environment to thrive and hang out.[1603] What would you do if you were a self-respecting bacteria? Wouldn't you go for this cushy, soft, warm, bloody, dark and nutrient-rich layer of irritated endothelium to set up shop? There is no question that infections may be aggravating heart disease, but the bacteria and viruses are only taking advantage of the inflammation already well under way.

The problem is not the bugs, nor the calcium, but a lack of the antioxidant vitamin K; this causes calcium to be poorly distributed in the body, ending up in the lining of arteries. This is one reason why supplementing vitamin K2 reduces heart disease by 57 percent[1604] and improves bone density.[1605] The other reason? Vitamin K lowers IR.[1606]

Since vitamin K2 reduces arterial calcifications[1607] by helping the hormone osteocalcin transport calcium out of the arteries to our bones,[1608] it would be foolish to refrain from supplementing calcium[1609] as some people recommend avoiding "arterial calcification from nanobacteria." The bottom line is that vitamin K lowers the risk of heart disease;[1610] antibiotics do not. A significant concession to the infection hypothesis of heart disease is the fact that an imbalance of GI flora may affect the immune system therein. For example, periodontitis has been linked to higher rates of heart disease.[1611] This is why supplementing probiotics . . .

" . . . Leads to a reduction in cardiovascular disease risk factors and could be useful as a protective agent in the primary prevention of atherosclerosis in smokers . . . The short change fatty acids formed in the human colon by bacterial fermentation of fiber may have an anti-inflammatory effect, may reduce insulin production and may improve lipid metabolism."[1612]

In other words, going after toxic gut flora reduces TOILing and gut permeability, resulting in less TOILing in the endothelium.

Funny Heartbeats

Even normal people have occasional funny heartbeats. I mean, *besides* those times when you see somebody who looks like Anne Hathaway or George Clooney. Also, the kind of foods we eat and associated insulin levels affect the autonomic or subconscious control of our heart rates,[1613] even in normal, non-obese, non-diabetic people. This is especially true when we start to show signs of metabolic problems.[1614]

Funny heartbeats could be a warning that we are developing IR,[1615] even when our hearts are fairly normal.[1616] This is particularly true when our job stress is a bit overwhelming[1617] and when we have metabolic problems worsened by low-level lead exposure.[1618] I see lots of patients with some kind of funny heartbeats. If they seem to be doing well, I don't send them on a wild goose chase to waste their time and money on fancy heart tests. By taking the time to reassure them, and showing them how to overcome sweet death and supplementing their diets with omega oils, minerals, and leafy vegetables,[1619] just about all of them see those worrisome heartbeats go away in time.

Some of these funny heartbeats may be due to a lot of stress and anxiety. Sometimes these folks need to get tested, just to reassure them quicker. And some of them may have more serious heart disease. How are you going to tell which is which? Well, you are not. I am, since I am the one who gets paid the big bucks . . .

Some of these funny heartbeats, like atrial fibrillation, may indeed signal early heart disease. Still, atrial fibrillation is more likely in those with IR[1620] and metabolic problems.[1621] Some patients do require those fancy tests. But, again, even these patients are likely to have some other clues that they are starting to have metabolic problems,[1622] which is particularly true in the obese.[1623]

Recently, I had a patient who refused to go to the emergency room. I was really worried about him because his heart rate was as low as a snake's belly, presumably, due to atherosclerosis. He begged me to give him IV magnesium in my clinic so that his day would not be ruined waiting around in the ER. He knew that a lack of magnesium not only overexcites muscles like the heart, but also increases IR. Still, I insisted that he go to the ER. After negotiating some more, I felt I needed to honor his request.

Having properly warned him of the risky nature of postponing more dramatic and effective treatment, I gave him a squirt of magnesium in the vein, as well as omega oils to help the heart's rhythm and variability.[1624] He left the clinic with me wondering how he could walk with a heart rate in the thirties. When I called him the next day, his heart rate was back up in the normal range. But, Mr. Tough Guy eventually ended up with a pacemaker, anyway. His heart was already too compromised for magnesium to rescue him. Needless to say, he had a belly that reminded me of Santa Claus.

Singing the Blues Over a Broken Heart

Patients with heart problems are often depressed. I would be depressed, too, if my ticker weren't in good shape. But the problem is stickier than that. It turns out that "IR [is] a metabolic link between depressive disorder and atherosclerotic vascular diseases."[1625] Remember the discussion on IR causing our neurotransmitters to be somewhat compromised with IR?[1626]

In chapter 34, we will talk more about the heart and our feelings. You could read more about all this from Dr. Dean Ornish who wrote the book, *Love and Survival.*[1627] This world-renowned cardiologist will touch your heart. He recommends meditation, which he practices himself, and he will tell you story after story about his patients healing their hearts by healing their relationships and avoiding a sweet death. For example, he documents how men with heart attacks have a greater chance of pulling through if they have a loving wife. Moral of the story: be nice to your wife.

Tired Heart

A failing heart, or congestive heart failure (CHF), is due to the muscles of the heart inefficiently pumping blood out to the lungs and body, resulting in pooling of fluids in the lungs and legs because of leaky blood vessels and higher pressure inside said vessels. Why would you guess the heart muscle is getting tired? What else, but E&I issues . . . Abnormal left ventricular energy metabolism has been associated with IR.[1628] The article, "Metabolic Mechanisms of Heart Failure," confirms IR as the central issue and adds that IR compromises ATP production in the mitochondria.[1629]

What we have here is pretty significant TOILing of the heart pumping muscles: the elevated glucose in the bloodstream also triggers oxidation of heart muscle cells.[1630] Air pollution, or the "T" in TOILing, can be significant enough to increase hospitalization of patients with CHF by 13 percent.[1631] The dysfunction of the heart muscle is worse as we age, but if we have IR we increase our chances of ventricular dysfunction.[1632] The bottom line is that higher fasting glucose in non-diabetic patients increases the sixty-day mortality rate in hospitalized patients with CHF.[1633]

Heart TOILing may be improved by a low glycemic index diet, fiber (fenofibrate), and the antioxidant, CoQ10, which improves mitochondrial function; the left ventricular chamber of the heart then gets better E&I to pump more efficiently.[1634] The fact that a healthy sugar, D-ribose, significantly improves cardiac muscle function[1635] should serve as a reminder of the necessity to keep sweet death at bay. And the fact that thiamine (B vitamin) also helps the heart muscle[1636] is a reminder to avoid bleached-out grains and toxic environments, since we need B complex to detoxify.

Fatty Cushion?

Obese people recover better than thin people after they have a heart attack.[1637] Odd, but the American Society of Echocardiography feels this may be so because obese people have strained their heart for a longer period of time; this stimulates the gradual thickening of their left ventricles, the part of the heart that pumps blood to our bodies. The stronger the left ventricle, the better we may cope with a heart attack. Think of a tree growing better as it fights for sunlight amongst taller timber.

It seems that one's fat butt may save one's fat butt . . .

Another study showed that 50 percent of overweight adults have a healthy heart, that is, normal blood pressure, cholesterol, and sugar levels.[1638] Some researchers feel that obesity may only be a "cosmetic problem" because obese people can have a healthy heart. That may be so, but I feel a follow up of these patients for a longer period of time would be helpful. Will those obese patients still have a healthy heart in a few years? Also, the study did not look for insulin levels; it would have been a more subtle marker than the three parameters mentioned above. Had they done so, could they have found that those obese patients already had some degree of IR that may be the first signs of future problems?

More Facts About Insulin Resistance

Below are some key points from the article, "Insulin Resistance: The Cardiovascular Aspect":[1639]

- "Vascular insulin sensitivity": Insulin binds to endothelial receptors to trigger *no* production
- Prolonged hyperglycemia results in ADMA accumulation that leads to more atherosclerosis.
- Calcium metabolism affected by abnormal Nitric Oxide function: more calcification of arteries.
- "A hyperglycemic environment provokes production of reactive oxygen species and switches mitochondrial-NOS from nitric oxide generation towards superoxide-production."
- AGE products are formed after long exposure to excessive glucose; they upset cell communication.
- "IGT individuals provide higher oxidative stress than constant hyperglycemia."
- Incretins are hormones released by intestines after a meal to induce insulin release.
- Atrial fibrillation results from the heart atrium being remodeled by IR.

Chapter 27

Metabolic Syndrome and Bone/Arthritic Problems

The bottom line, with respect to bone and arthritic issues, is pain. Sadly, chronic pain is affecting more and more people these days. In my opinion, the main reason is a dysfunctional metabolism.[1640] The excessive weight our joints, ligaments, muscles, and skeletons carry around is only part of the reason. The other reasons are poor communication of E&I due to TOILing; it leads to psycho-neuro-immune-endocrine network breakdown and to more inflammation and bone stiffness, not just in our joints and bones,[1641] but also throughout our bodies.

Not surprisingly, you will see in this chapter that most of said inflammation comes from the food we eat and how it is processed in our intestines.

Joy of Living?

Emile Zola makes two great points in his book, *Joy of Life*. It is the story of a self-absorbed family who whines incessantly about their perceived miserable life, all the while ignoring the father's intractable arthritic pain. He suffers in silence, but occasionally succumbs to legitimate wails of pain. At the end, when they find the body of the maid who has hung herself, the arthritic father has the last lines of the book: he is shocked that anyone would take their own life because he is so grateful to be alive, despite the

305

pain that he knows gets worse when he eats refined sugars.

Zola and most of our forefathers were keenly aware of both the connection between our attitude about life and pain and refined sugars making the pain worse. Today, we eat so much of it and it is such an accepted part of life that we have lost the clarity of mind to see the association there for all to see.

Our Savings Accounts

Our bones' functions are best understood by thinking of them as savings accounts where we deposit nutrients that may be needed at times of stress and starvation, especially when it comes to minerals. Thinking of our bones as rock-solid marble that never changes is not accurate. Bones are much more than racks to support our bodies' flesh. Watching too many Halloween movies with skeletons terrorizing kids may leave us with the impression that bones are cast in stone.

Our bones are totally renewed every year. Can you ever step in the same river twice? No, because its waters are always flowing. Bones have arteries and veins that are constantly bringing and taking nutrients to and from our bones. It is the same with the soft ligament tissues that connect bones together, our joints (not the ones some people smoke); they are even more susceptible to the factors outlined above. For example, carpal tunnel syndrome, a problem triggered by inflammation of the ligaments in our wrists, may be a harbinger of type 2 diabetes.[1642]

Soft, Sweet Bones

Osteoporosis and its precursor, osteopenia, are nothing but an overdrawn savings account: we eat so poorly that we end up tapping into our bones for nutrients not seen in our diets. A TOILing gut that cannot optimally absorb minerals worsens this problem.

Bone thinning afflicts almost 50 percent of American women.[1643] Why is there so much osteoporosis in Western countries, yet, hardly any in the Orient? Because osteoporosis is a "hidden tax on high-tech living" that is based on refined foods:[1644] dairy, meats, wheat, and soda.[1645] But the worst factor is high-sugar diets because they inhibit the absorption of calcium and magnesium in the gut.[1646]

Liquid candy is high in refined sugars and in phosphates. The former worsens IR and the latter bind calcium and magnesium out of our bodies.[1647] Refined sugars compound the problem of bone thinning by lowering the pH of our blood. Calcium is then mobilized out of our bones to buffer the low pH in the blood, thus "overdrawing our savings account" in the bones.[1648] Predictably, osteoporosis is worse in diabetes because the pH is already lower in diabetics.[1649] Some docs believe that the metabolic syndrome worsens even osteoarthritis.[1650]

When calcium and other minerals are released into our bloodstreams, they contribute to plaque calcification in the arteries, or they are eliminated in the kidneys, which may already have their filtration function a bit compromised by hyperinsulinemia. This may lead to kidney stones and gout. Remember that gout is also a rheumatologic problem initiated by uric acid not being filtered very well in the kidneys.[1651]

The hormones adiponectin and leptin, produced by our VATs, increase bone density in type 2 diabetics. In other words, a beer belly increases bone thinning.[1652] VAT is also associated with IR and an abnormal secretion of the parathyroid hormone in charge of bone turnover by regulating serum calcium.[1653] If IR results in hypoglycemia, the dysfunctional secretion of parathyroid hormone is worsened.[1654] The function of the parathyroid is further compromised when low serum levels of vitamin D3 compound IR.[1655] Yet another vicious cycle . . .

Overcoming IR, fixing intestinal absorption, and promoting physical activity—particularly lifting weights[1656]—are the best ways to prevent and treat osteoporosis. If you are still brainwashed by the dairy industry, this may come as a surprise to you: vegans have good bone health, even without dairy.[1657]

Vitamin Sunshine

A lack of vitamin D3 is emerging as a very important factor in the development of osteoporosis. Vitamin sunshine seems to be more important than minerals in the prevention of bone thinning, if our parathyroid hormones are healthy.[1658] Vitamin D improves the absorption of calcium and phosphorus from the intestines and at the same time it lowers IR.[1659] Again, I recommend that you take 1,000-2,000 IU. You may find that you need even more if you check your blood levels because genetically some people

307

don't process vitamin D very well: their receptors to vitamin D may not be functioning optimally.[1660] These patients tend to have more IR.[1661]

As stated above, vitamin K is also a very important factor in maintaining health bone density.[1662]

The Myth of Osteoporosis

The Myth of Osteoporosis is the title of a book favorably reviewed in the *Journal of the American Medical Association*.[1663] The author doesn't say that bones do not get softer, but that this is a normal process that is rarely associated with problems because the tougher type of bone, trabecular bone, takes over, thus preventing serious fractures. She feels that the problem of osteoporosis is a disease created by Big Pharma to sell drugs. I agree.

She also documents how drugs barely decrease the risk of the vertebral fractures we all get as we age (that is why I am getting shorter every year and I am already vertically impaired). But drugs do nothing for hip fractures, the biggest threat when our bones thin out. And whence hip fractures? IR and diabetes.[1664]

Interestingly, the hormone, osteocalcin, which is involved in bone maintenance, is also involved in modulating glucose metabolism.[1665]

Myth of the Sacred Cow and Strong Bones

Milk is a bit problematic. In my opinion, the dairy industry has done an amazing job convincing Americans that milk strengthens our bones. The dairy industry, as well as Big Pharma, is very interested in promoting the "myth of osteoporosis." I would like you to look up the article I will now faithfully outline for you. As you read this information, remember that milk promotes IR.

"Calcium, Dairy Products, and Bone Health in Children and Young Adults"[1666]

- Fifty-eight studies were reviewed. Most of them found no relationship between dietary calcium intake and measurements of bone health.

- Dairy consumption is among the highest in the United States, yet osteoporosis and fracture rates are also high. Animal protein, including milk, is associated with urinary calcium losses. Doubling protein intake increases loss of calcium by 50 percent.

- Physical activity in twelve to eighteen-year-olds strengthens bones more than calcium intake.

- "We found no evidence to support the notion that milk is a preferred source of calcium." The NIH does not say that milk is the preferred source of calcium. Only the industry interprets it to be so.

- "Calcium in dairy products is not as well absorbed as that in many dark green leafy vegetables ... Dairy products contain protein and sodium (the latter competes with calcium), and some dairy products, especially processed cheeses, clearly increase the urinary excretion of calcium as a result of the increased sodium, sulfur containing amino acids, and phosphorus content."

- "Although dairy products tend to contain more calcium in absolute amounts than calcium-rich plant foods, when absorption fraction is taken into account, the amount of plant food needed to get the same amount of absorbable calcium is modest. For example, one cup of cooked kale or turnip greens, two packets of instant oats, two-thirds of a cup of tofu, or one and two-thirds cups of broccoli provides the same amount of calcium as one cup of milk, as would one cup of fortified orange juice, soy milk, or Basic 4 Cereal."

Despite this article getting lots of press coverage when it was published, most moms, with a microphone in their faces, insisted that they would continue to give milk to their children to strengthen their bones. I suspect that most of you will do likewise. After all, milk ranks way up there, close to God, country, motherhood, and apple pie. It is, without a doubt, a sacred cow. Holy cow…

Pill Pushing

Big Pharma likes to create the impression that non-pharma-ceutical approaches not only don't work, but they may also be illegitimate or, God forbid, "alternative." The motivation is clear: more sales of its drugs legitimized by alleged scientific research.[1667] But there may be some behind-the-scenes hanky panky—both in pushing its pills and demonizing its competition.

A study came out reporting that padded hip protectors don't prevent hip fractures in the elderly.[1668] Three of the authors didn't reveal that they had been paid by Big Pharma to do research on bone-strengthening drugs in the past. The Associated Press dis-covered the potential conflict of interest. "A close reading of the *Journal of the American Medical Association*'s guidelines suggests that the fracture study authors' ties to drug makers are clearly relevant," said Daniel Callahan, the president of the World As-sociation of Medical Editors.

> "A consumer advocate with the Center for Science in the Public Interest agrees. Readers could easily interpret the study to say that because hip protectors don't work, 'I guess I better take the drugs.'"[1669]

Not surprisingly, there are some studies that find no use for vitamin D3 and supplementation of minerals in strengthening bones. It can't be good for business as usual to have these simple interventions widely known: 800 IU of vitamin D3 plus 1,200 mil-ligrams of calcium a day reduce the risk of hip fractures by 43 percent and the risk of non-vertebral fractures by 32 to 58 per-cent.[1670] Will Big Pharma try to discredit a study that showed the best way to prevent fractures is to help the elderly prevent falls? By the way, the very same study showed that 80 percent of pa-tients with fractures have no signs of osteoporosis at all.[1671]

Perhaps sex hormones are okay pills to push to treat osteopo-rosis, but this approach may create other problems like strokes, heart attacks, and cancer.[1672]

And the Winner Is...

Phosphonate drugs (i.e., Fosamax®) for osteoporosis have side effects. Some of them include atrial fibrillation or abnormal/inefficient beating of the upper chambers of the heart,[1673] a rare osteonecrosis of the jaw, and the fairly frequent reflux or heartburn. Also, they don't seem to be effective after five years of therapy.[1674]

Ironically, the drugs to treat reflux, like the "purple pill," cause osteoporosis.[1675] We have already talked about vicious cycles ad nauseam. This one gets the Oscar: the purple pill also blocks enough digestive acid to alter the pH of our intestines. This causes our intestinal flora to mutate;[1676] bad bugs get selected out, creating more inflammation in the intestines. This leads to poor absorption of minerals and that is how the PPI drugs (like the purple pill) increase the risk of osteoporosis. Furthermore, said intestinal inflammation contributes to poor metabolism of vitamin D, which is critical for mineral absorption and bone health.[1677]

Okay, take alendronate/Fosamax for your osteoporosis. "But, Doc, it gives me reflux . . ." Okay, take Prilosec. You get the picture. This is enough to drive you mad or make you depressed. Okay, take Fluoxetine/Prozac. "But, Doc, I just read that Prozac can give me osteoporosis . . ."[1678] It's enough to keep you awake at night—or laugh your head off.

Story Time

This one doesn't have anything to do with osteoporosis. It just reminds me of an ironic and sleepless night on call, caught in a vicious cycle. I got a call about 3:00 a.m. from a new patient I had seen that very day in clinic:

"Doc, I can't sleep," he said.

"But, didn't I prescribe you a sleeping pill just today?" I tried to hide my anger.

This guy had woken me up and during our daytime visit he had shown no interest in working on the roots of his insomnia. He was dealing very poorly with his stressful life.

"Yes, but I am afraid of the side effects," he said.

"Well, don't take it, then," I replied, feeling my annoyance

311

mount.

"But, Doc, I can't sleep," he complained.

"Okay, take the pill, then." I couldn't believe my ears.

"But, Doc, I am afraid of the side effects!" he cried.

"Don't take it, then!" I was losing it.

My ex-wife was awake by now, yelling through fogs of interrupted sleep: "Give *me* the f***ing pill so I can sleep!" she hissed.

By the way, sleeping problems have been associated with IR,[1679] in addition to morons calling in the middle of the night . . .

"Drugs for Pre-Osteoporosis: Prevention or Disease Mongering?"[1680]

- An already controversial condition has been expanded to increase market cut-off values for bone density "somewhat arbitrary" according to original WHO statement in 1994. Values intended for epidemiologic studies, not clinical treatment
- "Treating those at risk of being at risk? ... Impressive sounding reductions in relative risk can mask much smaller reductions in absolute risk." A 75 percent reduction of relative risk by raloxifene translates into 0.9 percent reduction of absolute risk. The true incidence of fractures is less than 1percent a year; this influences the results as above, when risk is overstated.
- We need to treat 270 women for three years to prevent one vertebral fracture.
- Focus on vertebral fractures, not hip fractures. Two-thirds of vertebral fractures are subclinical.
- Side effects of drugs are played down. Examples: diarrhea, GERD, clots, jawbone decay and more vascular, neurologic, and lab abnormalities.
- This data was analyzed mostly by docs with ties to drug companies.

Anti-aging Pill

Dehydroepiandrosterone, or DHEA, is an adrenal hormone that may be supplemented to help our bones by improving mineral absorption. Interestingly, it also helps reduce IR[1681] and it may help resolve depression.[1682] At this point in the book, you understand how it is that one single molecule can do so many things. No wonder the French call it the "anti-aging" pill and awarded the doc who promoted the safe use of DHEA in 1995 as "man of the year" in France. Despite his impeccable credentials as an endocrinologist in Paris, his work, upon crossing the Big Pond, became an "alternative."

Of course, this happens often, especially when natural products do not generate the huge profits that Big Pharma has grown accustomed to earning by marketing its drugs. The same thing happened with SAMe (S-adenosylmethionine, a derivative of B vitamins) and alpha lipoic acid, antioxidants now sold as drugs in Europe.

Rheumatoid Arthritis

Rheumatoid arthritis (RA) has also been associated with diabetes and with IR; it increases inflammation everywhere—not just in our joints and bones. There is also a clustering of autoimmune diseases that include RA and diabetes.[1683] In other words, diabetics are more susceptible to all types of arthritis, a result of an overall imbalance of the psycho-neuro-immune-endocrine system of cell communication.[1684] RA is even seen in pre-diabetics or those with an abnormal 2hGTT.[1685]

The article, "Inflammation, Insulin Resistance, and Aberrant Lipid Metabolism as Cardiovascular Risk Factors in Rheumatoid Arthritis,"[1686] integrates some of the concepts you have seen in previous chapters. In a practical way, we may simply say that the same factors that lead to heart disease are at play in RA and vise versa.[1687]

This is why drugs for RA seem to decrease the inflammation markers seen in the metabolic syndrome.[1688] The problem with said drugs is that they often have significant side effects. By the way, the PPAR drugs for diabetes increase the risk of fractures.[1689]

Inflammation Beneath the Surface

Arthritic problems start with inflammation in the intestines.[1690]

It's that simple: poor metabolism, or TOILing of the cells lining the intestines when we eat refined food, take too many antibiotics and/or get infected by toxic organisms are the main factors that lead to "inflammation beneath the surface."[1691] Of course, there are genetic tendencies, but again, don't forget nutrigenomics.

If the intestinal cells cannot absorb nutrients very well, our joints and bones don't get the minerals and other micronutrients necessary to maintain optimal function and structure. Also, toxins are poorly eliminated when our intestines TOIL; they get reabsorbed back into our bodies through the leaky gut mechanism. These toxins become "peroxynitrates" that are then attacked by our circulating immune systems, creating the inflammation we see in arthritis.[1692]

Remember our discussion on probiotics and the point that their mutations, or imbalances, lead to inflammation in the gut. Said inflammation tends to leak back into circulation and subsequently ends up in every tissue of our body, including our bones and joints. Microflora imbalances also affect the immune system based in the intestines. The food we eat is the main reason why this happens, as we learn from the article, "Gut-Joint Axis: Cross-Reactive Food Antibodies in Rheumatoid Arthritis."[1693]

The article, "The Clustering of other Chronic Inflammatory Diseases in Inflammatory Bowel Disease," leaves no doubt that intestinal inflammation is associated with inflammation in other parts of our body:

> "Both ulcerative colitis and Crohn's disease had a significantly higher likelihood of having arthritis, asthma, bronchitis, and pericarditis than population controls. An increase risk for chronic renal disease and multiple sclerosis was noted in UC, but not in Crohn's disease patients. The most common non-intestinal comorbidities identified were arthritis and asthma. The finding of asthma as the most common comorbidity increased in Crohn's disease patients compared with the general population is novel. These may be diseases with common cause or complications of one disease that lead to the presentation with another."[1694]

Some may argue that this little problem is only true when the intestinal inflammation is very severe, like in colitis. There we go again: our mind thinking "either/or." Lesser amounts of intestinal inflammation do cause systemic inflammation as well.

Henry C. Lin at the University of Southern California to congratulate him on a watershed article he published in the *Journal of the American Medical Association*. Again, I will let you read the main segment so that you don't think I am interpreting the results incorrectly, as I often hear from people who have not bothered to read the articles I present to them:

> "The clinical criteria for irritable bowel syndrome diagnosis do not include the extraintestinal symptoms that are common in these patients such as fatigue or myalgia. Instead, these complaints are viewed as symptoms of other diagnoses that coexist with IBS and fibromyalgia. This separation may be an artifact of medical specialization. As such, a unifying framework for understanding IBS that could account for both... gastrointestinal as well as extraintestinal symptoms would warrant serious consideration... The gastrointestinal and immune effects of small bowel bacterial overgrowth, SIBO, provide a possible unifying framework for understanding frequent observations in IBS, including postprandial bloating and distension, altered motility, visceral hypersensitivity, abnormal brain-gut interaction, autonomic dysfunction and immune activation."[1695]

Now you know why the best diet for arthritis is a low-glycemic index diet: vegan and no wheat.[1696]

Chapter 28

Metabolic Syndrome and Other Health Problems

The following is a list of problems that often don't find a sympathetic ear at doctors' offices: irritable bowel, syndrome, chronic fatigue, multiple chemical sensitivity, non-specific chest pain, premenstrual syndrome, non-ulcer dyspepsia, repetitive strain injury, tension headaches, TMJ, atypical facial pain, hyperventilation, globus syndrome, sick building syndrome, chronic pelvic pain, chronic whiplash syndrome, chronic Lyme disease, silicone breast implant effects, candidiasis, food allergies, Gulf War syndrome, mitral valve prolapse, hypoglycemia, chronic low back pain, dizziness, interstitial cystitis, tinnitus, pseudo seizures, and insomnia.[1697]

I believe these, and practically all other health problems, are manifestations of the simple principles of metabolism, E&I, thermodynamics, cell communication, and TOILing underlying all diseases. If doctors ignore the evidence pointing in that direction, they are likely to attribute the problems above and every other disease that they cannot explain by diagnosing and treating stress and depression with antidepressants.

The following is an incomplete listing of common ailments and their association to sweet death and metabolic issues:

- More infections in people with IR and high inflammation markers[1698]

- Abdominal obesity related to macular degeneration[1699]
- Obesity and underweight associated with infertility[1700]
- Obesity alters nocturnal blood pressure patterns[1701]
- High sugar in the blood associated with more clotting problems[1702]
- More deep venous thrombosis (DVT) is seen with "diabesity."[1703]
- Recurrent DVT risk higher in obesity[1704]
- The lower the GlycoHb, the fewer post arthroplasty complications.[1705]
- Periodontal disease is more prevalent in type 2 diabetes.[1706]
- Impaired fasting glucose boosts stroke risk[1707]
- Obese men have low-quality sperm.[1708]
- "Asthma and Obesity"[1709]
- Thyroid autoimmunity is associated with gestational diabetes.[1710]
- "Sleep-Disordered Breathing and Impaired Glucose Metabolism in Normal Weight and Overweight/Obese Individuals."[1711]
- "Sleep Apnea: A Proinflammatory Disorder that Coaggregates with Obesity."[1712]
- High-fat, high-sugar diets, and milk linked to acne: IR the common denominator"[1713]
- Type 2 diabetes increases risk of Parkinsonism[1714]
- A low-glycemic diet lowers insulin-resistance and improves acne.[1715]
- A low-glycemic diet has 30 percent more fiber than an average diet and substantially more polyunsaturated fats, both of which decrease androgen levels that worsen acne.[1716]
- "Obesity Brings Risk of Plethora of Skin Conditions."[1717]
- An increased stroke risk is seen in obese women.[1718]
- Pre-diabetics may have neuropathic problems, especially those with a bigger VAT.[1719]
- Growth hormone suppression is seen in children after a glucose load.[1720]
- "Metabolic Therapy for Early Treatment of Age-Related Macular Degeneration."[1721]

- A higher risk of cancer of the esophagus and stomach is seen with a high BMI.[1722]
- Resistin and adipokines in obesity associated with abdominal aorta aneurisms[1723]
- Sleep apnea is associated with diabetes.[1724]
- More colon and rectal cancer is found in the obese.[1725]
- IR worsens liver fibrosis in hepatitis C and fatty liver disease.[1726]
- Weight gain and waist circumference are risk factor for psoriasis.[1727]
- Metformin quells acne in Polycystic Ovarian Syndrome.[1728]
- More skin problems are seen in type 1 diabetics.[1729]
- Obesity and larger waist circumference increase the risk of psoriasis.[1730]
- "Psoriasis Independently Associated with Hyperleptinemia Contributing to Metabolic Syndrome." [1731]
- Ferritin and transferrin elevation (iron overload) is seen in metabolic syndrome.[1732]
- Obesity increases risk of Barrett's esophagus (severe reflux).[1733]
- More IR in HIV and . . .[1734]
- . . . more IR with HIV treatment.[1735]
- IR is associated with bone thinning in girls with anorexia nervosa.[1736]
- Poor glucose control, added to genetics, worsens cystic fibrosis.[1737]
- Obese men dilute PSA (marker of prostate cancer) value through higher plasma volumes.[1738]
- IR increases the risk of abortion after invitro fertilization.[1739]
- Overweight workers are at a higher risk for injuries on the job.[1740]
- Waist circumference, not BMI, is associated with pulmonary function.[1741]
- There is a link between obesity and headaches that is seen in children.[1742]
- Abnormal 2hrGTT is a risk factor for idiopathic axonal polyneuropathy.[1743]

- Green tea attenuates diabetic neuropathy in rats.[1744]
- A high-glycemic diet increases the risk of macular degeneration, light damage, and inflammation/oxidation of eye tissues.[1745]
- IR increases the risk of pancreatic cancer.[1746]
- Anemia in diabetes may signal kidney disease.[1747]
- Obesity and smoking increase the risk of psoriasis.[1748]
- IGT (Impaired Glucose Tolerance or Pre Diabetes) enhances liver cirrhosis.[1749]
- Seizures have been noted from reactive hypoglycemia.[1750]
- More skin rashes and allergies are seen in obese women.[1751]
- Impaired glucose autoregulation is associated with impaired lung function.[1752]
- Babies born to diabetic mothers have five times higher risks of heart defects than babies born to non-diabetic mothers.[1753]
- Reduced lung function is associated with IR.[1754]
- Acanthosis nigricans (skin rash around neck) and skin tags are associated with hyperinsulinemia.[1755] Up to 60 to 90 percent of children who develop diabetes have these issues. Acanthosis nigricans regresses when sugar is better controlled and insulin receptor antibodies disappear.[1756]
- More cataracts are seen with high-sugar diets.[1757]
- Refined sugars lead to acne.[1758]
- "Acne Vulgaris: A Disease of Western Civilization."[1759] It comes from processed food high in refined sugars and low in essential fatty acids and micronutrients. Acne is not seen in primitive societies eating the Paleolithic diet.
- Refined carbohydrates worsen asthma, sinus problems, and ear infections.[1760]
- Sugar weakens eyesight.[1761]
- Sugar increases risk of cavities.[1762]
- Sugar can make tendons more brittle.[1763]
- Sugar affects carbon dioxide production in premature babies.[1764]
- Sugar dehydrates newborns.[1765]

The "Dwindles"

When we get old, it seems like everything starts to sag southward and we just don't feel so good. Docs call this less-than-optimal consequence of aging "frailty." Some of them call this process "inflammaging,"[1766] which connotes increased TOILing as we age. I affectionately call it "the dwindles."

Anyone struggling with sweet death is likely to have a shorter life expectancy, especially when one has a genetic tendency to heart disease.[1767] IR and TOILing are the main reasons for the dwindles, or the kind of aging that increases your chances of ending up in a nursing home playing chess with some partner who insists on moving the pieces like checkers.[1768]

Does aging necessarily need to be so bad? No. Aging does not necessarily mean we will get the dwindles; we could be healthy until we cash in the chips. We should reasonably expect to die "with our boots on." (I hope they find me in some ditch, dead, with my running shoes on, or, better yet, I wouldn't mind dying in my nineties with a thirty-something-year-old or running away from her jealous boyfriend . . .)

Dr. J.F. Fries (what a name!) agrees; this poor doc was ridiculed in 1980 when he published an article saying that we could live longer if we ate well (avoided TOILing and IR).[1769] At the time conventional wisdom held that if people did just that, society would wind up spending more money because people would end up in expensive nursing homes. Approximately twenty years later, after meticulously following a group of old-timers who ate better than their peers, Dr. Fries showed less nursing home admissions and less money spent on health care overall. He called his follow-up study, "Compression of Morbidity."[1770] I would have called it, "I Told You So."

Because of dietary and public health advances and less stress in our lives, truly, the fifties are the new forties. At least that is what I keep telling myself . . .

Some people may say that it would be boring to live too long. They think we would have to create stimulating "virtual realities" to keep us entertained.[1771] In my opinion, this attitude reflects living in one's head instead of following one's heart. Being bored is a reflection of a life that cannot easily imagine anything beyond "bread and circus." Living from the heart, overcoming our egos, and living long lives to be of service to our fellowmen can keep us very well-entertained.

Part IV

Licking Sweet Death

Don't wait for a solution to your sweet death issues to come from the government, your spouse, your priest, or E.T. (yes, Drew Barrymore's partner in crime once upon a time). You must take the first step alone, unless you have special access to celestial spheres or light-beings more powerful than us mere mortals. Start by looking at the "man in the mirror" like the late Michael Jackson advised, and admit that you are a "sugara-holic." After that, others, especially your family members, may be able to help you overcome your addiction.

The best solutions to any problem are within us all. The best way to help the main victims of sweet death—our children—is for us to change first and become an example of good living to them.[1772]

Some folks may try to tell you that you should get used to wallowing in sweet death, since there is no solution for it, or for obesity, arguing that science has no answers for you.[1773] While this may be true for a minority of us, in my experience, most people willing to face their addictions to refined sugars may be helped. "Lifestyle *does* have long-term benefits."[1774]

Chapter 29

Fixing the Politics of Sweet Death

In the nineties, I found myself in India, Somalia, and Rwanda, working with medical non-governmental organizations trying to alleviate some of the medical problems those good people suffered in wars and economic deprivation. It was rather frustrating to give them pills to treat malaria when we knew darn well that they would get it back as soon as we left with our pills and bandages. Yet, we couldn't do anything about the stagnant waters and swamps where the mosquitoes carrying the malaria bug were breeding.

Still, we persevered and did what little we could with the resources we had.

Today, I see many kindhearted young people volunteer their time in places like Africa, Costa Rica, Haiti, Peru, and Bolivia—just like I did in my youth. They want to be part of the solution to the vexing problems developing nations are challenged with. After going around the block a few times, I wonder if "ambulance chasing"—running into these countries, laden with medicines, construction materials, seeds, and hygiene classes—is the best way to help. Either way, I'm sure they do help relieve a little bit of the suffering at those critical times.

In many ways, we are dealing with our own health care problems, particularly sweet death issues, in much the same way we treat their malaria with drugs and then go back home without having done anything about the mosquitoes.

I recommend that you read *The Secret History of the American Empire* by John Perkins. Believe it or not, people in those countries sometimes harbor resentment toward well-intended Americans. Many of them feel those Band-Aid solutions are part of the problem: they merely perpetuate the underlying problems in their societies. They may even pick up on certain feelings of superiority and condescension from some of the volunteers.[1775]

Awareness Rising?[1776]

Not everyone agrees that we have a problem with sweet death in the United States. A recent study by the CDC concluded that the percentage of children who are overweight or obese has remained stable since 1999. Some feel that focusing on children at risk of becoming obese adults neglects normal children and that research does not show that preventive efforts, such as fussing about their BMIs and talking about healthy foods, really help. They argue that such interventions have not been shown to be successful.

Fortunately, many people—including politicians like democrat Chris Dodd from Connecticut—are concerned enough to have introduced the Federal Obesity Prevention Act of 2008, which would create a federal interagency taskforce responsible for creating a strategy to address the epidemic of obesity. Most educators and parents do feel that there is enough data and research to justify an aggressive approach to save our children a lot more grief when they get older. As we have already seen, some of our obese kids suffer emotionally and mentally as much as a cancer patient does.

It won't be easy to turn the corner. Will you be part of the solution? You can easily start by being a good example.

Sweet Politics

As you may recall, we talked about the politics and economics of sweet death in chapter 6. I am sure you agree that we cannot lick our sweet deaths without addressing the corn subsidies; the incentives to process food; the stress and emotional issues that predispose our society to addictive behavior; our belief that only drugs constitute "mainstream care"; our disregard for simple solutions (like nutrition and prevention); our uninsured problems; our insurance companies pricing health care out of the range that most Americans can afford; and all the factors that make processed food so readily available and addictive.

Since I am not an expert in social or political reform, and I feel that I do not possess the talents necessary to singlehandedly bring change in those arenas, I leave others who would be more effective than me in finding potential solutions to these complex problems. *You* may be one of those people.

I will continue to do my thing through the Utah Medical Association, volunteering for the UMA's "Adopt A School Program," writing, lecturing, teaching, voting on who will become a doc in Utah, and bugging politicians and other people better positioned than me to bring about the changes we desperately need.

An Olive Branch

I have bashed Big Food and Big Pharma throughout this book. I don't believe doing so is particularly successful because it may antagonize them and make them more recalcitrant to change. After all, they are following the dictums of modern Darwinian capitalism and they are people, just like us, trying to make a buck

A better approach would be to help Big Pharma change: I am sure that some of them, deep in their heart of hearts, know their way of doing business is doomed. Surely they are reading in our business journals that in order to succeed in the markets of the future they need to focus on the triple bottom line: profits, social responsibility, and environmental responsibility.[1777] I could not say what I feel about Big Pharma and Big Food better than John Perkins, the author of "The Secret History of the American Empire" agrees:

> "We must insist that corporations become democratic and transparent. No longer will we accept imperialistic capitalism, where a very few rich men make all the decisions and most of the money and do so largely in secret. We will de-

mand that they abide by those principles we hold to be self-evident, as stated in our most sacred documents, principles of justice, equality, compassion, and governance with an eye toward providing peace and stability for future generations . . . and they must protect the communities and environments where all these people live."[1778]

Sweet Jobs

Our kids' schools are not going to solve our society's sweet death by themselves. Neither are our employers. They cannot be expected to do what we must do ourselves (remember Virchow vs. Bismarck?). Hopefully, our employments are not part of the problem.

It is not my field of expertise to work on employment issues. However, it seems obvious to me that we could educate employers and managers so that we may at least quit having doughnuts all over the place. I bet that where you work everyone is always bringing in junk like that and that there is a vending machine to assuage your work-related anxiety with a little sugar fix. I am sure I am going to upset a lot of the wonderful nurses who might be reading this book. But be honest: don't you agree that our nurse stations, both in clinics and in hospitals, are often generously sprinkled with junk food?

In today's Darwinian capitalism, businesses are aiming to perform at the speed of light. Companies are expanding very rapidly, which has been shown to create significant health problems in their personnel.[1779] The successful companies of the future will take better care of their workers:

"Solutions? Value people over profits? Recognize human capital as paramount? Depressed and anxious personnel are unlikely to be productive and absence from work costs employers and society money. The re-engineering of work ought to perpetuate fulfillment and productivity, not illness and disability."[1780]

It is becoming quite obvious that overweight employees suffering with sweet death are not going to perform as well. Besides, they are more prone to injury and to disabilities.[1781] The journal Business Weekly has reported that:

> "The notion that the financial health and competitiveness of a business depends on the health and well-being of its employees is gaining acceptance . . . The [United States] economy cannot remain competitive in the global marketplace if we don't take better care of our workforce's physical and mental well being . . . When people feel strong and resilient, physically, mentally, emotionally, and spiritually, they perform better, with more passion, for longer. They win, their families win, and the corporations that employ them win."[1782]

General Motors had to increase the price of its cars by $1,600 to cover health care insurance premiums for its employees. This is why, in view of mounting premiums, many employers and corporations are dropping health insurance coverage and even reneging on pension plans covering health insurance for their retirees. How odd is it that industries and corporations have to be reminded on a constant basis that their most important assets and tools are their employees?

Calvin Coolidge, and more famously George W. Bush have told us that, "The business of America is business." Such a myopic view will continue to sink our country into a morass of social and health problems that will contribute to losing our country's place at the top of the world's economies. Societies that understand the implications of this quote are quickly moving to the top of the heap, not only economically, but also in the parameters that monitor health in their citizens. The Romans warned us that neglecting their ancient wisdom would bring chaotic results: "Salus populi suprema lex,"[1783] not business.

For each dollar invested in preventive issues, employers may save $3 to $5. Now, why couldn't the health care system work on the same principles? Because each HMO is afraid that you will leave their system after they have spent money on you to help you with lifestyle and preventive issues. The benefits from all the money they spent on you would be accrued by the next HMO you end up with.

These are some of the reasons why an employer-based health insurance program is bound to fail. The rub is that the present system of multiple insurance companies is going to fight very hard to maintain the status quo. It has been shown that consolidating insurers may cut down on overhead from 15 percent down to 2 percent.[1784] American employers and our industries are at a disadvantage as they struggle to compete with countries that do not burden their employers with the responsibility of financing their citizens' health care coverage. Often, employers end up dismissing more employees who end up butt-naked out there with no health coverage.

Forced to Be Fit[1785]

The entire section is based on a presumably well-researched article published in the Salt Lake Tribune.

Several companies have begun charging employees if they don't shape up, but critics are saying these employers are turning the health care system into a police state. Many companies, citing growing medical costs tied to obesity, are offering fit workers lucrative incentives that shave thousands of dollars a year off health care premiums. An Indiana-based hospital chain will charge employees up to $30 every two weeks unless they meet weight, cholesterol, and blood pressure guidelines the company deems to be healthy.

UnitedHealthcare insurance introduced a new plan where a typical family's yearly deductible may be reduced from $1,000 to $5,000 if an employee isn't obese and doesn't smoke. A similar plan was offered to county workers in Arkansas. The county's benefits administrator said the plan had seen about a 30 percent drop in claims and significant changes in the workplace, thanks to weight reduction classes and competitions between departments to see which department is "the biggest loser." "When we have birthday parties now, people don't want sugar-laced cake and candy; they want fruit and deli trays." The results? The county didn't have to raise its insurance premiums the last two years.

Sixty-two percent of 135 executives responding to a survey in 2008 said that unhealthy workers, such as those who smoke or those who are obese, should pay higher benefit costs—compared to 48 percent of executives in 2005. This is likely due to the explosive rise of health care premiums that are growing twice as fast as the rate of inflation.

In January 2007, the United States Department of Labor released final clarifications of the Health Insurance Portability Act of 1996 that ruled that employers may use financial incentives in wellness programs to motivate workers to get healthy. Still, critics of these measures feel that these programs are infringing on employees' civil liberties, especially when the obese are already being paid $1.20 less per hour than slim workers.

"It's reprehensible to punish and emasculate someone for having a disease, like obesity. Anyone who penalizes workers for being overweight should brace themselves for a backlash," said the director of the Obesity Law and Advocacy Center in Chula Vista, California.

The president of the National Workrights Institute in Princeton, NJ, agrees. "[This is a] very dangerous road that could lead to employers controlling everything we do in our private lives. To penalize for things that are beyond some people's control is just wrong. Some people are fat because that is how God made them," said.

"This is a fight that is likely going to be dealt with in the courts," said a principal in a famous health law firm. Indeed. But, this is what we get when we insist on an employer-based health care system. In my opinion, these are the complications we see when we choose the wrong system. Isn't it the American way to give power and control to whoever signs the check? If we go to single-payer system run by the government, we will likely see similar demands to punish or motivate beneficiaries. It is the same can of worms we get into with tobacco-related diseases or insurance coverage for drivers with a history of drunken driving.

The fact that Alabama has already started to penalize state employees who are overweight is a sign that civil liberty issues will likely give way to health issues. The state has given its 32,527 employees a year to start getting fit or they will have to pay $25 a month for insurance that otherwise is free. Alabama already charges workers who smoke and will do so to those who do not get routine health screenings starting in 2010.

It's going to be fun in the courts. I predict the lawyers will win.

A Game as Old as Empire[1786]

A Game as Old as Empire, by Steven Hiatt and John Perkins, is a book on an alternative view of America's dealings with countries that are not as strong economically. Don't read it if you feel there is nothing wrong with our way of doing business.

In my opinion, understanding the economics and politics running our markets, including food and agriculture, may help us lick sweet death in our own country. I feel special interests have created the conditions that lead to sweet death. Applying the same business solutions that developing countries need to lift themselves out of poverty may help us save our children at home. To only deal with sweet death in clinics—without addressing the politics/economics causing the problems—is the same as leaving the swamps not drained and the mosquitoes untreated.

The Debate Over Subsidizing Snacks

THE DEBATE OVER SUBSIDIZING SNACKS was the title of a newspaper article that filled me with hope. It came out on July 4, 2007. I was home with the flu, watching the History Channel's ten-hour summary of the Revolutionary War while also finishing reading *Founding Brothers,* a Pulitzer Prize-winning book by Joseph Ellis.[1787] I got out of bed only to buy the *New York Times* and get a cup of coffee. Reading it was, for me, some of the best "fireworks" I have enjoyed since immigrating to the United States as a sixteen-year-old boy. I want you to enjoy it as much as I did; here are the bullet points:

- Every five years, the farm bill that has perpetuated subsidies to farmers growing corn, wheat, soy, rice, and cotton comes up for renewal. Only farmers and their lobbyists have been paying attention in the past. This year is different.

- The Bush administration, the American Heart Association, Environmental Defense, Taxpayers for Common

Sense, and GMA/FPA (food industry association) are teaming up to make changes in the farm bill, arguing that the subsidies are behind the growing epidemic of obesity, the increase in food poisoning, and the disappearance of the family farm.

- "This is not a farm bill. It's a food bill, and Americans who eat want a stake in it." (Senator Tom Harkin, D-Iowa; chairman agriculture committee.)

- The lack of subsidies for fruits and vegetables has made these preferred foods more expensive than the snacks made from subsidized crops. Between 1985 and 2000, the cost of fruits and vegetables has gone up by 40 percent while the cost of soda pop went up by 25 percent.

- Some of the bills before Congress are aimed at helping growers of fruits and vegetables, especially those who produce locally. The development of more farmers' markets and local processing plants should be encouraged to compete with far-away producers. There are lots of advantages on energy consumption, too.

- Grants may be given to minority and immigrant farmers to start new local farms, including organic farms. Preservation programs will be financed, too, as well as renewable energy sources. Those farmers who are already doing these things would be rewarded.

- Those farmers who get paid $5.2 billion to grow nothing ("fixed direct payments") would be eliminated. Even dead farmers are still getting this money. Why did we ever start such a program? Too much food being produced? Sure, but that was a result of government policies that encouraged corporate farming, which is energy-intensive and relies heavily on pesticides. The result was the decimation of family farming.

- According to the Environmental Working Group, one giant cotton farm collected $2.95 million through crop subsidies in 2005. Former President George W. advocated eliminating subsidies to any farmer making more than $200,000 a year. Some folks in Congress have proposed eliminating subsidies altogether.

Failing Programs

I am often invited to hear well-intended teachers, parents, businessmen, concerned citizens, and government workers discuss new programs to curve our children's sweet death, or epidemic of obesity and diabetes. Generally they aim at teaching kids about physical activity, vegetables, and taking junk food out of our schools. These are good issues to discuss, but I am afraid they don't strike at the root of the problem.

Invariably, my opinions on what needs to be done are dismissed as too radical. Yet, I plan to continue saying that we will never solve the problem until we work on the politics and economics driving the marketing, consumption, and the addicting nature of junk food. I think that it is naïve to ignore these issues by claiming that we must not confront the "powers that be." Any approach that leaves out these harsh realities is likely to be based on the participants trying to feel good about doing something.

People who want to see some changes often concentrate only on nutrition and exercise programs and campaigns to change our kids' eating habits. I am not saying these efforts are worthless. Nevertheless, we now have good evidence that this approach is not working. After the federal government's $1 million worth of school programs on nutrition education, the Associated Press documented that fifty-seven such programs have yielded mostly failure.

For example, one of the programs offered free fresh fruits and vegetables. But, at the end of the program, kids were "eating less of them than they had at the start." In Pennsylvania, researchers gave out awards to kids who ate more fruits and vegetables, "but when they came back seven months later, the kids had reverted to their original eating habits: soda and chips." The studies that recorded the kids' self-assessment that they were eating better found "no changes in blood pressure, body size, or cholesterol levels; they want to eat better; they might even think they are, but they are not."

Not surprisingly, the Associated Press study listed three of the many reasons that have already been discussed in this book to explain why these programs are not working. One, parents have the most say and often they, themselves, are addicted to junk food. Two, the advertisement from Big Food is too much to over-come. And three, low incomes force families to eat the cheapest and most convenient foods available. Sadly, the Associated Press study still did not propose that we address the politics and eco-nomics fueling our sweet deaths. Instead, they wonder if the an-swer might be to take our fat kids to special clinics where their obesity is managed aggressively.[1788] That won't work, either.

A study in the Netherlands reported that preventing obesity and smoking can save lives, but it doesn't save money, because sicker people die sooner, thus saving the system more money.[1789] In my opinion, this study did not consider issues like more pro-ductivity from people who are healthier. Remember Dr. Fries' work?

School Report

My home state (Utah) got an "F" in 2006 from the Center for the Public Interest for allowing so much junk food to be sold in school vending machines. Embarasing reports like this one have recently motivated, schools throughout the United States to cut down on some of the factors that lead to sweet death in our chil-dren. They understand they have lost track of what it means to be healthy; they have to correct this problem and teach kids to eat better.

Responding to the crisis, the Office of Education came up with recommendations such as banning foods with minimal nu-tritional value, selling only foods with no more than 250 calories and 35 percent fat, or selling those with no more than 10 percent of total calories from fat and 20 grams of carbohydrates. Also, the Office of Education wants to ban cheese, yogurt, fruit, and any drink with more than 300 calories per package. Drinks also are to be smaller than 12 ounces. These recommendations are under-standably the result of a genuine desire to do something about sweet death.

But I feel the Office of Education is misguided. In my opin-ion, kids will buy multiple servings until their sugar addictions are taken care of. Unless we address their addictions to sugar, no interventions will help.

"Bee" Part of the Solution

According to the New York Times, Mary Kay Thatcher, a policy specialist with the largest lobbying group for farmers, thinks that "it is highly unlikely that we will see huge changes [in sweet death]." However, Gus Schumacher, Jr., a former under secretary of agriculture under former president George W. Bush feels that:

> "Congress and the administration have a unique opportunity to begin reforms providing a sustainable, community-linked food system . . . Will they take this opportunity to start or will it be business as usual?"[1790]

I hope Thatcher is wrong and Schumacher is right; our politicians must muster the courage to do what is right for our children. But, after making so much political noise, I need to reiterate my belief that the main changes must start within us, not without. Conventional group psychology maintains that:

> "Crowds tend to be wise only if individual members act responsibly and make their own decisions. A group won't be smart if its members follow fads, or wait for someone to tell them what to do . . . A honeybee never sees the big picture any more than you do . . . if you are looking for a role model in a world of complexity, you could do worse than to imitate a bee."[1791]

Chapter 30

Licking Sweet Death with Drugs

The health care system is focusing mostly on the consequences of sweet death, that is, diabetes and its devastating effects. Millions of dollars are so spent, but very little is being done to prevent sweet death itself.[1792] In the past six years, the money spent on drugs for diabetes has doubled—a result of more diabetics and more expensive new drugs.[1793]

Fortunately, docs are waking up from the pharmaceutical hangover of the last few decades. A landmark article appeared in the *Journal of the American Medical Association*, titled, "Promoting More Conservative Prescribing."[1794]

> "Given the well-documented prevalence of medication-related harm and inappropriate prescribing, such educational reform is necessary but not sufficient to ensure that patients are optimally treated . . . trainees need guiding principles to inform their thinking about pharmacotherapy to help them become more careful, cautious, evidence-based prescribers."

The article goes on to say that docs would do well to focus more on the roots of diseases, rather than the symptomatic treatment with pharmaceutical drugs.

The answer to sweet death lies within us. Changing our lifestyles is the key.[1795] Before we do that, we must explore the "standard of care," which is nearly 100 percent pharmaceutical. Sometimes we have no choice but to use drugs to help patients. The fact that only one-half of them take the drugs prescribed may be a passive way for patients to show their dissatisfaction with the pharmaceutical approach.[1796] Said treatment is highly organized and mapped out for better results,[1797] but as helpful as it is in many cases, it is fraught with side effects and misinformation about nutrition.

Hamsters on a Treadmill

Most docs are aware of metabolic issues in their patients, but they often refer them to a dietitian for instructions on how they should eat. In my opinion, punting like that quickly conveys the lack of urgency and importance that docs put on nutrition issues. Still, we would do better if we did not automatically place all the blame on docs for this state of affairs. My poor colleagues are simply too busy. I will never forget a medical meeting where doctors complained they didn't have the time to get their "normal" patients to take the 2hGTT because they were too busy caring for the patients who already had diabetes.

Consider what the article, "Improving Primary Care for Patients with Chronic Illness,"[1798] had to say:

> "Chronic disease care programs save money, reduce hospital admissions . . . This results in fewer Medicare dollars, so they are abandoned . . . Hospitals have no incentives to reward physicians for cost-saving chronic care improvement . . . Visionary clinical leaders are needed for chronic care improvements and the financial environments must either help them or at least not hinder them . . . Physicians who are working faster and faster like hamsters on a treadmill do not have time to improve chronic care . . . Delivery systems must be redesigned to rescue physicians from the hamster syndrome . . . Some physicians have an overly positive view of the quality of their chronic illness care and do not see the need to change practice systems."

Some docs get a little too close to Big Pharma to promote its agenda. Of course, most docs do legitimate research on drugs, but some merely get kickbacks for prescribing these drugs. This practice is a significant enough problem for the states of Maine, Vermont, and Minnesota to have enacted laws to have docs report the money they get from Big Pharma. Iowa Senator Chuck Grassley has introduced a bill in Congress to have the same laws apply nationwide.[1799]

Let us now look at the pills you could end up getting from your doc . . .

Fat Pills

It makes perfect sense for our busy docs to quickly reach for their prescription pads; the fast draw only takes a few seconds. Besides, most patients get inpatient with their docs after five minutes into the interview because they already know what they want: the drug they saw on a TV commercial.

Most patients are not ready to change their lifestyles; they are perfectly willing to rely on a drug that will allow them to continue living the way they have grown accustomed to. Big Pharma knows this. It has done its homework and it merely provides "a service" to the vast majority of Americans. Many patients' sweet deaths are too advanced to reverse them without drugs.

Before we develop diabetes and need a drug for that, most people struggle with their weight. They would love to find a drug to help them lose the rings around their waists. But, in my opinion, these type of drugs are not worth the side effects and it is unknown if they decrease the morbidity and mortality associated with obesity.[1800] In other words, you may lose some weight, but you will still suffer sweet death because these drugs do nothing for IR.

For example, sibutramine helps teens lose weight, but it increases their heart rates.[1801] Xenical has significant absorption problems, which is why patients prescribed this drug are advised to supplement vitamins.

In June 2007, Alli/orlistat was launched as an over-the-counter drug with a $150 million ad campaign. Too bad that one-half of patients have side effects, like diarrhea, that may be mitigated a bit if you eat less than 15 grams of fat a day. Well, why don't we start there in the first place? It sounds just like the drug, Antabuse, which one takes before drinking to assure the patient of a nasty reaction if he or she falls off the wagon. If you decide to take Alli anyway, carry a cork around with you . . .

In my opinion, taking any drug to enable you to continue with your addiction to refined sugars and saturated animal fat is not a wise approach. Yet, I understand the desperation that leads to this type of behavior; I see it in alcoholics, too.

Pushing Sweet Pills

The dismal track record our health care system has in treating metabolic syndrome is compounded by some of the drugs that are used to treat diabetes. Metformin/glucophage may cause a B12 deficiency.[1802] Remember that B complex deficiency compromises the liver's detoxification function (methylation), DNA copying, and the production of neurotransmitters. All other oral drugs for diabetes cause weight gain, except for metformin, which may be used in obese children[1803] and those who need to lose weight.[1804]

Metformin's relative safety may be due to the fact that it is a derivative of Galega officinalis, an herb used in Europe for centuries to treat diabetes,[1805] a fact that Big Pharma chooses not to advertise. We wouldn't want Joe Blow to know that metformin came from an herb because "herbs are not supposed to be any good."[1806] In chapter 32, you will see that this is not true.

Metformin, while helpful in preventing diabetes,[1807] is not as effective as lifestyle modifications in the prevention of diabetes from early pre-diabetes or IGT.[1808] When metformin is combined with sulfonylurea drugs (Glucotrol, DiaBeta, etc.), they increase the risk of heart problems. Metformin alone does not do that.[1809] Sulfur-based drugs have the annoying problem of losing their effectiveness after patients have been on them for a while.

Still, metformin and the second generation of these sulfonylurea drugs appear to be as safe and effective as the newer, more expensive and more questionable drugs like the PPAR drugs rosiglitazone/avandia and pioglitazone/actos;[1810] they reduce cell membrane IR by working on receptors on the cell and mitochondrial membranes.[1811] They also work on serum cholesterol,

339

the endothelium, and blood pressure.[1812] These drugs work the same way essential fatty acids do;[1813] this is why they are now discussed as valid treatment to prevent diabetes in people with IR or IGT.[1814] Rosiglitazone/avandia reduces the risk of diabetes by 62 percent.[1815] PPAR drugs appear to be more effective and more active for longer periods of treatment than other available drugs, such as metformin and glyburide.[1816] Too bad PPAR drugs are synthetic enough to cause side effects like weight gain, congestive heart failure, heart attacks, and water retention. In fact, rosiglitazone is no longer recommended:[1817] it has more of these risks than pioglitazone does.[1818] Other than that, these drugs are pretty safe . . .

The risk of heart attacks increases by 50 percent with rosiglitazone, a fact that, although hotly contested by Big Pharma, was known to some researchers before the drug was marketed in 1999. Out of about four thousand patients, approximately forty of them were shown to have heart attacks back then.[1819] Dr. John B. Buse, a leading endocrinologist and researcher, claims he was harassed and called names by Big Pharma executives when he objected to the soft-pedaling of the data showing the serious nature of the side effects of these drugs before they were released to the public. Big Pharma even threatened to sue him, arguing that his "attitude" would seriously undermine its profits.[1820]

After the report came out in the *New England Journal of Medicine* implicating rosiglitazone with heart attacks, the incidence of cardiac problems tripled, once docs started paying more attention to this drug's side effects.[1821] Because of all these problems, an FDA committee felt that rosiglitazone should not be used in patients with heart disease and those taking insulin.[1822] But, after further deliberations, the FDA finally decided to go against its own advisory committee's recommendations and settled for only a black box warning.

Newer types of drugs, like sitagliptin, seem to be working okay, so far. It is a dipeptidyl peptidase-4 enzyme inhibitor in the pancreas that reduces the hormone glucagon and increases insulin production.[1823] As an old doc, I am going to wait a while before I rush to prescribe sitagliptin. Who knows what side effects will be discovered after they go around the block a few times?

Another new drug is exenatide/byetta, which works on our

cells-signaling network. It has been shown to trigger pancreatit-is.[1824] Because it's given via an injection, I have not been too keen on prescribing it to my patients. I suppose these new drugs are fine when diabetes is hard to control. Even using malaria pills (hydroxychloroquine) may be needed if nothing is working for diabetes.[1825]

Big Pharma is now very interested in "new diabetic drugs [to] target gut hormones."[1826] Incretins are gut hormones secreted when we eat sugar. Another hormone, glucagon-like peptide 1 (GLP-1), will help diabetics lose weight, too.[1827] These drugs are going to focus on our VATs and the connection to our fat thermostats. Let us be patient and keep an open mind. Because of the many instances we have gotten burned by new and improved diabetic drugs, the FDA is raising the bar on the requirements and assurances of safety before the newer drugs in the pipeline are turned loose on the market.[1828]

Pills for Other Metabolic Issues

Simvastatin used to treat high cholesterol may reduce the risk of heart attacks, but it increases IR. Fortunately, adding vitamin A and CoQ10 prevents this problem and potentiates the cholesterol-lowering effect of the drug.[1829] Those two supplements heal the TOILing cell membranes, particularly oxidation and mitochondrial dysfunction.[1830] As we saw above in the article, "Are Lipid-Lowering Guidelines Evidence-Based?"[1831], these drugs are not what they are advertised to be. It turns out that total mortality is not reduced by statins, according to pooled data from eight randomized trials. These drugs are especially less effective in women.[1832] Too bad that most people have forgotten that fermented red rice (monascus purpureus) from which Big Pharma got the statin drugs lowers cholesterol just as well.[1833]

Fenofibrate binds cholesterol in the intestines so that it is not absorbed as much. Interestingly, this drug also reduces the oxidation and inflammation seen in the metabolic syndrome.[1834] The bile acid sequestrant-cholesterol-lowering drug, colesevelam, also helps diabetics control their blood sugars by blocking intestinal absorption.[1835] Many drugs that have been helpful in treating metabolic problems turn out to have IR-lowering effects to explain their action. For example, drugs to treat high blood pressure, like valsartan, decrease toxic glycoxidation.[1836] Carvedilol/coreg, a drug to slow down the heart, has also been shown to decrease IR.[1837]

Amlodipine (a calcium channel blocker) plus perindopril (an ACE inhibitor) reduce IR, thereby cutting the risk of new onset of diabetes by one third. The herb hibiscus sabdariffa works better that the ACE type of drugs in lowering high blood pressure and with no side effects.[1838] ACE inhibitors to lower blood pressure like lisinopril are also used to delay diabetic problems in the kidneys.[1839]

The fact that telmisartan, an ARB type of drug that also works in the kidneys to treat high blood pressure, "shows an equivalent effect of vitamin C in further improving endothelial dysfunction"[1840] points to TOILing as the underlying mechanism of blood pressure elevation. The same may be said of the new drug for angina, Ranolazine: it lowers the GlycoHb A1c.[1841] Other drugs for the metabolic syndrome, like atenolol, a beta blocker, plus thiazide diuretics do not show the same benefits.[1842]

Etanercept, for arthritis, lowers inflammation and the CRP. Not surprisingly, it also improves the markers for the metabolic syndrome because it reduces TOILing.[1843] Arthritis and heart disease are very much linked[1844] like all diseases are.

On the other side of the ledger, several drugs seem to elevate blood sugar. The water pill hydrocholothiazide (for blood pressure), the antibiotic ciprofloxacin, and the antidepressant lexapro have been shown to do so. While taking cipro, patients' sugar levels rise 112-fold in diabetics and ten-fold in non-diabetics.[1845] Perhaps the sugar goes up because of the fluoride inserted into the fluoroquinolone family of antibiotics like cipro.

The Cure May be Worse than the Disease [1846]

It is common knowledge that drugs have significant side effects that often may be quite problematic. Dr. Steven Nissen from the Cleveland Clinic has become a controversial crusader for drug safety. He was the main doc who alerted us to the problems with Vioxx® and Avandia.

"Compounding" the potential problems of pharmaceuticals

is the "bitter pill" that a significant number of drugs sold in pharmacies are counterfeits from countries like Colombia, India, and China. Drugs to treat the metabolic syndrome like Viagra, Lipitor, Plavix, and Norvasc are particularly vulnerable to counterfeiting. Besides missing the active compound, these drugs may be even more harmful because of the toxins used to make them: lead paint, drywall fabric, and road-paving materials.

Many reports are emerging about people being harmed, and even dying, by taking these fake drugs. United States drug enforcement officials are already expecting fake Tamiflu to treat bird flu to flood our country. But that little problem may pale to the possibility that terrorists may use these bitter pills to harm Americans.[1847] Worrying about fake Viagra ruining your hot date is the least of your problems; if your date is taking fake birth control pills, you'll soon have some real problems.

Problems with drugs don't stop there: read the main points in the article, "Hidden Disruptions in Metabolic Syndrome: Drug Induced Nutrient Depletion as a Pathway to Accelerated Pathophysiology of Metabolic Syndrome":[1848]

- Magnesium is lost with diuretics/water pills, which worsens atherosclerosis, hypertension, strokes, and heart attacks. A lack of magnesium contributes to muscle cramps, nervousness, insomnia, IR, depression, fatigue, abnormal heartbeats, migraines, constipation, bone thinning, and kidney stones.

- The antioxidant CoQ10 is depleted with statin drugs to lower cholesterol, diuretics, beta-blockers, and second-generation sulfonylureas for diabetics. Statins may decrease CoQ10 as much as 54 percent. COQ10 is needed in the mitochondria of cells to produce energy. A reduced amount may result in heart muscle problems, high blood pressure, angina, strokes, fatigue, abnormal heart beats, gingivitis, mitral valve prolapse, IR, leg weakness, and decline in immune and cognitive functions.[1849]

    CoQ10 in reduced amounts may increase the risk of Alzheimer's disease by reducing IR. Excess insulin in the brain increases the formation of inflammatory plaques called beta amyloid. In other words, CoQ10 sensitizes cell membranes to receive insulin more efficiently.[1850] Consuming 225 milligrams of CoQ10 helped 51 percent of patients get off 103 medications for high blood pressure within six months.[1851]

- Zinc is reduced with water pills. This may trigger loss of taste and smell, poor wound healing, anorexia, immune problems, depression, photophobia, night blindness, skin/hair/nails problems, joint pain, alterations in hormones, kidney disease, celiac, malignant melanoma, macular degeneration, prostate problems, and IR.

- B complex vitamins are depleted by acid blocking drugs, antibiotics, metformin, and hormonal replacements, including birth control pills and water pills. Low levels of B complex vitamins raise the levels of homocysteine, a toxin associated with practically all diseases. It also increases the risk of cancer, IR, heart disease,[1852] depression, abnormal pap smears, anemia, fatigue, and birth defects.

- Melatonin levels are decreased by beta blockers used for high blood pressure, which increases the risk of IR, insomnia, inflammation, and cancer.

The bottom line is that "medications are not as effective as lifestyle changes and it is not known if treatment with these drugs is cost-effective in the management of impaired glucose tolerance."[1853] Many now feel that "the pharmaceutical revolution of the fifties and sixties has petered out."[1854]

Insulin Treatment

Type 1 diabetics cannot produce their own insulin in the pancreas. This means that it is very unlikely that they will ever stop needing to inject it. Inhaled insulin was discontinued because of problems with lung inflammation. Transplanting pancreatic cells is another possibility, but sometimes the host rejects these beta cells that produce insulin. In those cases, administration of seaweed and iron capsules has been shown to increase the chances of the transplanted cells being accepted.[1855]

Often, insulin administration leads to blood sugar dropping too low. Most people are told to eat candy, which is hard to fault in life-threatening situations. The prevention of hypoglycemia (when one uses insulin) with the sugar-elevating hormone glucagon holds promise in these cases.[1856]

There are cases where patients may have been misdiagnosed as type 1 diabetics; they may end up taking insulin like some type 2 patients do because of poor control. These are the patients who may be able to get off insulin, or at least reduce the amount they need. **Never try to stop taking insulin on your own.**

Trimming the Fat

Gastric bypass surgery is recommended for the morbidly obese. Before we rush into it, it would be wise to try less aggressive treatments, or at least improve the surgery techniques. As it is now, 2 percent of people die within the first thirty days after surgery, 2.8 percent within ninety days, 4.6 percent within the first year[1857] and 40 percent of people have complications.[1858] Still, these surgeries have been shown to reduce overall mortality.[1859] Gastric banding also has been shown to help control type 2 diabetes.[1860]

In my experience, most patients who have this surgery end up regaining their weight. (Think of Al Roker, the weatherman on the *Today* show.) Could it be that these patients don't learn to face and overcome their addictions to sugar? Changing our lifestyles trumps gastric bypass surgery in the long run.[1861] Many of the patients who undergo this surgery find new addictions, like gambling, compulsory shopping, alcoholism, and smoking. Some of them even "outfox the procedure by taking in calories in liquid form."[1862]

Sweet death is becoming such a problem that now these surgeries are being recommended for children[1863] and teenagers; it helps reduce their chances of developing diabetes.[1864]

Liposuction does not correct patients' underlying metabolic problems; patients who undergo this procedure do not reverse their IR. Neither do the patients who undergo gastric bypass.[1865]

I understand the mental turmoil that morbid obesity brings. I don't blame patients for trying whatever they can find to mitigate the effects of their sweet deaths. But, as professionals, I feel it is our duty to help them understand that these are often nothing more than cosmetic Band-Aids. To sell them these procedures as a final cure-all is not in their best interest. Any of these fat-trimming procedures is bound to fail if their addictions to sugar are not honestly addressed.

Prevention? Follow the Money

As crude as it may sound, allowing docs to share the money saved by Medicare has been shown to be successful: the more docs emphasize prevention, nutrition, and lifestyle changes to their patients, the more money docs may make.[1866] Someone please tell me why this is not the case in Utah . . .

Trying to pass for prevention, recently a panel of experts rounded up by the FDA proclaimed that cholesterol levels should be much lower in diabetics. This is likely true, but the fact that most of the panel members were taking payments from Big Pharma raised some eyebrows. The panel argued that diabetes presents a greater risk for coronary disease; consequently, statin drugs should be used more aggressively in these patients, despite the evidence that statin drugs to lower cholesterol do not alter the progression of TOILing of the lining of the arteries (intima media thickness) in diabetics.[1867]

In other words, their endothelium, or lining of the arteries, does not improve with these drugs. You know why not: cholesterol is not the problem. It is oxidized cholesterol due to IR and TOILing in the liver where we process cholesterol.[1868]

Lionizing True Prevention

The Lyon Diet Heart Study showed fewer heart attacks, high blood pressure, strokes, and angina in people eating the Mediterranean diet compared to the American Diet—despite both groups having the same blood pressure, weight, and LDL cholesterol of 160. The Mediterranean diet, having more antioxidants than the SAD diet, showed a "70 percent reduction in all-cause mortality and non-fatal sequelae."

> . . . At a time when health professionals, the pharma-
> ceutical industries, and the research funding and regulatory
> agencies are almost totally focused on lowering plasma cho-
> lesterol levels with drugs, it is heartening to see a well con-
> ducted study finding that relatively simple dietary changes
> achieved greater reductions in risk of all-cause and coronary
> disease mortality than any of the cholesterol-lowering stud-
> ies to date . . . [This] unprecedented reduction in risk for cor-
> onary heart disease was not associated with differences in
> total cholesterol levels between the control and experimental
> groups." [1869]

This "unprecedented reduction in risk for coronary heart
disease was not associated with differences in total cholesterol
levels." Remember that both groups had an LDL of 160, a much
higher number than the LDL of 70 recommended by the panel of
experts. Yet, did Big Pharma look at this evidence? For that matter, did Big Pharma look at the article that showed that we lower
cholesterol better with a low-glycemic diet instead of a low-fat
diet?[1870]

Better Approach: Nutrition

We have already talked about the polymeal and how a low-
glycemic, Mediterranean diet is better than the polypill, or the
lumping of several drugs together to treat metabolic problems.
It turns out that "the preventive polypill [is] much promise [but
with] insufficient evidence"[1871] while forty-three studies on the
Mediterranean diet have shown how well it works[1872] through
its main mechanism of action: reducing inflammation or TOIL-
ing.[1873] The Mediterranean diet "has the most desirable attributes,
including a lower content of refined carbohydrates, a high content of fiber, a moderate content of fat (mostly unsaturated), and
a moderate-to-high content of vegetable proteins."[1874]

Chapter 31

Food is the Best Medicine

Ilove to read history books. It is remarkable how we continue to repeat the same mistakes our forefathers made and fail to learn from the good things our beloved departed ones had done. For example, before we had insulin and oral drugs to treat diabetes, many people were able to control their sweet deaths with diet alone.[1875] But, low-tech treatments are often ignored when there are huge profits to be made by marketing the latest and greatest treatments. While the latter bring relief in many cases, the rejection of simple and efficacious modalities is based on profits—not efficacy or safety. I am not saying that we should do without insulin, but that we don't need to reject diet as the cornerstone of treatment.

It turns out that lifestyle changes and good diets are just as effective as pharmaceutical methods in preventing the progression from pre-diabetes (impaired glucose tolerance) to full-blown diabetes.[1876] Lifestyle changes are also the key to treating every facet of the metabolic syndrome.[1877] It is imperative to reinforce these changes by continual social support to avoid regaining the weight by falling off the wagon, especially in children.[1878] The best approach to sweet death is prevention.[1879] It is not easy, but a steady and realistic commitment to changing our lifestyles and overcoming our sugar addictions can help us escape sweet death and thereby dodge the diabetic bullet.[1880]

There is considerable evidence that a diet low in refined carbohydrates is best for our metabolisms.[1881] In a major shift from old, entrenched dogma, the American Diabetes Association is now recommending "either a low-carb or a low-fat diet" for pre-diabetes.[1882]

Even though pharmaceutical agents have been mapped out in detail to manage patients, endocrinologists are now of the opinion that it is best to individualize treatment and emphasize lifestyle changes and prevention while avoiding "cookbook approaches."[1883] Some doctors now refer to sweet death as "diabesity"; they propose a color-coded approach to nutrients to teach patients which foods to emphasize in their lives.[1884] But for this preventive approach to work, it needs to be drummed up by docs at each visit and be discussed face-to-face with the patient instead of punting the idea over to a dietitian.[1885]

People need to become aware how stressful lifestyles are contributing to IR and they need to be empowered to choose their meals after good education from the medical community.[1886] Public health and environmental policies are needed to clean up our environment and reign in Big Food and its brainwashing of Americans. What we do in these areas in the next few years will determine whether our country can get out of this spiraling sweet death. These problems will get worse before they get better. Our health care systems will continue to be overwhelmed by the burden of hyperinsulinemia. With the economic events of the summer of 2008, it is likely that true health care reform will yield to insurance reform. But we can make noise and demand change in our communities. The critical step to initiate any change:

> "Will be active engagement of policy makers and the reimbursement systems, which share responsibility for putting into place the necessary incentives for identification and treatment of pre-diabetes, particularly the behavioral interventions that will likely need to last a lifetime."[1887]

Let's Be "Hippocrites"

Hippocrates, the father of ancient medicine, Maimonides, a philosopher in medieval Spain, and Sir William Osler, the father of modern medicine, all said "food is the best medicine." And if this is too testosterone-y for you, so did Hidegard of Bingen, a German nun in the Middle Ages. They are examples of how we fail to learn from history. Dr. Osler holds a special place in my heart. He was also the president of the American, Canadian, and British Library Associations; he was a "synthesizer."

If we could only train our docs to be more like Osler. Then, they would base their practices on these historical principles of proven wisdom. We would see an integrative emphasis in public health, prevention, nutrition, and less harm would come to patients; "primum non nocere" or "first, do no harm" is often violated as the 100,000+ deaths each year from adverse pharmaceutical outcomes attest. Inculcating Osler's teachings would emphasize, what one article calls, "The Medical Humanities, For Lack of a Better Term."[1888] In my opinion, we urgently need to apply these concepts to develop docs' skills in interviewing and motivating children to avoid their sweet deaths.[1889] The book, *A Clinical Guide for Management of Overweight and Obese Children and Adults*,[1890] by Caroline M. Apovian and Carine M. Lenders, could become an introductory text for students and clinicians who wish to be more "hippo-critical":

> "Behavioral change is the major component of therapy and prevention of further weight gain. Many clinicians have not been trained in the application of motivational interviewing and other techniques used to lead patients to maintain a healthy diet and increased physical activity. [We must] empower clinicians with the tools needed to meet the new demands presented by this major public health epidemic."[1891]

Malnourished Docs

Despite volumes of evidence, nutrition is still considered an "alternative" by the National Institute of Health. Sadly, docs are not getting enough nutrition classes in medical schools. Approximately one hundred medical schools teach nutrition, but the range of hours spent varies from two to seventy, with an average of twenty-four hours in the four years of medical school. This malnourishment of our medical students must be corrected

> "As more and more Americans are afflicted with chronic diseases in which nutrition plays a key role, the need for improved nutrition training of physicians has never been more evident . . . Even though medical technology continues to make advances in the pharmacologic and surgical management of these chronic diseases, the evidence is that much of the morbidity and mortality associated with these conditions may be preventable through dietary and lifestyle modifications."[1892]

The Man Behind the Curtain

Poor articles on nutrition are often given a lot of publicity; this confuses docs, patients, and the public at large. For example, a study reported that no matter what diet people tried, they would not stay on it for more than a year.[1893] Even though its results are valid, the study did not address the real problem behind the failure of any diet to maintain weight loss. It discusses inactivity, preference for high calorie foods, increased IR, obesity compromising our endocrine functions, and nutrigenomics, suggesting that each patient should find his or her own type of diet. These are all good points, but the study didn't say anything about "the man behind the curtain": the politicians, farmers, and food companies working to produce cheap, subsidized, and highly refined foods that are addictive. These are the reasons why people cannot stay on any kind of healthy diet.

Let's imagine that you are addicted to cocaine and that you are able to withdraw from it in a controlled clinic. You leave that environment and on your way home you see advertisements for cocaine everywhere; you see people using it right in front of you, even at home and in churches. You also find schools making cocaine readily available to your children. Will you stay clean for very long?

We will never solve this epidemic of obesity until we adopt

351

policies and marketing practices that go after the source of the problem.[1894] We need to address the problem of marketing to keep people addicted to bad processed foods. We need to educate people about the reason for their addictions to toxic foods. But, can we succeed in doing so with:

> "This little pamphlet with no money behind it to publicize it, and you are up against $34 billion worth of marketing that uses health claims like they are going out of style."[1895]

In my opinion, our food politics and ads are designed to make money, without regard for the truth or our health. The USDA compounds this state of affairs, since it is in charge of promoting the interests of Big Food and, at the same time, it is supposed to educate Americans about food. The end result is that people are so confused that they give up trying to learn and just eat what is convenient. One has to wonder if this was not the outcome envisioned by Big Food . . .

Even organizations like Weight Watchers promote refined and convenient foods, like trans-fats.[1896] A diabetic patient once told me that he had been advised by a hospital dietitian to eat muffins as a source of good oils. And how confusing is the following? An attempt to expand the rule that fast food joints list the amount of calories in their servings to include all restaurants is likely to be deemed illegal by United States District Judge Richard J. Holwell. Why?

Nutrigenomics and Metabolomics

"Nutrigenomics and Metabolomics Will Change Clinical Nutrition and Public Health Practice" is the title of a remarkable article[1897] that encapsulates much of what this little book has been trying to say. "Methods of profiling almost all of the products of metabolism in a single sample of blood or urine are being developed" because each of us has a different way to handle E&I in food. The future lab evaluation of our metabolisms will focus on pinpointing glucose concentration, insulin activity, and IR. Sound familiar?

But medical practices have not taken into consideration these principles resulting in a "one size fits all" approach to nutrition. If these metabolic and genetic tendencies were considered, each of us would be given optimal advice on what to eat and what to avoid. More than two thousand molecules are involved in the human metabolome, which is the grouping of all the factors that influence how we metabolize E&I. The number goes up by the thousands when we include the bacterial metabolites that come from the gut:

> "Eventually, nutrition scientists will use measures of gut microflora metabolism to develop a better understanding of the role of gut microflora in human nutrition. For example, the altered availability of the micronutrient choline caused by metabolism by gut microflora was associated with fatty liver in IR."[1898]

Mediterranean Roots

The Mediterranean diet should be the main way to treat metabolic problems.[1899] It is based on whole grains, olives, nuts, fish, fruits, vegetables, lemons, garlic, onions, cruciferous, lean meat, and wine. By eating this well, people who are between seventy and ninety years old have a 50 percent reduction in mortality.[1900] How does this diet work? Check out this article title: "Effect of a Mediterranean-Style Diet on Endothelial Dysfunction and Markers of Vascular Inflammation in the Metabolic Syndrome."[1901] That is how the Mediterranean diet, high in antioxidants and fiber, lowers CRP, a marker of inflammation.[1902] It also improves adiponectin, a hormone from our fat in diabetic women.[1903]

Fortunately, there are some signs that our health care system is beginning to understand that nutrition and supplements are not "alternative" practices. The 2003 Annual Meeting of Teachers of Family Medicine in Fort Lauderdale, Fla., emphasized that the main treatment of the metabolic syndrome should be nutrition. By so doing we reduce our risk of type 2 diabetes later in life,[1904] but it may not prevent obesity as kids age[1905] because they very likely will fall prey to Big Food's disinformation.

353

Food: E&I and "Foreign Control"

We already discussed the concept that food contains foreign molecules that greatly influence how our cells work. This is so because humans have adapted to these micronutrients after millennia of ingesting said substances. Plants have developed those molecules to adapt to their own environment. For instance, antioxidants have helped plants cope with stressful conditions, like droughts and excessive heat. When we ingest said micronutrients, we accrue the same benefits for practically the same environmental conditions. This concept has been christened "xenohormesis," or foreign control.[1906]

Earlier, we discussed xenohormesis as a way to explain why toxins in food can be so deleterious. In this chapter, we will see that the same applies to benign molecules in food. The minutest amount of food or toxins may have extremely important effects on cellular function. You may want to review the main point in the article highlighted in chapter 16.

Dieticians' Dilemma

This will need a bit of sugar to go down: most dietitians cannot tell you what I am about to recommend for you. They are taught in school that *all* foods are good, including processed foods. As you saw in the "xenohormesis" article, processed foods give us subpar E&I, which messes up cell signaling and metabolomics. Why then, don't dietitians come out against food processing? It is because Big Food contributes to their education. If you wish to read more about this issue, remember the book, *Food Politics*.

Please, don't conclude that I am saying dieticians don't care. I happen to be an adjunct professor at the University of Utah in the Department of Nutrition. Every one of my colleagues is deeply troubled by this sweet death epidemic and they would like to help as much as they can.

Practical Advice to Lick Sweet Death

What can a busy physician do to help patients understand these concepts and get them to change their toxic diets? What can patients do themselves? After reading many books and thousands of medical journals that address these issues, I have condensed my approach to patients in very simple terms. It has to be simple. After all, we are not talking about rocket science.[1907] If we complicate things too much, people lose interest and diets become unsustainable. These are the points I cover:

First, I give patients a "state of our society" talk, so that they understand the forces at play that drive them to eat poorly. Without such understanding, they are not likely to succeed. I show them that they are likely addicted to refined/processed foods, especially sugar. I pull no punches: they come to hear the truth about their health problems. I remind them that alcohol is nothing but fermented sugar and that their diets have the same addictive hook as the booze most of them avoid for different reasons.[1908]

Second, industries processing food intentionally place addictive substances, like advanced glycosylated end-products and HFCS, to increase consumers' addictions to their foods.[1909]

Third, fats have been demonized unnecessarily,[1910] causing people to avoid fats of all types. As a result, they have turned to sugar. The fats we need fear most are the "trans-fat: the latest and worst fat on the block,"[1911] and saturated fats.

Fourth, the food industry spends over $33 billion dollars to promote its agenda, which is based on profits, not on maximizing our health.[1912] In contrast, farmers only spend $5 million a year to advertise fruits and vegetables. As a result, American's are eating one-and-a-half vegetables a day on average. These "vegetables" tend to be French fries and ketchup; sad but funny, no?

Fifth, politics and economics have created wicked incentives leading to more profits and more production of cheap processed sugar.[1913]

Sixth, our perverse economic incentives push them to go to McDonald's restaurants. It is cheaper for them to eat there than to buy fruits and vegetables. Rushed lifestyles make it very hard to eat fresh produce. Yet, people end up spending a lot of money on soda, candy, and other addicting foods. If they were to change that, they may have more money to eat better.[1914]

Seventh, I tell them they will not get better until the regain ir ternal control (see below). I cannot help them unless they assv responsibility and stop ingesting kilograms of bad food. I out that it is not logical to expect milligrams of drugs to correct the imbalances created by kilograms of bad E&I from processed foods. I will help them with education, motivation and moral support, but I will not enable their addiction to sugar.

I cannot help them unless they assume responsibility and stop ingesting kilograms of bad food. I point out that it is not logical to expect milligrams of drugs to correct the imbalances created by kilograms of bad E&I from processed foods.

After this talk—it should not take very long; it is critical to motivate them to change—I give them very simple directions to change their diets:

In the first two weeks: eat only vegetables, nuts, and lean meats like fish, chicken, turkey, sardines, and tuna (eggs are fine). Eat lots of asparagus, leafy greens, colorful vegetables, and cruciferous vegetables (Brussels sprouts, broccoli, cabbage, cauliflower, collard, kale, turnips, water crests). Avocados and tomatoes (fruits) are great, too.

Eat with a shovel; don't even think about going hungry.

The following salad dressings are permitted: olive oil, vinegar, pepper, lemons, tarragon, and garlic.

The following drinks are permitted: water with lemons and vegetable juices (using a juicer is best).

If an item is not on the list, it is to be avoided.

Fasting for one day each month helps reduce TOIL.[1915] Why use this approach?

Participants are reducing their storages of glycogen, reducing IR peripherally and centrally in the hypothalamus, and they are changing the way their taste buds perceive sugars—which must be done for their metabolisms to start changing. Their appetite thermostats are disrupted; they will never succeed unless it is fixed.[1916]

They are ridding themselves of their sugar addictions, which must be done aggressively, just as we do with alcohol addictions.

During the second two weeks: add all fruits. Fruits juices are okay if they are organic (don't get Ocean Spray, Snapple, etc.), but dilute them in one-half water. Eat lots of grapefruits; they decrease IR.[1917]

In the third two weeks: add legumes: peanuts, peas, lentils, soy, and beans.

During the fourth two weeks: add brown rice, corn, and whole grains. Be very observant when you get back on wheat, since many people react differently to it. The most common reactions to wheat or gluten are gstorintestinal and neurological. Don't eat white grains or rice again.

Helpful Tips

- No refined foods, soda, or white flour (breads, pasta, candy, cakes, etc.).

- Participants will have to decide if they will introduce red meat, pork, dairy, and coffee back into their diets. I feel the latter is okay if consumed only in moderation. Red meat increases metabolic problems and inflammation.[1918]

- Indiscretions: will participants stop at one or two or will they relapse, like an alcoholic? They will need support when or if they fall off the wagon; they need to be encouraged to keep trying.

- Stress management: many people have personalities that cause their eating habits to be driven by stress. They must become aware of this to deal with those issues more responsibly. I advise Tai Chi, meditation, etc.

- Look into HPA axis dysfunction. Most abused children have a disruption of this axis that creates significant metabolic problems.[1919] They must address these issues through counseling or any other technique that will increase their sense of control and forgiveness.[1920]

- Never go hungry. This will cause patients to eat what is convenient (fast food, refined food, etc.). Participants should be proactive: carry nuts, vegetables, and other healthy convenient foods. People should be so full that they will pass on that stale doughnut at work. Filling up on the foods listed above (fruits, vegetables, nuts, legumes, lean meats, and whole grains) will never cause patients to have waist issues.[1921]

- Stop the emotion-laden practice of monitoring weight; monitor the waist.

- Don't count calories. Restrictive diets don't work. While counting calories may succeed in weight loss for some people, this approach requires an iron will, which is rare in our society. Most people will have abandoned such diets within a year.[1922]

- Why would one stop eating when one is still hungry? Counting calories only makes sense when participants have not yet fixed their fat thermostats. Addicted people cannot stop eating on their own. Their metabolic signals are so disturbed that their hunger is not slaked, unless the addicted substances (refined sugars) are consumed. A vicious cycle is perpetuated. Counting calories is their only hope, unless they fix their thermostats and rely on their "healthy hunger" to guide their choices.[1923] Keep it simple: cooking is okay, but not necessary. My dad, a French cook, would not be happy I said this.

- Have you ever heard the saying, "Eat breakfast like a king, lunch like a queen, and dinner like a pauper"? Skipping breakfast causes more IR[1924] and increases the risk of obesity.[1925] If you eat a big breakfast, you may have to force yourself to eat lunch and dinner. You will likely end up eating less if you do this. Your need to snack to satisfy the "munchies" will be greatly reduced. I think that an overwhelming need to snack is driven by poor breakfasts and by consuming processed foods or empty calories that just don't satisfy normal hunger. The food industry knows this; it's really good for its business.

- Okay, you still need to snack? Plan ahead so that you don't get caught with your pants down. Your snacking should not be driven by some stupid vending machine or convenience store along the way. Carry lots of nuts and fruit. I have even carried sardine cans that have an easy key to pull. Be creative and proactive with your meals.

- If you cannot eat those three meals like that, try to eat six small meals a day. It is really better for us, because that way we don't overload our insulin levels and metabolisms as much. By spreading the amount of food throughout the day, we lower IR.[1926] Don't be afraid of good fats (fish, sardines, tuna, olives, nuts, avocados). If the fats are veggie-based and unsaturated or monosaturated, your hormones associated with energy regulation will work better and you will increase your ability to thin out.[1927] If you are a doc, for best results, ask your patients about their diets "at each visit". This simple intervention would be a good start to turn back the

    > "Insufficient awareness on the part of physicians of the benefits of dietary treatment. Although dietitians do have an important role in patient care, the key to dietary changes is the repetition of dietary education by the primary care provider at each visit."[1928]

- Don't inhale your food; eat slowly. I tell my patients to chew their food at least a dozen times before swallowing. In fact, chewing almonds forty times significantly reduces hunger and lowers cholesterol.[1929]

- Eating out: there are plenty of restaurants that serve great salads. Order more than one if you feel you may not fill up with just one. Add liberally to it. Restaurants love to make more money by adding extras like avocados, tomatoes, mushrooms, etc.

- Better eating out: find the restaurants that have organic food. In Salt Lake City, Utah, I often eat at One World Café, located downtown. It's best to avoid food processing, additives, and contaminants. At least, find restaurants like Souplantation & Sweet Tomatoes.

- Traveling: I know it's hard to eat good food while on the road. My speechifying takes me to many cities in the United States and around the world. (Chances are, I have been to your hometown.) I cope by asking hotel staff about the best restaurants close by. Also, I find a grocery store and buy sardines in those cans you easily peel back, nuts, fruit, and whole grain bread. If you are asked to eat with business contacts that are still battling sweet death, remember that the best restaurants are flexible and will help you build your own super-salad.

Lots of Protein and Fiber

The diet above is high in veggie-protein and low in sugar and saturated fats; it will lower IR.[1930] The dogma that high-protein diets are harmful is only true when we over-emphasize animal protein, which doesn't have as many micronutrients as veggie proteins do to protect the kidneys and stimulate protein metabolism in the liver. A study found that supplementing veggie-protein powder in childhood resulted in adults whose health was significantly better; they also had higher wages.[1931]

Since high-protein and fiber diets have been shown to control hunger and appetite a lot better,[1932] it is best to emphasize veggie and fish protein ad libitum, or at will. This allows you to get full with low-glycemic foods, which lower your risk of IR and obesity.[1933]

A vicious cycle may be perpetuated with a high-sugar diet because such diets may interfere with the absorption of proteins.[1934] So, the more sugar you eat, the hungrier you are. The more energy-dense and low in fiber your food is, the fatter you get, especially children.[1935]

You will also get a lot of fiber with this diet; this improves intestinal function so that you may optimize the rate and quantity of glucose and cholesterol absorbed. This is why fiber decreases the risk of developing type 2 diabetes[1936] and improves your metabolism.[1937] Low-glycemic diets tend to have more fiber; those two factors lower the risk of diabetes 2 best.[1938] But, if one is to choose, the glycemic index diet seems more beneficial than a high-fiber diet.[1939]

Since most of our immune systems are in the intestines, fiber also decreases inflammation, or TOILing of cell membranes.[1940] Simply put, diets based on legumes, vegetables, and fruit are best to lower the risk of disease—particularly metabolic disease and cancer.[1941]

Don't Be Full of It

You may have heard that it's okay to have two to three bowel movements a week. Anyone who thinks that is "full of it." Ideally, we need to have two to three bowel movements *per day*. If we eat as outlined above, we will have very good bowel function, especially if we supplement fiber and friendly bacteria, or probiotics.[1942] By normalizing intestinal function, we not only absorb E&I better but we also detoxify better, all of which helps resolve TOILing. These are some of the reasons why I take constipation very seriously. But we don't have to be "pampered," too serious, or "stuffy" about constipation all the time:

> "Why are you worrying about
> You-know-who
> You should be worrying about
> U-no-poo
> The constipation sensation
> That's gripping the nation."[1943]

Story Time

Dr. Denis Parsons Burkitt, whose name is attached to an infamous type of pediatric lymphoma, did a lot of work in Africa where he noticed that people who produced the biggest piles of stool had less cancer. This reminds me of that scene in Jurassic Park, when actress Laura Dern digs through dinosaur poop,

---

looking for a radio. Hey, I am a doc: I have a licence to talk about poop. Sadly, this story ends on a constipating note: when Dr. Burkitt presented his observations in the United States, his peers ridiculed him.

What a shi*** deal . . .

More Substance

Fiber is so dramatically helpful in the treatment of E&I/metabolic[1944] issues, as well as in the prevention of type 2 diabetes,[1945] that I include a whole article on one of the most studied fibers, "Guar Gum: A Miracle Therapy for Hypercholesterolemia, Hyperglycemia, and Obesity":[1946]

> Guar gum is an annual legume crop mainly grown in India and Pakistan. It can be eaten as a green bean, fed to cows, or used as green manure. Its galactomannan gum forms a gel when mixed with water. It is used as thickener and binder in sauces, salad dressings, ice creams, noodles, pet foods, processed meats, bread improvers, and beverages. It is also being used to replace flour from grains.
>
> Guar gum is 75 percent soluble fiber, which is why it acts like a gel. Insoluble fiber (7.6 percent) adds bulk and feeds probiotics. This action also lowers cholesterol.
>
> An increase of 10 grams of fiber a day reduces coronary death by 17 percent
>
> Diet with 5 percent guar gum significantly lowers cholesterol. Ten grams a day reduced LDL by 12 percent, triglycerides by 42 percent, and raised HDL by 6 percent. Most people use 8 to 36 grams per day.
>
> Guar gum reduces peak postprandial glucose and 2hGTT by 10 to 35 percent. It is also helpful in obesity, since it increases satiety, reduces IR, and helps with the absorption of glucose in the intestines.

Insoluble fiber also helps reduce appetite and reduces the glycemic response to foods consumed seventy-five minutes later;

this means that you may want to eat lots of fiber before you must indulge on some high-sugar treat.[1947] When indigestible fiber is high in evening meals, and followed by a healthy breakfast, IR diminishes considerably.[1948] Fiber is also high in sterols, which have been found to be quite beneficial for the regulation of cholesterol absorption in the intestines, since they compete for the same absorption mechanisms in the gut.

The Religion of Soy Haters

If you are one of those people who think soy is terrible for you, please, skip this section. I have no hope of dissuading you, nor do I want to.

Soy haters have a religious-like fervor against soy despite clear evidence that soy is quite beneficial (see below). Inadvertently, they fall prey to the propaganda disseminated by Big Pharma and the dairy industry; they are losing millions of dollars to soy. How on Earth did a God-given crop all of a sudden turn bad? How is it that billions of people throughout the world eat soy and have nothing but good reports for their troubles? The blind attacks on soy are often based on (1) questionable soy subsidies. (Why take it out on the crop?) (2) Genetically Modified soy that has pesticides introduced into its DNA; (but, again, why blame soy?) and (3) misinterpreted and old information.

For example, a report showing that soy consumption is linked to longer life was spun to say that soy caused dementia. The authors of the study warned that such a conclusion would be erroneous: people who live longer by eating soy do end up with an older brain that appeared smaller in CT scans. The Honolulu Star Bulletin was the only newspaper to publish the twisted logic demonizing soy.[1949] I wonder how soy haters would interpret a much more recent report that showed soy and fish to increase the production of an insulin-degrading enzyme, which eliminates beta amyloid in patients with Alzheimer's disease . . .[1950]

If we were to believe that soy messes up our sex hormones and thyroid because of soy's phytoestrogens, we would have to give up on all the foods that have such micronutrients. There are three types of phytoestrogens: (1) isoflavones, like soy, nuts, tea, coffee, beans, and licorice; (2) coumestans, like alfalfa and broccoli; (3) and lignans, like oil seeds, linseeds, and berries.

Soy haters also ignore the fact that soy is an adaptogen: its effect on our livers is quite flexible.[1951] If we need more or less estrogen, soy will have the beneficial effect needed on our livers' glucoronidation pathways of detoxification. In other words, estrogen goes up or down after soy consumption, depending on the need of the person consuming it.[1952] (The same goes for our thyroid functions.) Soy is a natural selective estrogen receptor modulator (SERM) whose adapting function was copied by Big Pharma to make drugs, like tamoxifen and raloxifene/Evista®—both of which have been found to decrease the risk of breast cancer.[1953] In other words, soy reduces the risk of breast cancer.[1954]

Another worn-out argument against soy is that it has phytates that may block the uptake of minerals leading to many diseases. What they fail to consider is that all grains and legumes have phytates. Should we eliminate them, too? I wonder what they say about the fact that soy ferritin is a good source of iron.[1955]

Perhaps the claims that soy causes breast and prostate cancer are the most tiresome of all. I hope you read the report on the "Fifth International Symposium on the Role of Soy in Preventing and Treating Chronic Disease."[1956] The truth is that soy reduces the risk of these estrogen-driven cancers. Again, this is due to soy's function as an adaptogen.

Do soy haters have any valid concerns about soy? Absolutely; let's examine them. "Soy has GMO pesticides in its genome." Yes, but so does 60 percent of the food we eat in America. "Soy shouldn't be consumed at all, but if one is going to pollute one's self with it, it is best to eat it fermented." Yes, but this is true of all foods. "Soy may cause severe allergies." True, but so could any food, particularly legumes and nuts eaten too early in our infancy. "Soy is a subsidized crop used to make trans-hydrogenated fats." Correct, but that doesn't mean soy, itself, is bad. Would you hate corn because it is used to make HFCS? Better yet, would you condemn sex because it may be used to hurt people?

I tire of arguing about this issue. Truly, "they are taking the joy out of soy."[1957] Often, my fatigue from having Bible-bash-like arguments with soy haters makes me give up and simply advice people to drink almond or rice milk and forget about soy.

Let us look at the evidence on soy and metabolic issues from reputable and very recent medical journals starting with the research that soy reduces IR.[1958]

- Soy decreases non-small cell lung cancer growth in female mice.[1959]
- Soy isoflavones increase NOS vasodilatation in menopause.[1960]
- Soy and tomatoes lower the risk of prostate cancer.[1961]
- Soy improves liver and adipose tissue metabolism.[1962]
- Soy protein isolate lowers biomarkers in prostate cancer.[1963]
- Soy protein isolate ameliorates atherosclerosis in mice with lipid problems.[1964]
- Genistein improves nitric oxide function in endothelium: it lowers blood pressure.[1965]
- Genistein lowers blood pressure in salt-sensitive rats.[1966]
- Isoflavones improve endothelial function and lower risk of carotid atherosclerosis.[1967]
- Isoflavones decrease cardiovascular risk in type 2 diabetes.[1968]
- Soy reduces arterial stiffness and blood pressure in people with metabolic issues.[1969]
- Soy improves metabolic syndrome issues in postmenopausal women.[1970]
- Soy reduces Fatty Liver and improves lipid profile.[1971]
- A high-soy, low-fat diet helps weight loss and preserves muscle mass.[1972]
- Soy reduces glucose toxicity in ventricular myocytes (heart muscle).[1973]
- Soy inhibits fat formation.[1974]

Will all that evidence settle the issue? Don't hold your breath . . .

The Right Sugars

Remember that all foods have polysaccharides, or good, natural sugars. When these sugars combine with proteins, they are called glycoproteins. When combined with lipids (fats), they are called glycolipids. The general term for sugars combined with other molecules is glycoconjugates. Glycoconjugates coat the surfaces of cells; they are found freely in bodily fluids and in many other locations in the body. A glycoconjugate may contain as little as one sugar or may contain chains of sugars. Some are branched and very complex. Specific sequences of sugars in a glycoconjugate control its recognition and communications with other molecules.

Glycoconjugates on the surface of one cell bind to receptors on another cell, allowing the cells to communicate with one another. This cell-to-cell communication process allows the body to carry out the many complex functions necessary for health. Glycoproteins that are formed by the cells in our bodies play roles in building enzymes, hormones, immunoglobulins, and antibodies. Some autoimmune conditions are related to improperly formed glycoconjugates on the surfaces of cells. Immune system cells may not recognize abnormal glycoconjugates as "self" and may attack them as if they were foreign cells.[1975]

It's pretty easy to find refined sugar. Just walk out the door if you have not already stacked your pantry with all the addicting, HFCS-rich foods that you crave. This type of diet muscles out the right sugars. But, when we eat the Mediterranean and Low-Glycemic Index diets, we get these natural sugars easily. How many of you will be able to lick this massive addiction to refined sugars?

Two of the glyconutrients, glucose and galactose, are found readily in the average diet. However, the other six sugars may be missing, or in short supply. Modern food harvesting processes and diet choices may have an impact on the availability of these important nutrients. Our bodies are capable of synthesizing each of these eight sugars, but this synthesis process may not always function optimally. A series of enzymatic steps are necessary to convert one sugar into another. This is why it may be prudent to supplement the eight natural sugars we discussed above. There are two brands: glyco-8 (Nature's Sunshine Products) and ambratose (Mannatec).

Marooned

Tom Hanks found himself marooned on a deserted island in the movie, *Castaway,* much like Robinson Crusoe. If we were to contemplate the same fate for ourselves, and we were told that we could take only one item with us, what would you take? Sigmund Freud would have a field day analyzing our answers. Would you pick an "aspirin" like marooned docs on a TV commercial?

They can keep their aspirin. I would pick Olive Oyl, Popeye's girlfriend, and kill two birds with one stone.

Bird #1: This would be the need for company, even though Olive Oyl is a bit too skinny for my taste. Popeye would no doubt sail the Seven Seas to find us; this may mean I could be rescued if I survived his jealous spinach-overdeveloped muscles.

Bird #2: This would be omega oils. At this point in the book, you understand the importance of healthy cell membranes: their main component is phospholipids, or healthy fats. Omega oils are indispensable for the correct structuring and function of our cell membranes for the optimal use of E&I through cell communication. Omega oils are, in my opinion, the most important nutrients to avoid TOILing. This is one of the reasons why the nutty Mediterranean diet is so good for us.[1976] It is high in vegetables, fish, and lean meat oils, which are the best sources of omega oils. Essential fatty acids significantly lower the risk of getting the metabolic syndrome, especially in those of us with genetic tendencies.[1977]

There are several kinds of omega oils. The most important are omega-3s, omega-6s, and omega-9s. The latter two are found in abundance in our Western, processed diets. It's the omega-3s that are lacking, which is why I recommend to everyone, including those who eat well, to supplement omega oils. The best supplements are EPA and DHA. The latter is particularly helpful for neurologic function. The evidence for omega oils is vast. There are many books available to review these concepts.

Selling Snake Oil

A symbol of quackery, snake oil has nevertheless been found to have significant benefits because of its high omega oil content. Significantly, it lowers IR.[1978] Could it be that those old cowboys did find some benefit in snake oil while taming the Wild West, working under very difficult conditions and away from the marine products that would have helped them with their omega oil needs? Could it be that snake oil reduced their TOILing and IR? Their hard drinking may have had a synergetic effect on their snake oil levels.[1979] You be the judge.

I am often hired by nutraceutical companies to talk about their products. I believe that they have a lot to offer because they market E&I in the form of nutraceutical supplements. I applaud their efforts, which, in my opinion, have more worth than pharmaceutical products in chronic, but not in acute, conditions. Nobody is going to recommend omega oils when someone is having a heart attack. This is the time for the best doctors available and for the best drugs to keep you alive.

As well intended as nutraceuticals are, I am afraid they are picking up the same bad habits that corporate Big Pharma has perfected. I hardly blame them because any business in America is going to play by the same "legal" rules. I emphasize "legal" because there is nothing wrong with "doing business at the speed of light." However, as we have seen above, the best businesses are beginning to adopt the "triple bottom line" of profits, social responsibility, and environmental responsibility.[1980] Hopefully, the health care system will reflect the ethical higher ground that physicians have sworn to uphold:

> "For-profit industries do not share the same ethical norms to which physicians and other health care professionals must adhere. Their primary commitment is to create shareholder value, not maintaining an altruistic commitment to patients. But at some point the leadership of the pharmaceutical industry and their board of directors must begin to recognize that growing public and professional mistrust could substantially detract from their value."[1981]

We may as well replace "pharmaceutical" with the word "nutraceutical." I am afraid that many nutraceutical companies are going to lose the public's trust if they maintain profits ahead of "an altruistic commitment to patients." People are not dumb. They are starting to laugh at any product claiming to "cure every-thing." There are so many supplements claiming to be the very best that it is becoming embarrassing.

I do mention their products as adjuncts to a good diet, or as an insurance policy to lower TOILing as much as possible. My main message to nutraceutical agents is that we need to empower peo-ple to heal themselves and avoid looking at any "outside prod-uct" as the final answer.[1982]

You might think that this attitude limits my speaking en-gagements from nutraceutical companies. Perhaps, but the more enlightened nutraceuticals have embraced this approach whole-heartedly. I find it interesting that their sales are booming. They also have more credibility and public trust when they stop attack-ing Big Pharma and its questionable marketing tools. You know the saying: "What is good for the goose is good for the gander." If we are going to continue to insist that Big Pharma clean up its act, we—those who support more natural products—must live by the very principles we demand from the pharmaceuticals. In other words, we must put the "health of the people as the supreme law of the land" as the overriding concern of the business, besides profits, of course.

Because of my role as a lecturer and adjunct professor, I have chosen not to sell any products myself.

Graduate-Level Nutrition?

I am a fish-eating vegetarian. While it is not necessary to give up meat altogether, there is no question that vegetarians are healthier. I will not bother you with a ton of references, but if you care to read more about this, get the book I mentioned earlier: The China Study. The main problem I see with so-called vegetarians is that they eat too much sugar because they are often hungry, hav-ing eliminated a lot of convenient food. In my opinion, they go from the frying pan to the fire. Also, vegetarians need to supple-ment B-complex vitamins, particularly if they don't do the work of optimizing intestinal function.

Another graduate-level suggestion is to eat as organic as possible. They can be more expensive and harder to find, but organic foods do have many advantages: more micronutrients, like antioxidants, and less toxins, like pesticides and heavy metals. Despite more awareness about these issues, the FDA recently announced that genetically altered and enhanced animal products will be allowed in the market without any labeling.[1983] One has to wonder how much lobbying it took to get such bonehead decision to pass through the government-business revolving door.

You may be interested in "PhD level" nutrition. If so, read Barbara Kingsolver's book, Animal, Vegetable, Mineral.[1984] It's about eating only locally produced food. I wholeheartedly agree with the author, so much so that my family and I are in the process of looking for a little place in rural Utah to soon retire far from the maddening crowd . . .

Then, there are those who recommend eating certain foods at certain times and specific combinations of foods while prohibiting other combinations at other times. While there may be some advantages to these suggestions, I find them to be impractical and obsessive. People seldom stick to these regimens. In my opinion, 99 percent of the battle is won by getting off processed foods, especially sugar and trans-fats. But, if you still have some energy and motivation left to undertake these micromanaging programs, go ahead.

Future Shock: Codex

Ongoing legal battles will soon change the future of nutraceuticals. There are those who would like to take away your right to obtain nutritional supplements freely. The whole concept is being called "Codex alimentarius." I recommend that you become more educated about this issue by logging onto the American Holistic Health Association's Web site and clicking on its "Codex" section. If these laws pass, we may not be able to supplement nutrients at all without a doc's prescription. I leave you to figure out whom this sad state of affairs would benefit.

When you delve into this issue, you will see that the main reason given to legislate these supplements out of existence is "quality control." While this is an extremely worthy goal, the claim that all nutraceuticals are deficient in this area is ludicrous. I am sure that some of them are not selling good products. But I assure you the top names in the industry take pride in producing "pharmaceutical-grade" products.

The other worn-out argument against supplementation is that we don't need "expensive urine," meaning that quantities of micronutrients above the RDAs are a waste. One, they ignore that approximately 90% of prescription drugs are also eliminated in the urine unused; two, they ignore the fact that some people require more of some nutrients because of differences in the enzymes that process said nutrients.[1985] In other words, some of us need more vitamin D because of the way kidney enzymes activate it, like me.

Now you are ready to look at more evidence for nutrition and supplements and their role in optimizing E&I.

In Defense of Food

I can think of a couple of patients who have given me honest and liberal feedback about the nutrition advice I gave them. Surely other patients have quietly agreed with these good folks. One family was upset that I told the mother to only change her diet and quit refined foods. She had been too many docs trying to find relief for her arthritis because powerful drugs had failed. As a last resort, she came to my clinic having heard that my team could help her. They were disappointed that their initial "homework" was so . . . pedestrian.

Another patient felt that our discussion on her request to become vegetarian was "treating her like cattle," or like just another patient. She told me she had special needs about "her relationship with food" in rather metaphysical terms. I felt this was an invitation to delve deeper into her "mind-body" issues, which she repeatedly expressed a desire to do during our first visit. After a few questions about her life, she was offended when I asked her about her childhood . . .

I remain open to the possibility that these patients and I did not get off to a good start. Perhaps I was entirely at fault in both encounters. After all, a professional relationship between a patient and a doctor is just like any other. Occasionally, the first interview goes so poorly that both parties would do well to acknowledge that it would be wiser to abort right then and there.

But in Michael Pollan's book, *In Defense of Food,*[1986] this is not rocket science: get off refined foods, eat lots of fruits and vegetables, and stop eating when you are full. The results are nothing short of miraculous. If anybody tells you more than that, they are likely trying to sell you something.

Ideally Speaking

If we weren't so addicted to sugar, I would say we would do best to be vegetarians for many reasons. But, realistically, many of us may not be able to resist the temptations of refined sugars without some dead meat. Most people who profess to be vegetarians turn out to be relying too much on the convenient garbage they find everywhere. Real vegetarians (they are few in numbers) are committed to healthy living and avoid a sweet death by staying away from refined sugars. But, if one were to become as self-sufficient as possible and eschew agribusiness, one would have to raise one's own poultry and cattle in an organic and self-sustainable way. In that case, I feel meat is a necessity, given that crops cannot be harvested year round nor stored easily if energy or power is not readily available. Sadly, I feel those circumstances are not farfetched, given the chaotic state of our economy in the fall of 2008.

Growing meat is very hard on the environment when done in the slash-and-burn manner that agribusiness pushes onto us to maximize their profits. In that fashion, the resources used to feed meat to one person may feed seventy vegetarians. Animal meat raised full of chemicals, hormones, and antibiotics, grain-fed and made to wallow in its own feces, has been shown to increase the risk of chronic diseases. There is no question that vegetarianism is the healthiest way to eat when we cannot avail ourselves of gently and sustainably raised meat.[1987]

Another problem is the shipping of food across the world. It is not only energy-inefficient and more expensive, but it leads to diets that are not in keeping with nutrigenomics concepts. We descend from people who ate only food available in season in their part of the world. By eating local food in-season only, we are a lot better off and we are more likely to get real organic food without pesticides. Besides, we support our local economies rather than heavily subsidized (with our own taxes) corporations that take money away from small local businesses.

Big Food is trying to cash in on the higher demand for organic foods, but its products leave a lot to be desired. By emphasizing profits over health, Big Food cuts corners. I would much rather get locally grown food from a local farmer who looks in my eyes and tells me that he or she is committed to sustainable farming without chemicals and invites me to his or her little farm to see for myself.

But, realistically, we need to fight one battle at a time. I often run across food-fanatics, who end up turning off other people with their extreme ideas, like never eating fruits and vegetables at the same time or not eating certain foods unless it is a specific time of the day. While they may have a point here and there, they end up alienating themselves and losing credibility. This is why I wish to keep it simple for you: if you stop eating refined foods, you have the most important battle won. If, in the future, you choose to "go to the next level," that would be great. But, first things first, don't you think?

Proof of the Pudding

"Your diet is too restrictive." I hear this sometimes; I disagree. Patients are eager to hear from their doctors what to do to overcome their chronic health problems. My patients are thankful that someone has shown them the way out of their sweet deaths and their consequences. This simple approach works. I see the results in my clinic every day. You will find a whole chapter on how their specific problems are handled nutritionally. Their metabolic issues are corrected or improved, their cholesterol levels improve, IR decreases or disappears altogether, and practically all problems they face improve. Pre-hypertension is resolved by these simple interventions[1988] and their blood pressure drops 10 to 60 points just by following this diet, which is practically the same as the Dietary Approaches to Stop Hypertension (DASH) diet. The DASH diet has been thoroughly shown to work, yet few doctors recommend it.[1989] It has many other benefits, including lowering the risk of stroke in middle age women.[1990]

Most people get very discouraged trying to lose weight. It is true that it is not easy, but it can be done if we are patient and stop expecting miracles overnight. At the last Annual Meeting of the Endocrine Society in Toronto, experts reported that 20 percent of people are able to lose at least 10 percent of body weight and keep it off for only one year.[1991] A report from the CDC added that nearly 60 percent of people who lost 10 percent body weight were able to keep it off for that long.[1992] "Weight maintenance following weight loss is doable," they concluded. I agree, but I add that it is a certainty, *if* you don't fall off the wagon and start eating refined sugars again.

In the past, some folks believed that the resting metabolic rate was lowered when we lost weight, which would have led to more storage of fat. This is partially true, but the effect is transitory: "the idea that your body is fighting you doesn't hold out in the literature."[1993] Another bad idea is to become anorexic, a disease that requires psychiatric care. Unfortunately, many Internet sites and fashion magazines promote this eating disorder; it has led France to pass a law against this practice.[1994]

Please, don't lose hope. You may lose the weight that keeps you from getting into your swimsuit; if you so choose, you may even skip the swimming suit and go swimming naked in the future; I am only thinking about your vitamin D levels.

Chapter 32

Mother Nature's Bounty: Herbs

"The search for natural products is currently not an approach to drug discovery that the larger pharmaceutical companies are pursuing with vigor. By ignoring nature's bounty, these companies may be missing out."[1995]

That's according to the *Journal of the American Medical Association*. True, but I don't believe herbs are some magic remedy. On the contrary, they are nothing but foods that have higher concentrations of polysaccharides, essential oils, amino acids, antioxidants, anti-inflammatory micronutrients and E&I. By now you know how powerful nutrition is; herbs are part of the package.

Doctors are beginning to listen to patients who for some time now have been interested in herbs. The article, "Herbal,"[1996] offers sound advice:

Honor patients' choices
Encourage proven practices
Read about integrative issues
Be honest about what you read
Avoid criticism
List integrative items on chart

Since the metabolic syndrome involves just about all diseases, it is not surprising that practically all herbs may be used for some aspect of this syndrome. They all work by improving E&I, metabolism and cell communication. Here is some of the evidence:

"Guggulipid May Combat Metabolic Syndrome":[1997] Taking 2,000 milligrams, of guggulipid, three times a day, lowers cholesterol via thyroid stimulation; it reduces glucose by 6 points and insulin by 2 points. It also lowers CRP (marker of inflammation) by 31 percent and it lowers blood pressure by 4 points. Guggulipid is a drug in India.

"Complementary and Alternative Treatments of Diabetes" was one of the topics at the 2004 Annual Meeting of the American Diabetes Association in Orlando, Florida. Before a packed audience, evidence was presented to justify the use of chromium, alpha lipoic acid, and vanadium. Also, the following herbs were highlighted: gymnema silvestre, fenugreek, bitter melon, aloe vera, ginseng, prickly pear (nopal), minnamon, and ivy gourd. In addition, the drug metformin was recognized for being derived from the French lilac.

"Herbs that Affect Blood Glucose Levels"[1998] lists the following herbs:

- Panax ginseng lowers IR.[1999]

- Fenugreek[2000] also lowers the risk of cancer and it helps the adrenal glands.

- Bittermelon (momordica charantia)[2001] is better than the drug, tolbutamide, for decreasing the production of sugar in the liver (gluconeogenesis) and sugar absorption in the intestines.

- Garlic[2002] also keeps vampires and prospective dates away. (Vampire books seem to be hot again.)

- Catechins (polyphenolic antioxidant plant metabolites. They belong to the family of flavonoids) [2003]

- Other herbs listed in this article: aloe, blueberry leaf, guayusa, grifola mushroom, shiitake mushroom, and mistletoe. The last one may also reduce your stress levels if you stand long enough under it . . .

Chapter 33

Get Off the Couch

Since there are so many books out there about exercising, you could try lifting them and get a pretty good workout, or you could read one of my personal favorites, *Sports Nutrition: Energy Metabolism and Exercise*,[2004] by Ira Wolinsky and Judy A. Driskell. Then again, you could wait for the drug that is being developed that could help you gain some of the benefits of exercise without even getting off the couch: no exercise? No sweat![2005] Isn't it amazing, the power of the human mind to deceive itself and make money at it?

I wish I could say something profound to get you off the couch, but only 40 percent of you would get it done.[2006] Maybe the fact that endurance exercise mitigates the ill effects of a meal too high in sugar will motivate you to get off the couch.[2007] Can anyone say "indulgences"?

There is no question that even minimal exercise will greatly improve glycemic control, lower IR, reduce glycosylated hemo-globin levels,[2008] improve practically every aspect of our health, decrease morbidity and mortality,[2009] improve cognitive function in the elderly,[2010] *and* lower the risk of having metabolic problems.[2011] Even walking three to four hours per week lowers mortality in diabetics.[2012] The French prefer strolling to running or jogging. They feel that it is not dignified to exert oneself so strenuously in public. They have even objected to their leader, President Nicolas Sarkozy, showing his knees while jogging[2013]. . . This may be why Lance Armstrong won the "Tour de Lance" seven years in a row. (Don't tell them I said that; it's a touchy topic over there.)

The references on exercise are too numerous to list, but the following ones are too good to leave out. In only three weeks of walking and eating more fruits and vegetables, people lost weight and reduced their blood pressure by 14 percent. They reduced cholesterol by 19 percent, free radicals by 28 percent, insulin levels by 48 percent, and blood glucose by 7 percent.[2014] The better our treadmill testing looks, the lower the risk of metabolic syndrome, hypertension, hypercholesterolemia, and diabetes.[2015]

Perhaps this will help motivate you more than anything else: walking briskly for thirty minutes a day saves $600 a year on drugs.[2016] It's never too late to begin an exercise program. Even if we feel we are already doomed, we could think about starting just so that we may be a good example to our children; they too may lower IR early in their lives with exercise.[2017] Still, there is much to be said about more gentle activities:

> "If you would exercise, go in search of the springs of life. Think of a man swinging dumb-bells for his health when those springs of life are bubbling up in far-off pastures unsought by him."[2018]

Chapter 34

Is it All In Your Head or In Your Heart?

I had the privilege of interviewing Dr. John C. Nelson, the 2004 American Medical Association president, on my radio show. He told us a very sad story: when he was training as an intern at a hospital, he found himself at the bedside of a patient who had just passed away. He was overcome with grief watching the widow crying by her husband's remains. Not knowing what else to do, he embraced her and they cried together. His ranking resident happened to go by; seeing Dr. Nelson so shook up, he called him out in the hallway and chastised his "weak intern," Dr. Nelson, "for acting like a woman."

Why is medicine so . . . "male?" Enter Dr. William Osler and Abraham Flexner.

Osler is considered to be the father of modern medicine. Flexner was the director of the Carnegie Institute in the early 1900s when he was commissioned by the Feds to tune up medical education in the United States. At the time, many docs attended questionable schools and some were getting diplomas from mail courses, which may not have been any better than the ones anyone could get from a Cracker Jack box. (No, that is not how I got mine.) The implementation of Flexner's report made our medical schools much like German schools, that is, very scientific. There is nothing wrong with that, but Osler sounded a warning at the time. He felt that docs would not get enough "humanitarian training."

A hundred years later you may have an opinion on the balance between Flexner's reforms and Osler's warning . . .

"Because She is Below Him"

In my opinion, just about everything that ails our society stems from a poor understanding of who we are, and the rejection of the feminine nature in us all—males and females. We minimize the feminine while we overvalue logic and the intellect. It is not that one aspect of our nature is better than the other, but that an imbalance is quite harmful to us all. If we were to restore the feminine in our belief systems, we would better much better off. (Remember Lao Tsu?)[2019]

I am not saying that women are superior, but that our feminine aspect, our intuition, our feelings, and our caring natures in both men and women will always win the day over cold-blooded logic. Many will disagree. Let me ask you a simple question: is our society today doing well under the leadership of Ivy League-trained graduates?

Oscar, the Cat

In our intellectual arrogance, we may feel vastly superior to animals. While we do have superior brains, animals share in our capacity to feel and emote. Arrogance may be why some believe that we may be "anthropomorphizing," or attributing human qualities to animals. But, the argument cuts the other way, too:

> "The real problem underlying many of the criticisms of anthropomorphism is actually "anthropocentrism." Placing humans at the center of all interpretation, observation, and concern—and placing dominant men at the center of that—has led to some of the worst errors in science, whether in astronomy, psychology, or animal behavior."[2020]

Because of their relative lack of intellect, animals rely more on their so-called "instincts." In my opinion, we choose to call "instincts" that which we don't understand very well. I would not be surprised if animals are able to tap into E&I fields that may only be accessible to us when we humble ourselves. Oscar, the cat, would agree. He lives in a nursing home where he doesn't fail to curl up in bed with those who are about to pass away in a few hours.[2021]

Does Oscar feel something we cannot feel? Does this cute gray-and-black cat tap into a realm we are too proud to access? Does he merely pick up on clues from staff and docs? We don't know. Maybe we need to humble ourselves and admit that our intellect only goes so far.

Jay Leno thinks that Oscar may be killing the patients himself.

"Bugging" You

Throughout history we have tried many ideologies and philosophies to govern our societies. Would you agree that our track record is not so hot? We still pit capitalism against communism as if the answers were "either/or." This is characteristic of intellectual approaches that are often ego-driven. One of these days we may be able to see past such divisiveness and govern ourselves from the heart, seeking to put our fellowman's welfare first and foremost.

You may think this is too quixotic. Touché; it turns out I was the lead in a neighborhood rendition of "Man of La Mancha." (As a child I wanted to become a Jesuit priest to indulge my love of learning, books and service under the banner of a spiritual quest. For better or worse, I abandoned that quest when my hormones hit the fan . . .)

These ideas are hardly wishful thinking, but cutting edge science: ants and bees don't "think" like we do and may have no clue why they do what they do individually, but they are still able to govern themselves quite successfully for the good of the colony. By simply following their pheromones or instinctive behavior ("from the heart"), they get it right:

> "The bees' rules for decision-making—seek a diversity of
> options, encourage a free competition among ideas, and use
> an effective mechanism to narrow choices—so impressed [a

researcher] that he now uses them at Cornell as chairman of his department . . . Almost any group that follows the bees' rules will make itself smarter . . . even in the face of exceptionally complex decisions."[2022]

I will never forget the line from the latest 3-D dinosaur movie where the narrator makes the point that dinosaurs with brains smaller than walnuts were able to live on Earth for millions of years in peace and harmony. Will Homo economicus be able to match that feat? If you wish to read more about these concepts, read the book, *The Wisdom of Crowds,* by James Surowiecki.

"Your Money or Your Life"

That is the choice we need to make in our lives—and not just at the point of a knife in a dark alley. Isn't it amazing how we tend to make the right choices under those circumstances? Would we make the same choice otherwise? Are you working as hard as you do by choice? Some of us have to work two or three jobs just to make ends meet. I find that to be deplorable given that a substantial portion of the fruits of that labor end up in someone else's bank account.[2023]

When we work too hard by choice, we are choosing "money over life." I am very happy with my choice of "life over money," which I can afford because I am blessed with a job that is remunerated handsomely. I do feel bad that some of you have to work much harder . . .

Your Money or Your Life is a great book by Vicki Robin, Joe Dominguez, and Monique Tilford.[2024] It will help you simplify your life so that you are not consumed by consumerism. It's not funny that we took the old word for tuberculosis, "consumption," to denote our compulsive need to shop. When we do that, that is, work hard so that we may shop more we end up with "TB." No, not tuberculosis: "tired butt."

Stress is having a huge impact on our sweet deaths. The daily grind worsens the metabolic syndrome.[2025] We already discussed how the adrenal glands, or the HPA axis, are overburdened by our fast-paced lifestyles. We may have an excuse when we must work hard to provide for our loved ones' basic needs. But, please, don't bring it on yourself.

The mind-heart-body connection is very strong in diabetes. Any form of "stress reduction" will greatly improve your glycemic control,[2026] as will psychological interventions.[2027] There are many ways to deal with stress. Ultimately, it is not the stress that causes problems, but how we handle it or how we allow it to affect us. You may choose Tai Chi, yoga, meditation,[2028] sports, gardening, biofeedback,[2029] and even "watching submarine races" with your favorite companion.

McDonald's restaurants' efforts to bring more serenity to their establishments through Feng Shui[2030] may be a step in the right direction for some, but to me this seems to be a cynical attempt to cash in on people's surging rise in awareness about the mind-body connection by maximizing consumption; they just want you to stick around longer while you wax your coronaries a bit. At any rate, don't confuse Feng Shui with Sinn Fein or worse . . . with Sean Penn.

Humor is the Best Medicine

Sigmund Freud said, "When confronted with unrelenting suffering, the only sane response is humor."

According to the journal Lancet, "Clown doctors remind us of so many things: to take our work seriously but ourselves lightly; the value of a smile and a laugh; that it is okay to take a minute to play."[2031]

Norman Cousins, a reporter who developed ankylosing spondylitis, a disease somewhat like lupus, cured himself with high dose IV vitamin C and watching Groucho Marx movies.[2032] Please, think about watching fewer movies about depressing and intellectualized calamities. Isn't real life depressing enough that you have to be entertained by someone else's misery? I get it: you want to understand others' suffering. Great, but please, take a break to watch funny movies more often. Read funny books, too, and hang out with happy and "lighthearted" people.[2033] Remember the feather and the heart?

No doubt it may be hard for some to give up philosophizing. If that's the case, I recommend you check out my favorite philosophers, Calvin and Hobbes.

Love is All You Need

True, but in my opinion, we cannot love until we lighten up, overcome our egos, and see others as an integral part of ourselves. To do that, we have to stop taking ourselves so seriously and see the ego for what it is: a wonderful survival mechanism that *you* are blessed with. The ego is not really you. Once we are able to "put off the natural man" (the ego) we are able to love our true selves deeply, the selves that are divine and a part of the whole. Then, and only then, we are able to love others.

The myth of Narcissus is about self-love. The common negative interpretation of Narcissus's self love is not what the myth intended. If you hang around until the whole story is told, you may see that Narcissus is "transformed" into a flower as he tries to reach down in the river to touch his reflection. As a flower, Narcissus becomes "part of the whole," and eventually overcomes his ego. The negative aspect of Narcissism describes the love of the ego, which is not our real self. The positive aspect of Narcissism means that we overcome the ego and love ourselves as part of the only consciousness that exists in the universe.[2034] When we do the latter, we may then love ourselves, and everyone around us.

Self-hate is often the result of bruised egos that overload us with emotional baggage and brain programming we may carry from our childhoods. The toxic effect of these problems is potentially so severe that many docs feel that childhood maltreatment should be handled as a disease.[2035] Facing early childhood traumas through our adult eyes, instead of perpetuating infantile memories about them,[2036] may help us forgive others, abandon self-defeating and victimizing programming, and regain a sense of fairness about life—a very important key to good health.[2037]

Forgiving and forgetting are a must to maintain health, especially in our intimate relationships. Defending our roughed up egos by perpetuating our rights to feel victimized and slip into apathy about life makes us more likely to struggle with IR. The more hostility we harbor, the higher our blood glucose levels; this may be mitigated by a good marriage.[2038] Apathetic diabetics have a harder time controlling their blood sugars.[2039]

Story Time

A priest was trying to figure out if a little girl's claim to speak with God was true. Every test or question he designed could not provide the proof he wanted. In desperation, he told the girl to ask God what he himself had asked God to forgive him about in his last personal confession. When the girl came back from talking to God again, the priest anxiously asked what God had said about his confession. The little girl replied that God had forgotten all about his confession.

That's What Friends Are For

The more we belong to a community, the less preoccupied we are with self-pity and self-aggrandizement. The ego thrives when we feel lonely and isolated. The more socially-oriented we are, the less we dwell in our own little corner of the universe. As we commune with our fellowmen, we become more exposed to their suffering and we then get to see that our own suffering is either not as bad as we thought and/or we are able to see that all suffering is part of life.

> "Excessive assertion of a philosophy of self-interest with belonging, and excessive expression of relational philosophy forfeits individuality; we have to keep both in check."[2040]

A balance of individuality and being part of a community is best. The problem is that in the United States we are leaning a bit toward pathologic isolation. The case of Roseto, Penn., is a good example. From its beginnings, Roseto's population was made up of mostly Italian-Americans who had immigrated from the same town in Italy. They maintained very close community ties, pretty much like we see in the movie *Mediterraneo.* Despite eating diets high in fat and pasta, they had nearly half the incidence of heart disease compared to other counties in Pennsylvania. When the citizens of Roseto started to lose their close community ties in the sixties and seventies, their incidents of heart problems increased and matched those of other typically disconnected American cities.[2041]

Scratching Our Backs

Altruistic behavior is hardwired in our brains, like any other survival behavior.[2042] "Selfish altruism" realizes that the best way to take care of one's self is to advance the interests of the community.[2043] Sadly, human nature with its "either/or" mentality thrives in splitting these two balancing principles and contributes to the polarizing of our society. On one side, we have those who preach Darwinian capitalism; on the other side, we have those who feel that government involvement will fix all our problems. Why is it so hard to see that we may have the cake and eat it, too?

When Gandhi was asked whether his reasons for serving the poor were purely humanitarian, he replied, "Not at all. Rather, I am here to serve myself only, to find my own self-realization through the service of others." This is a concept I struggled with when I was a missionary in my youth. After much soul-searching, I came to terms with "selfish altruism"; the more we give, the more we receive. But, growing older has necessitated this simple principle to be constantly relearned.

Our giving-nature may be thwarted by emotional trauma early in our childhoods, leading to egocentric attitudes clear into adulthood. Of course, we may change this, but only if we are aware that this may be a problem. As you saw in the chapter about our adrenal glands, often our metabolisms are less efficient when our HPA axes are compromised, making the chances of developing sweet death later in life more likely.

Story Time

I wasn't able to see my dad for what he really was until after he died. My emotional issues from a rather traumatic childhood kept me from seeing the goodness in him. Perhaps your own story is a better example of how early emotional trauma may keep us from actualizing our giving nature. My story probably

---

pales in comparison to yours. So, forgive me for indulging in it. I do so to illustrate a few points.

My dad was a French-Chilean who was raised feeling more French than Chilean. On more than one occasion, he told my mother (Chilean-Basque) that he resented the fact that she had given birth to a child with dark skin, me; maybe he was mad at her because she left us repeatedly, shortly after I was born. My overwhelmed mother was just fourteen years old. I had to come to terms with that, too . . .

My dad had records of Edith Piaf and Maurice Chevalier playing all the time in his bistro. I will never forget the night he read to me from his favorite book, *Les Miserables*, by Victor Hugo. Fighting back tears, he struggled through the part when Jean Valjean puts his cover as the mayor of his little town in jeopardy. Valjean lifted a runaway cart off the body of the only man who hated him in that town. Inspector Javert watched in disbelief as Valjean accomplished the feat, bringing back memories of the only "other man" he knew who was strong enough to lift such a heavy load: the parole-breaker 24601.

Valjean had been imprisoned because he had stolen a loaf of bread to feed his nephew. After seventeen years in jail he broke free, but he was still a prisoner of intense hate. He became a saint after being redeemed by a priest and henceforth dedicated his life to serve the less fortunate and his adopted daughter, Cosette. I cried with my father that night. I still cry every time I watch the play, "Les Mis," —even the tenth time when I watched it with my wife and my six-year-old, little Cosette.

May we all stop suffering from our bruised egos and hearts and dedicate our lives to serving others. And may we overcome the dire consequences of a past stuffed with bad, refined sugars and bad "bread."

"Resistance is Futile"

If you are familiar with the Borg from *Star Trek*, you know that nanotechnology is advancing quite rapidly, making that science fiction show a not-too-distant reality. Many health problems will likely be addressed by replacing body and brain function with nanochips. No doubt sweet death issues will also be addressed by trying to turn us into cyborgs—part man and part machine. The allure of a future where we may live forever aided by machines is too hard to resist. In his book, *The Singularity Is Near,* Dr. Ray Kurzweil predicts that we will become something beyond Homo economicus, when we will "mutate" into a higher being that likely will conquer death itself.

I am sure that science will take us so far that we will be pushing the envelope of our very nature. However, I feel our poor track record on how we deal with advanced technology makes it likely that such advanced science will be used to inflict more pain and suffering on each other. I also feel that if these lofty scientific concepts become reality, they will be for the benefit of the rich and famous, not the common man. In my opinion, cyborg-like goals are yet another reflection of the ego which refuses to yield to the finality of its own demise.

Still, I believe that we can develop more understanding and a greater capacity to love one another.[2044]

Munching Together

A survey of 527 teens aged twelve to eighteen showed that those who ate a meal with an adult in their family an average of five days a week (versus three days a week) tended to smoke and abuse drugs less, drinks less alcohol, were more motivated in school, and more optimistic about the future.[2045] People who laugh more at dinnertime have lower glucose levels.[2046]

Children of breastfeeding moms with a sense of humor "had markedly reduced [eczematous] reactions." These moms had higher levels of melatonin in their milk, which is lower in people with eczema. Their milk was tested while they watched Charlie Chaplin movies or boring weather footage.[2047] Remember the gut-brain connection? Most serotonin, the happy neurotransmitter and a cousin to melatonin, is found in the intestines—a key factor in our sweet deaths. (The link between eczema and intestinal health is well proven.)[2048]

Everything about the universe is creation-destruction. Our bodies are no different. They need E&I from our food to fuel the massive recreation of every molecule in our bodies. Eating is a sacred activity whereby we incorporate the universe, or God, into ourselves. This is why eating together is a sacrament in most religions.

In *The Upanishads*, Eknath Easwaran writes, "I am the food of life, I am, I am; I eat the food of life, I eat, I eat."[2049]

I Link, Therefore I Am

The mind-body-spirit connection gets a lot of attention in more spiritual and psychological fields. I feel that the heart-body-spirit connection is just as important. I am not poo-pooing logic and intellect, but I do belong to "intellectual anonymous." I often see people who over-rely on their logic only to atrophy their feelings. I feel that they will not heal until they realize that our intellect may be fooled, but our hearts always see clearly.

"What is important is invisible to the eye;
it is only with the heart that we see clearly."[2050]

The Frenchman René Descartes famously declared, "I think, therefore I am," and thereby started the modern era of logic as king. In my opinion, this is when feelings, intuition, and the heart were relegated to second banana status.

I was amused to read that the new French government led by President Sarkozy has come out saying, "Enough thinking, already." Of course, the intellectuals in France who think that the French president should not show his knees while jogging are very upset with these developments.[2051]

Logic got us to the moon, but we are not able to solve our social ills on Earth. While we need a strong ego and logic to get along in this world, it is the heart that wins every time. After years of struggling with intellectual pursuits, and being quite proud of my intellect, one day I was able to renounce all that and surrendered my life to the mystery of creation. Since then, I have been very happy and at peace. As a synthesizer, I now say, "I link, therefore I am."

Heartdroppings

We are light beings highly sensitive to the E&I that exist all around us. Some of you surely call these things God and his Gospel. Others have different beliefs that I venture say mirror these concepts, but the doctrines may be stated slightly differently. Please, don't be offended. Don't let my "karma run over your dogma."

Immersed in the mad rush of our busy lives, often we cannot find a few moments of solitude to recharge our batteries and seek the divine within us through meditation or prayer. We may learn from Odysseus who, after being assaulted by the singing of sirens and becoming shipwrecked, says, "Alone, alone at last." When we slow down enough to still the waters, to see clearly the bottom of our spiritual ponds, we catch a glimpse of what the wise man said about living a simple life:

> "When an ordinary man gets knowledge, he becomes a
>   sage.
> When a sage gets understanding, he becomes an ordinary
>   man."[2052]

This sweet realization cannot come to us unless we are quiet enough to cultivate awareness. Once we see how simple life is, we understand the words of The Prophet; we are filled with gratitude and we sing of it at every waking moment:

> "Take no thought for your life, what ye shall eat, or what
> ye shall drink. Which of you by taking thought can add one
> cubit unto his stature? Consider the lilies of the field, how
> they grow; they TOIL not, neither do they spin: and yet I say
> unto you, that even Solomon in all his glory was not arrayed
> like one of these."[2053]

As long as we are above ground (and vertical), it is a good day. Awakening to the beauty of simplicity and non-striving, we see that our suffering—like our sweet deaths or our addictions to refined sugars—is but an opportunity to heal by humbling ourselves, live by our hearts, and hear their whispers saying that life is a transitory step to living in unity with all. Lots of books have been written about our minds and hearts influencing our physiology, and vice-versa. They have been written by better minds and hearts that specialize in these topics. Perhaps you would like to read some of their work. But, then again, must you always intellectualize everything? You may want to start with a few of my favorites:

- *Why Zebras Don't Get Ulcers*[2054] by Robert Sapolsky is about the harmful physiology of stress.

- *The Biology of Belief*[2055] by Dr. Bruce Lipton is about emotional and psychological issues contributing to cell membrane TOILing. Dr. Lipton also demonstrates how it is that our heart/mind may modulate our body functions and our perception of the universe.

- *The Intention Experiment*[2056] by Lynne McTaggart is about modern research in paranormal phenomena. You would be surprised to read that there is lots of research validating those experiences.

- *Cell-Level Healing*[2057] by Dr. Joyce Whiteley Hawkes is like Dr. Lipton's book, but more "touchy-feely."

- *Full Catastrophe Living*[2058] by Dr. Jon Kabat-Zinn is great to learn to relax and meditate.

- *Living from the Heart*[2059] is Gandhi's autobiography.

- *Space, Time & Medicine*[2060] by Dr. Larry Dossey is written by a medical doctor who has a lot of clinical experience on mind-body healing.

- *Love & Survival*[2061] by Dr. Dean Ornish documents that heart disease is often a result of a wounded heart.

- *Self-Efficacy: The Exercise of Control*[2062] by Dr. Albert Bandura teaches readers to regain control by focusing on "heart issues."

- *Les Miserables*[2063] is by Victor Hugo. I dare you read this long, long book. Don't wimp out with the condensed version if you love history.

- *The Little Prince,*[2064] by Antoine de Saint-Exupéry, is my other most favorite literature book. It won the Nobel Prize in 1945. I don't want to tell you what it is about so that you may be thoroughly delighted and touched by reading it in less than ninety minutes.

- *Jitterbug Perfume,*[2065] by Tom Robbins, is about repressed sexuality. It is raunchy, funny, rebellious, and full of sex and passion—just the stuff you want to read.

Sleep On It

When I was a little boy in Viña del Mar, Chile, I was bummed when naps were done away with so that people wouldn't have to go home in the middle of the day from work. Economists argued that productivity would go up. Did it? No, says a recent article that showed the annual loss of productive time worth $136.4 billion annually in the United States may be reduced by 34 percent if employees take a nap.[2066] Talk about sawing too much wood without letting the saw cool down. If you still don't feel like napping, check this out: naps reduce the risk of dying from a heart attack by 37 percent.[2067]

"Vitamin S" or sex, also helps us relax. Most women find it a bit annoying how relaxing sex can be for men. While women would like to hug or cuddle post-romp, most guys just roll over and start snoring. Did you know that the average woman burns 500 calories when she makes love? Too bad the average guy only lasts 5 calories. Don't have a heart attack, okay? If you do, you don't have to worry about your ticker when you resume sexual activity.[2068]

I Have a Dream

Dreaming is the best way to understand reality according to many traditions, including Buddhism and Judeo-Christianity. Too bad that dreaming has not been accessed very often to help people heal. But hope is on the way: many docs are getting into dream work with their patients.[2069] I will never forget a little old German lady who told me that in a dream she had been told that she had a "fistula" in her intestines. She didn't even know what the word meant. Thanks to an understanding gastroenterologist who performed an urgent colonoscopy, she survived a potentially fatal bleeding episode in her intestines; a fistula is a pathologic connection between an intestinal loop and a blood vessel.

I found out through a dream that I had ankylosing spondylitis. In my opinion, any health problem including TOILing, IR, and the metabolic syndrome may be helped if we just open our hearts to the power of dreaming. If you wish to know more about this, read *The Healing Power of Dreams* by Dr. Patricia Garfield.

Chapter 35

Other Forms of Treatment

Once you understand the basic concepts of E&I, cell communication, metabolism, and the effects of TOILing you may see why rather "odd" interventions seem to help us lick sweet death. It is worth considering non-pharmaceutical treatments of sweet death, particularly when the TOILing is so advanced that people suffer in a lot of pain, like we see in diabetic neuropathy. After all, "only about a third of patients with painful diabetic neuropathy respond to conventional pharmaceutical therapies." With such poor results, it seems logical for more than 40 percent of patients try things like alpha lipoic acid, biofield therapies, infrared phototherapy, and pulse-magnetic field therapies.[2070]

Pushing the Envelope

There is a lot of energy on information about stem cells. The Bush administration vetoed funding for this type of work, despite clear evidence that we may harvest stem cells without "killing an embryo." Just about every other country has given the green light to their researchers to investigate potential cures for every disease, including type 1 diabetes by transplanting pancreatic cells. A study showed that fourteen out of fifteen patients got off insulin with stem cell work.[2071]

Please, Google "umbical cord stem cells" for your state for more information. You may be able to store some of your baby's cells at birth for "future use." Several other non-embryo sources of cells seem to be developed each year, like bloodlines and skin cells.[2072] In my opinion, it would be a terrible loss if we didn't explore this form of treatment further. I understand the concerns that some of us have about genetic work. I agree that we could overstep an ethical and moral line.

Nanotechnology is progressing by leaps and bounds.[2073] Some feel that soon the lines between machine and man will be blurred. But the potential gain in health-related fields like E&I issues, cell communication, and TOILing is limitless. Nanochips to record dietary patterns will soon be available; we will know exactly what foods each of us does better with.[2074] But the chances that we may screw up are significant, as we have frequently done in the past.

"Flab jabs," or shots of chemicals to dissolve fat, are not FDA approved—yet.[2075] Since obesity is so hard to treat, anything, including flab jabs, is likely to be seriously considered, especially if there is money to be made. The safety of this intervention will probably be kicked around for a while.

I am sure I am missing many other approaches to overcoming sweet death. If you find them, and they have scientific evidence to back them up, or if they have very little, if any, side effects, try them, provided that you don't get ripped off in the process. A good test would be to see if they match the simple concepts of E&I outlined in this book.

Detoxification

Once you understand TOILing and the "T" that stands for "toxicity," you may see why detoxification treatments help in sweet death. It all boils down to thermodynamics: any engine, including our cells' mitochondria, needs good fuel and a method to rid itself of the products of combustion to operate optimally. Genetically, we have different capacities to detoxify; some do it more efficiently than others.[2076] Think of the cars you have owned: some performed better than others because of their engines' thermodynamics and exhaust performances.

Still, there will be some who will try to tell you that detoxification diets don't work.[2077] I feel they ignore the basic E&I and TOILing principles you now are familiar with.

> "Food-derived chemicals, [like] cruciferous vegetables and fruits, modulate CYP expression and the expression of genes that encode cytoprotective phase 2 enzymes. Indoles and flavonoids activate CYP1A expression either by direct ligand interaction with the AhR receptor or by augmenting the interaction with xenobiotic response elements in target genes."[2078]

Huh? I know; that was a bit too technical. I threw that in for the benefit of those who still doubt that food is the best way to detoxify our cell membranes. These delicate structures need the right nutrients to function properly. Besides, all the organs involved in detoxification need proper E&I to carry out their detoxification functions. In my opinion, the best and simplest way to detoxify is to eat good food and improve intestinal function with lots of fiber and probiotics. (The latter also unburdens the liver.)

If you want to do more, start by sweating a lot through exercise. And if you are really ambitious, take coffee enemas. They are still being used in Europe. The other day I saw people forming a line to get out of Starbucks. Odd, I thought. But, after a second look, I realized they were backing into the store.

Other forms of detoxification may be considered, like colonics and several special nutrition-based formulas. While they all have merits, they may tend to enable you to continue to eat poorly. Why have a hose rammed up your butt when you still labor under your sugar addiction? Besides, anything from outside that ends up used all the time does not empower you. It would be sad to depend on a Roto-Rooter tech just to have a bowel movement. The "bottom line" is that you may reduce TOILing by detoxifying and thereby reducing IR and sweet death.

Sweating It Out

In my youth, I worked out to do better in soccer. As I got older, my motivation began to change. Not so long ago I worked out mostly out of vanity and to maintain my weight. Now, it's a combination of all those things, plus sweating out the toxins. As you choose some form of exercise, I hope you pick one that will make you sweat a lot. Now, why do you stink so badly after a workout? (At least I do.) It's because of the toxins being excreted.

More natural societies seem to have detoxification rituals, such as sweat lodges. They also feel that maintaining a healthy body through decreasing toxicity has a lot to do with better cognition and spiritual awareness. If you wish to try a sweat lodge, consult your doctor and avoid drugs alcohol while doing it.

Modern sauna practices with radiant heat have been shown to help with several conditions: multiple chemical sensitivity,[2079] rehabilitation from non-acute heart attacks,[2080] high blood pressure,[2081] congestive heart failure,[2082] and anorexia.[2083] I suspect that saunas are likely to help in practically all conditions (remember TOILing). We just don't have much evidence along those lines yet. But the fact that hot baths reduce IR is a good indication that this is the case. Hot baths help detoxification issues and increase circulation to our muscles; they use up glucose more effectively.[2084] There are some contraindications to saunas, however, including high-risk pregnancies, severe aortic stenosis, unstable angina, and recent heart attacks.

Cancer Prevention

While this book cannot address cancer issues in detail as this frightening topic deserves, I would like to throw in a few pearls. Cancer, in my opinion, is an immune-detoxification problem heavily impacted by the E&I we process, particularly in our DNA. Sweet death has a lot to do with these issues, as you saw in chapter 24. Besides, cancer is not a very good way to lose weight . . .

It turns out that proper nutrition may prevent two-thirds of cancers as proven by the article, "Apoptosis by Dietary Factors."[2085] And wouldn't you know it: the authors zero in on two vital concepts to manage cancerous cells:

"The two major pathways that initiate apoptosis are extrinsic (receptor-mediated) and intrinsic (mitochondrial mediated). Mitogenic and stress-responsive pathways are involved in the regulation of apoptotic signaling. Noteworthy is the crosstalk between some of these pathways."

Hmmm, that sounds a lot like energy and communication of information, don't you think? This is exactly what we find in two articles recently published in the *Journal Science:* "Tumor Biology: How Signaling Processes Translate to Therapy," and "Metabolic Targeting as an Anticancer Strategy: Dawn of a New Era?"[2086] A good nutrition program to decrease the ravages of sweet death and maximize our immune-detox pathways may reasonably be expected to help a lot of us with cancer issues. I can be very categorical with respect to prevention of cancer and this approach. But I have to be somewhat more circumspect when it comes to treating cancer already developing. Still, I have seen a lot of my patients do very well when thus afflicted. However, I cannot make any promises. Cancer, as you know, is not easily treated.

"A new paradigm for diet, nutrition, and cancer prevention can be developed using multidisciplinary approaches that include lifestyle and environmental changes, dietary modifications, and physical activity consciousness to reduce the burden of cancer for high risk patients and general public as well."[2087]

"An obsession with curing advanced disease has blinded cancer researchers to the promise of prevention . . . The concept that people with cancer are healthy until a doctor tells them that they've got an invasive lesion makes no sense at all."[2088]

Chapter 36

The Proof of the Pudding

Pudding is full of processed sugar and toxic dairy. Still, the proof is in eating it. Some may say what follows are a bunch of testimonials as if this line of evidence was not acceptable. I disagree, especially after we have herein reviewed more than two thousand references from reputable medical journals. I believe my patients' experiences and those of wise and more experienced practitioners have value; we would do well to duplicate them. To feel otherwise makes me wonder if opposing beliefs may be influenced by whoever is signing their checks. If this were true, no amount of evidence will convince them to open their minds:

> "Physicians trying to individualize clinical decisions have been forced to rely on judgment, empathic communications, and informal rules of thumb. Might this time-honored approach be improved if decision analysis were used not just to assess clinical strategies for groups of patients, but also as a tool to support decision-making at the level of the individual patient? [We must understand] the cognitive processes of those master clinicians who consistently make superb decisions without recourse to the canon of evidence-based medicine."[2089]

Do we have all the evidence we need to pass judgment on the positive experiences of those who, with nothing but the nutritional tools available to all of us, have healed 90 percent of what afflicts the common man?

> "[The] amount of information published in the medical journals far outpaces the ability to organize it . . . we don't know a whole lot anymore about too many topics . . . This dumbing down is not ideal for medical education . . . A broad glimpse of recent medical findings may help some of us retreat from reductionist ways of thinking that have been ingrained as we become increasingly specialized. Such cross-fertilization can stimulate new avenues of research."[2090]

Critics of "testimonials" often argue that "there is not enough evidence to justify the use of non-pharmaceutical approaches" as if what they usually practice, that is, the "standard of care" were 100 percent sanctioned by solid evidence. They should read the cover story to the J. Business Weekly, May 29, 2006. The article "Medical Guesswork: from heart surgery to prostate care, the health industry knows little about which common treatments really work", written by Dr. David Eddy, an expert in evidence medicine (a term he coined himself) tells us that about 75 percent of what docs do routinely lacks clear evidence. Talk about the teapot calling the kettle black.

A Note Before Getting Personal

Despite the best efforts from caretakers and patients, some people will need medication. This might be offensive to purists who maintain that drugs are never justified. I disagree with this extreme view. In my opinion, some conditions are too entrenched and too genetically loaded. Besides, some patients may not be able to motivate themselves to change their toxic lifestyles. Also, some situations require immediate pharmaceutical attention at a time of crisis. This is why we must have pharmaceutical drugs available.

The problem is that these lifesaving pharmaceuticals are often marketed for common day-to-day ailments, too. In other words, some diseases are created for the sole purpose of selling drugs. Think of ADD, osteoporosis, reflux, etc. We often watch TV commercials with happy, good-looking actors showing their dentures and frolicking in meadows where butterflies are pollinating to beat the ban.[2091] These ads never address the *cause* of the problem; unfortunately many people don't seem to feel this is important or necessary. Just pop a pill and continue living the way that got them in trouble.

Finally, we are ready to hear about my patients getting better. All of them get supplementation, but only after they change their diets and overcome their sugar addictions.

Metabolic Syndrome

For practical purposes, I am referring to the narrow definition of the metabolic syndrome, that is, the clustering of high blood pressure, high cholesterol, obesity, too much clotting, uric acid elevation, and diabetes/pre-diabetes. Most of these patients take L-arginine, omega oils, ALA, CoQ10, vitamins B, D3 and K, "SugarReg" (trademark containing chromium, vanadium, and gymnema sylvestre), calcium, magnesium, potassium, carnitine, and panax ginseng.

Their blood pressure drops anywhere from 10 to 60 points.[2092] Did you know that any of the $100+ drugs only drop blood pressure by 10 points? If you needed to lower your blood pressure by 60 points, you would need six drugs. Most of these patients stop taking oral diabetic pills. Some of them are able to stop insulin injections and virtually all of the patients still requiring insulin cut down on the amount they need. Most pre-diabetics return to normal.

Most of them reduce their waist sizes (remember we don't worry about weight). Most of them get rid of their dysrhythmias (funny heart beats), chest pain, and lower their risk of future heart disease. Some of them get proof of reversing plaque in the coronaries. Most of them lower their cholesterol without medications. For these patients I use a lot of fiber, like guar gum, fermented red rice, and "Heart Plus" —Dr. Linus Pauling's formula of amino acids and vitamin C to lower cholesterol.[2093]

Hormones

Most women shrink their breast lumps, uterine fibroids (over-growth of muscle tissue due to poor detoxification of xenoestrogens), resolve their PMS/PMDD problems, ease menopausal symptoms, and even become pregnant (if they were infertile) by changing their diets and supplementing most of the following items: I3C, MSM, curcumin, B-complex, omega oils, calcium, magnesium, and vitamin D. Some of them require items necessary to work on hyperinsulinemia more aggressively (ALA and perhaps metformin).

Thyroid dysfunction is a tough one because environmental toxins are causing a lot of thyroid dysfunction.[2094] Remember that thyroid problems are not just due to hyperinsulinemia. I noted before that many patients cannot get off prescription medications. But for those who don't want any drugs at all I supplement the herb, dulce, along with thyroid support: omega oils, iodine, selenium (Brazil nuts), and/or guggulu. The adrenal glands must always be supported when working on thyroid issues since these two hormones are very interrelated. Some patients get licorice, DHEA, and panax ginseng, too.

Testosterone deficiencies get better when IR is corrected (see above). Still, most patients need prescription replacement. Testosterone function may be supplemented with the herbs, maca and yohimbine. DHEA is a precursor to testosterone and it is very safe to supplement. A more flexible mind that is willing to explore lots of fun things in the privacy of one's bedroom may also help. For best results, the participants are communicating and relating to one another very well and maintain each others' well being as their main concern.

Kidneys

Kidney stones stop being made when people overcome their sweet tooth and use the supplements listed above for diabetes. Kidney failure is extremely challenging, but I do see kidney function improve with N-acetyl-cysteine, CoQ10, omega oils, asparagus, stinging nettles, and "Kidney Support," a trade name for a combination of herbs and micronutrients.

Immune System

Any patient with immune problems is put on a program to maximize intestinal function (see below). Most patients get rid of frequent infections. Children stop having ear infections, particularly when they get off dairy. Most people stop having so many colds and, if they get the flu, it does not last as long. Even people with autoimmune disorders, such as rheumatoid arthritis (see below), find significant relief; some are totally cured.

Dr. Paul Farmer's experience in Haiti is worth relating here. He has been able to successfully treat drug-resistant tuberculosis by putting together (with donated money) a cocktail of five or more drugs. This was considered a modern miracle, given the devastating nature of the problem and the overwhelming problems faced by that poor country. Interestingly, we never heard much about his follow-up act: he cured 98 percent of patients by providing good nutrition for them . . .[2095]

Most of these patients get IgG 2000 DF™, which is more powerful than colostrum. They also get elderberry for their colds. Most of them learn to lavage their sinuses with sesame oil and/or xylitol. After that, they are no longer tortured by frequent sinus infections. All of them get high doses of antioxidants, even by injection and sometimes through their veins. Uva ursis and cranberry juice are very helpful in urinary infections.

Cancer

This is a tough one, especially when we are losing our battle with this disease. Since this is also an immune problem, I put cancer patients on an intestinal cleanse (see below). The danger here is to give cancer patients too many supplements. I feel this is unfortunately a very common occurrence. I often see desperate patients being sold too many things because they are desperate to try anything. Might this be the same reason behind that fact that some patients tend to get too much chemotherapy in their last three months of life?

I advise patients suffering from cancer to take a regimen of supplementation that is realistic, evidence-based, and financially feasible (remember that I do not sell any products) such as: digestive enzymes, probiotics, fiber, IV vitamin C, omega oils, SAMe, vitamin D, the herbs pawpaw and anamu, and more specific antioxidants depending of what type of cancer is involved. If nothing else, I feel that this approach at least lowers our chances of relapses and of getting cancer in the first place. While my record in curing cancer is just as spotty as the pharmaceutical approach, I do see people living longer and in better shape.

Unfortunately, their oncologists who often dismiss any improvement in the patients' laboratory markers by attributing such good news to "spontaneous remissions" often discourage these patients. Some patients are even told that anything non-pharmaceutical is placebo.

I must tell you about Betty who told me I could use her name: she had stage IV ovarian cancer, which is pretty bad. She was very aggressive with diet and supplementation; she stunned her oncologist by surviving much longer and in much better shape than younger patients. She even had rosy cheeks. Despite all these good news, she was summarily told to stop all her supplements. Betty eventually passed away, but she and her family were grateful to have spent those extra years together.

Mind/Brain

All patients with Parkinson's disease, multiple sclerosis, and Alzheimer's disease improve with a change in diet. Some of them see their symptoms totally eliminated. They use a great book by Dr. David Perlmutter, *Brainrecovery.com,* to guide them through the principles we discuss. All of them follow the intestinal protocol because most neurotransmitters are found in the intestines. Most of them get omega oils (especially decosahexanoic acid, or DHA), phosphatidylserine, B-complex, glutathione, CoQ10, L-arginine, carnitine, the herbs huperzine A and sage, calcium, magnesium, and vitamin D. Some of them get other supplements according to their individual presentation.

For depression, which most patients overcome without drugs they mostly get SAMe, L-tryptophan, melatonin, B-complex, DHA, DHEA, CoQ10 and Panax ginseng. Some of them get St. John's wort, which is to be used with caution in patients taking prescription drugs. Of course, all of them get a pep talk on changing their views of the world. Most patients suffering from depression need to become more flexible and learn to forgive and laugh more, even in the face of misery.

For insomnia, most people find relief with l-tryptophan, gotu kola, gaba, passion fruit, and melatonin. Did you know that the newest drug to treat insomnia, ramelteon/remeron, is really melatonin? After people change their diets to low-glycemic programs, take some supplements, and adopt healthier lifestyles the majority of them are able to get off antidepressants and even improve their sleep patterns.

The Second Brain: The Intestinal Tract

This is where I find the most success. Irritable bowel syndrome, ulcerative colitis, and Crohn's disease are virtually *cured* when people follow an intestinal cleanse program. I have had many patients avoid recommended surgery to rip out their colons and part of their small intestines by following an intestinal protocol that involves probiotics, or friendly bacteria, digestive enzymes, lots of fiber and omega oils, glutamine, IgG 2000 DF, whey protein, and in some cases, selected antibiotics to go after ever-present organisms that may mutate and become more toxic.

These antibiotics must not be absorbed into the body. This is especially true in people with bad diets, taking too many antibiotics, and drinking chlorinated/fluoridated water. Thankfully, non-prescription items often suffice in ridding the intestines of parasites, excessive fungus, and mutating bacteria. These trade name items are very helpful: Silver Shield, Paracleanse, Yeast Detox, and Gastric Health.

People with gall bladder stones do very well ridding themselves of many stones by doing cleanses that must be closely supervised. Most hepatitis problems will improve with ALA, selenium, milk thistle, glutathione, whey, SAMe, and MSM. Most patients normalize their liver enzymes by following these recommendations. Ulcers and reflux are virtually cured in almost all patients just by changing their diets and adding some supplements in some cases: cayenne pepper, glucosamine, cabbage juice, ginger, bromelain, and licorice DGL.

Remember that patients with brain and immune issues also benefit from this approach.

Bone/Arthritic Problems

As noted above, most patients with rheumatoid arthritis will improve by doing an intestinal cleanse. Some are even cured. I will never forget a patient who came in with rheumatoid arthritis and evaluated his pain as ten on a scale of one through ten. His ESR, a marker for inflammation, was 90 mm/hr (normal is 15-20). He was extremely stiff and could not ambulate well; his hands were deformed. After treatment, his pain dropped to zero out of ten and then went up to three out of ten when he got in and out of a chair. His ESR came down to 30 and he was able to walk with no discomfort; his hands became functional. Was he happy with these results? No; he got mad when I refused to sign his disability papers.

For cases of rheumatoid arthritis, I add high dose omega EPA oils, glucosamine, chondritin, MSM, SAMe, boswellia, lots of avocados, and in some cases, hormonal support, as mentioned above.

For osteoporosis patients, most people will do just fine with calcium, magnesium, and vitamin D3. The latter is the most important and often it needs to be supplemented up to 5,000 IU a day. Exercise, weight lifting, and avoiding refined foods are also beneficial.

Gout responds to a low-glycemic index diet. Most of these patients do very well with the diabetic type of supplements that are listed above.

Asthma and Allergies

As noted above, these problems respond to intestinal cleansing, particularly when H. pilory is present.[2096] The majority of patients get off their medications by doing so. In some cases, I add the herbs, stinging nettle and lobelia, in addition to N-acetylcysteine (even in inhaler form) and omega oils. I also recommend a sinus lavage with sesame oil and/or xylitol, colloidal silver, and MSM.

Conclusion

Since 1998, most of the Nobel Prizes in medicine and biology have been awarded to research on cell communication of E&I. What we have discussed in this book are the practical applications of such work, which validates the holistic approach we have intuitively embraced. Still, cell communication, as esoteric a concept it might be, is totally dependent on the basics of classical medicine: nutrition, the environment, and the mind-body connection. These are the common sense, layman's way of describing metabolomics.

Everything is creation-destruction—even capitalism—which, in the hands of special interests, will do anything to keep from being overtaken/destroyed by competing forces. Think of the tremendous pull and resources put into motion to perpetuate a worn-out paradigm of treating symptoms with drugs, instead of addressing the simple concepts found in this book.

I am keenly aware that I may have given you "too much information." I did so to empower you to fight the forces that seek to deny the validity of these concepts. Even with all these references before their eyes, they will more than likely not concede that there might be some merits to a non-pharmaceutical approach to health care.

Let's Communicate E&I

In my opinion, an integrative approach to health is the best way to cope with our society's sweet death. When we come to an integrative table to discuss each other's ideas and talents, we must do it with an awareness of how our egos and financial interests may blind us to the merits of unfamiliar ideas. If these "alternative" ways have valid scientific evidence, they must be allowed at the table for the benefit of our patients.

Integrative thinking will continue to grow because it is correct and it is what people want. My heart has been committed to integration since I was a child when I taught myself to become a "lefty" to do better in school, on the basketball court, and on the soccer field. Today, I see the collective wisdom of integrative minds and hearts far surpass that of any single, isolated person. A great example is George Washington; his main domestic policy was "unity." He understood that if the fledging United States was to survive, he and other politicians needed to leave their egos at the door and transient party politics. Washington even had Thomas Jefferson, a republican as secretary of state and Alexander Hamilton, a federalist as secretary of the treasury in his cabinet. They were the founders of very antagonistic political parties whose venom almost doomed our nation at its inception. Abraham Lincoln also assembled a *Team of Rivals*[2097] to compose his cabinet; he called on the very men who ran against him.

For the good of our patients/clients, we must leave our narrow interests, our egos, and the influence of whomever butters our bread at the door as we humbly sit at the integrative table I envision. There, we may partake of E&I to keep our children and ourselves from suffering a sweet death.

Our Mission

We will not be successful in motivating our patients, loved ones, and the public at large unless we engage, as one article calls it, "The Most Powerful Therapeutic Force."[2098] And, what could that be? The personal relationship we have with our patients and clients.

Do you wish to be of help in our society? You may start by helping loved ones overcome their sugar addictions. We cannot do this unless we become aware of the forces at play keeping us addicted. To maximize profits, Big Food is hooking our children, and us, with billions of dollars worth of advertisement: do like the guy in the movie, *Network*. Open your window and shout at the top of your lungs: "I am mad as hell and I am not going to take it anymore!"

You must become the change you seek in health care. You must be empowered within yourself to change and develop healthy habits of mind, body, and spirit. The legend of the Holy Grail and King Arthur pulling the sword from the stone are allegories of finding truth within; *that* is enlightenment.

As we wrap up this book, I wish you the power/energy to find information within you to find what you seek: maximizing your health.[2099]

Story Time: Parting Words

1. On Air Force One, a certain president of the United States, on his way to give a speech in Florida to promote dietary and physical fitness, had his "lunch menu printed on gold-edged cards for all passengers [offering] corned beef sandwich, steak fries, and strawberry cheesecake."[2100]

2. A mother went to seek Gandhi's advice to get her child to stop eating refined sugar. Gandhi thought for a moment and then said, "Bring your child back tomorrow." The puzzled mother did so; Gandhi then told the child, "Stop eating candy." The perplexed woman then asked, "Why didn't you tell him that yesterday?" Gandhi replied, "Yesterday, I was eating candy myself."

It is your relationship with your loved ones, your patients, and your clients that will win the day. It is by your personal example that you will be most successful. Do you truly want to help people, or do you only wish to sell something? Your answer will greatly influence the degree of success you will have in treating sweet death. If you truly want to help people, stop eating candy.[2101] May the "force" be with you, so that you, too, can communicate this information with the power of conviction and through leading by example.

References

1   *Nature,* Dec. 14, 2006

2   *Metabolism—Clinical and Experimental* 2008; 57: 1345

3   *Archives of Pediatrics and Adolescent Medicine* 2008; 162: 764

4   "Impaired Fasting Glucose and Impaired Glucose Tolerance, as Well as Known Diabetes, Increased Risk for Death Within Five Years," *Circulation* 2007: 116: 151

5   *New York Times,* July 25, 2008

6   Seth Lloyd, *Programming the Universe,* 2006, (Alfred A. Knopf Press: 2006)

7   Bruce Lipton, *The Biology of Belief* (Mountain of Love/Elite Books: 2005)

8   Paul Pearsall, *The Heart's Code,* (Broadway Books: 1998)

9   "The Finnish Diabetes Risk Score is Associated with Insulin Resistance and Progression Towards Type 2 Diabetes," *Journal of Clinical Endocrinology & Metabolism* 2009, 94: 920

10 "You Are What You Grow," *New York Times Magazine,* April 22, 2007, page 15

11 *Archives of Surgery,* August 2008

12 "Understanding and Addressing the Epidemic of Obesity: An Energy Balance Perspective," *Endocrine Reviews* 2006; 27: 750

13 *New England Journal of Medicine* 1998; 338: 171

14 Stephen Wolfram, *A New Kind of Science* (Wolfram Media, Inc.: 2002)

15 "The Puzzle of Complex Diseases," *Science* 2002; 296: 605-792

16 *Nature Genetics,* September 2007

17 "The Conflict Between Complex Systems and Reductionism," *Journal of the American Medical Association* 2008; 300: 1580

18 *Archives of Internal Medicine* 2007; 167: 750, 766, 774

19 Edward O. Wilson, *Consilience: The Unity of Knowledge* (Alfred A. Knopf Press: 1998)

20 J. Lancet 2003; 362:93

21 "Homo Obesus: A Metabotrophin-Deficient Species, Pharmacology and Nutrition Insight," J. *Current Pharmaceutical Design* 2007; 13: 2176

22 *New England Journal of Medicine* 2007; 356: 213

23 "Fat Inc," J. *Readers Digest,* August 2007, page 104

24 Daviid C. Johnston, *Free Lunch: How the Wealthiest Americans Enrich Themselves at Government Expense (and Stick You with the Bill)* (Portfolio Books: 2007)

25 Centers for Disease Control and Prevention, *Morbidity Mortality Weekly Report* 2006; 55: 656

26 "The Runaway Weight Gain Train: Too Many Accelerators, Not Enough Brakes," *British Medical Journal* (USA) 2004; 4: 597

27 *New England Journal of Medicine* 1989; 320: 733

28 *Diabetes Care* 2008; 31: 1433

29 *Lancet* 1996; 347: 949

30 *Diabetes Care* 2000; 23: 1278

31 Centers for Disease Control and Prevention study; *Salt Lake Tribune,* Oct. 31, 2008

32 *Cell* 2007; 15: 1097

33 *Journal of the American Medical Association* 2001; 286: 1427

34 *New England Journal of Medicine* 2002; 346: 802

35 *John Hopkins Advances in Medicine* 2005; 5: 122

36 *Clinical Pharmacology & Therapeutics* 2007; 82: 509

37 *Atherosclerosis, Thrombosis, and Vascular Biology* 2006; 26: 1958

38 *American Journal of Clinical Nutrition* 2007; 85: 35

39 *Family Practice News,* April 15, 2008, page 9

40 *Journal of the American Medical Association* 2008; 299: 2401

41 *American Journal of Clinical Nutrition* 2006; 84: 449

42 *Metabolism — Clinical and Experimental* 2008; 57: 1315

43 *British Medical Journal* 2005; 330: 1363

44 *Journal of Clinical Epidemiology,* March 2008

45 *Pediatrics* 2008; 153: 845

46 *American Journal of Clinical Nutrition* 2006; 83: 3, 36

47 *Lancet* 2007; 369: 2059

48 *American Journal of Clinical Nutrition* 2007; 86: 549

411

49 *Medical Hypotheses* 2004; 63: 783

50 *New England Journal of Medicine* 2008; 359: 2105

51 *Salt Lake Tribune,* June 15, 2008

52 *Family Practice News,* Jan. 1, 2008, page 31

53 *Lancet* 2005; 366: 1640

54 *European Journal of Endocrinology* 2007; 156: 655

55 *American Journal of Clinical Nutrition* 2007; 72: 2sup

56 *Rapid Communications in Mass Spectrometry,* October 2006

57 *The Journal of Biological Chemistry* 1997; 272: 7759

58 *Journal of Diabetes and its Complications* 2002; 16: 72

59 *European Journal of Clinical Investigation* 2002; 32: 14

60 *Nutrition Journal* 2001; 131: 2074

61 *American Journal of Clinical Nutrition* 2004; 80: 337

62 Thomson Medstat Health Care Research, Aug. 2, 2006

63 *Diabetologia* 2007; 50: 1418

64 *Journal of the American Medical Association* 2008; 300: 2631

65 "Effects of Olive Oils on Biomarkers of Oxidative DNA Stress in Northern and Southern Europeans," Federation of American Societies for Experimental Biology (*FASEB*) 2007; 21: 45

66 *Archives of Internal Medicine* 2008; 168: 1791

67 Journal of the Federation of American Societies for Experimental Biology (*FASEB*) 2005; 19: 1602

68 *Journal of Internal Medicine* 2003; 254: 401

69 John Hopkins University, March 8, 2003

70 *American Journal of Clinical Nutrition* 2004; 80: 1478

71 *Science,* April 26, 2007

72 *New England Journal of Medicine* 2008; 359: 2558

73 *American Journal of Clinical Nutrition* 2007; 86: 55

74 "Personalized Nutrition: Nutritional Genomics as Potential Tool for Targeted Medical Nutrition Therapy," *Nutrition Review* 2007; 65: 301

75 *Salt Lake Tribune,* June 7, 2007

76 *Internal Medicine Journal* 2003; 254: 114

77 *New England Journal of Medicine* 1985; 312: 283

78 *Hormone and Metabolism Research* 2006; 38: 650

79 Loren Cordain, *The Paleo Diet* (John Wiley & Sons, Inc.: 2002)

80 *Circulation* 1975; 52: 146

81 *Internal Medicine Journal* 2003; 254: 114

[82] *Archives of Internal Medicine* 2003; 163: 2787

[83] *Internal Medicine Journal* 2003; 254: 114

[84] T. Colin Campbell and Thomas M. Campbell, II., *The China Study* (Benbella Books: 2002)

[85] *Journal of Allergy and Clinical Immunology* 2007; 120: 1300

[86] *British Journal of Nutrition* 2007; 97: 912

[87] *Archives of Internal Medicine* 2008; 168: 1500

[88] *American Journal of Clinical Nutrition* 2003; 78: 1053

[89] *American Journal of Clinical Nutrition* 2003; 78: 1053

[90] *American Journal of Clinical Nutrition* 1999; 70: 456

[91] *Circulation* 2004; 109: 2; *New England Journal of Medicine* 2001; 345: 790

[92] *New England Journal of Medicine* 2001; 345: 790

[93] "Endocrine and Nutritional Fegulation of Fetal Adipose Tissue Development," *Endocrinology* 2004; 179: 293

[94] *Journal of Clinical Endocrinology & Metabolism* 2007; 92: 624

[95] *New England Journal of Medicine* 2004; 350: 865

[96] *New England Journal of Medicine* 2007; 356: 2053

[97] *Journal of Family Practice* 2008; 57: 409

[98] *Journal of the American Medical Association* 2004; 292: 789

[99] *Journal of the American Medical Association* 2007; 297: 796

[100] *American Journal of Clinical Nutrition* 2007; 85: 4405

[101] *Endocrinology* 2008; 149: 3067

[102] *Family Practice News*, Sept. 1, 2008, page 33

[103] *Journal of Clinical Endocrinology & Metabolism* 2007; 92: 624

[104] Annual Scientific Sessions of the American Diabetes Association, Chicago, Ill., 2007

[105] University of Exeter study, *Salt Lake Tribune*, April 24, 2008

[106] *Journal of the American Medical Association* 2008; 300: 2877

[107] *International Journal of Obesity*, July 2008

[108] European Congress on Obesity; Amsterdam, The Netherlands, 2009

[109] *American Journal of Clinical Nutrition* 2007; 85: 346

[110] *American Journal of Clinical Nutrition* 2006; 84: 1033

[111] *Journal of the American Medical Association* 2004; 293: 43, 96

[112] Gary Taubes, *Good Calories, Bad Calories* (Ancho: 2008)

[113] *American Journal of Clinical Nutrition*, 2007; 85: 346

[114] *Journal of Nutrition* 2003; 133: 4260

413

[115] *British Journal of Nutrition* 2006; 95: 659

[116] *Diabetic Medicine* 2003; 20: 451

[117] *Diabetes and Metabolism* 2003; 23: 15

[118] *International Journal of Obesity and Related Metabolic Disorders* 2000; 24: 451

[119] *Journal of Internal Medicine* 2003; 254: 401; *International Journal of Obesity and Related Metabolic Disorders* 1996; 20: 1051

[120] *American Journal of Human Genetics* 1998; 63: 1271

[121] *British Journal of Nutrition* 2007; 97: 847

[122] *Journal of Clinical Endocrinology & Metabolism* 2007; 92: 386

[123] *Journal of Clinical Investigation* 2005; 115: 1431

[124] "Effect of a Low Glycemic Index Diet with Soy Protein and Phytosterols on Cardiovascular Risk Factors in Postmenopausal Women," *Nutrition,* 2006; 22: 104

[125] "A Low- Glycemic Index Diet Reduces Plasma Plasminogen Activator Inhibitor-Activity," *American Journal of Clinical Nutrition* 2008; 87: 97

[126] "Dietary Management of the Metabolic Syndrome Beyond Macronutrients," *Nutrition Reviews* 2008; 66: 429

[127] *Nutrition Journal* 2006; 22: 104

[128] "What Role Has Nutrition Been Playing in Our Health? The Xenohormesis Connection," *Journal of Integrative Medicine,* 2007; 6: 22

[129] *Scientific American* report 2006; 16 #4: 19

[130] *American Journal of Clinical Nutrition* 2006; 84: 1365

[131] *Diabetes* 2006; 55: 2986

[132] *Endocrinology* 2005; 146: 4192; *American Journal of Clinical Nutrition* 2006; 83: 74

[133] "The Effects of Fat and Protein on Glycemic Responses in Nondiabetic Humans Vary with Waist Circumference, Fasting Plasma Insulin, and Dietary Fiber Intake," *Nutrition Journal,* 2006; 136: 2506

[134] "The Nutritional Phenotype in the Age of Metabolomics," *Nutrition Journal* 2005; 135: 1613

[135] "Nutrigenomics, Proteomics, and Metabolomics, and the Practice of Dietetics," *Journal of the American Dietetic Association* 2006; 25: 1109

[136] "A Faithful Translation," *Genome Technology,* February 2007, page 22

[137] *Nutrition Journal* 2005; 135: 1613

[138] "Defective Lipolysis and Altered Energy Metabolism in Mice Lacking Adipose Triglyceride Lipase," *Science* 2006; 312: 734

[139] *Proceedings of the National Academy of Sciences* 2008; 105: 1420

[140] Thomas Kuhn, *The Structure of Scientific Revolutions* (University of Chicago Press: 1962)

[141] *American Journal of Clinical Nutrition* 2005; 82 #1(s)

[142] *American Journal of Gastroenterology* 2006; 101: 70

[143] *American Journal of Clinical Nutrition* 2007; 86: 625

[144] *American Journal of Clinical Nutrition* 2006; 83: 211

[145] *Journal of Endocrinological Investigation* 2007; 30: 771

[146] "Ghrelin: Novel Regulator of Gonadal Function," *Journal of Endocrinological Investigation* 2006; 28: s26

[147] *European Journal of Cardiovascular Rehabilitation* 2007; 14: 438

[148] *American Journal of Cardiology,* June 8, 2008

[149] *British Medical Journal* 2004; 329: 1447

[150] *American Journal of Clinical Nutrition* 2005; 81: 380

[151] "Bacterial Invasion in the Small Intestine," *Geriatrics* 2006; 61: 21

[152] *American Journal of Clinical Nutrition* 2008; 88: 894

[153] "Microbiota: A Factor in Energy Regulation," *Nutrition Reviews* 2006; 64: 47

[154] *Nutrition Journal* 2007; 137: 1944

[155] "Scientists Probe Microbe 'Communitites,'" *Journal of the American Medical Association* 2008; 299: 2265

[156] *Journal of the American Medical Association* 2008; 300: 1989

[157] *Journal of Proteome Research,* October 2007

[158] *Journal of the American Medical Association* 2008; 299: 2770

[159] *Salt Lake Tribune,* Aug. 20, 2007

[160] "Microbiology, Obesity and Probiotics," *Current Opinion in Endocrinology, Diabetes and Obesity* 2008; 15: 422

[161] *British Journal of Nutrition* 2006; 96: 820

[162] *New England Journal of Medicine* 2006; 355: 1952

[163] "Effects of Probiotics and Prebiotics," *Nutrition Journal* 2007;137 #3S-II; "Metabolic Diversity of the Intestinal Microbiota," *Nutrition Journal* 2007, page 751S

[164] *American Medical News,* October 2005, page 42

[165] *Family Practice* 2007; 56: 101

[166] *Journal of the American Medical Association* 2007; 297: 986

[167] *Journal of the American Medical Association* 2009; 301: 924

[168] Federation of American Societies for Experimental Biology (*FASEB*) 2007; 21: 3431

[169] *Free Radical Biology & Medicine* 2007; 42: 775

[170] *Nature* 2006; 444: 337

[171] *Trends in Molecular Medicine* 2007; 13: 64

172 *American Journal of Clinical Nutrition* 2007; 86: 7

173 "Sirtuin Functions in Health and Disease," *Journal of Molecular Endocrinology* 2007; 21: 1745

174 "Nutrient-Sensitive Mitochondrial NAD+ Levels Dictate Cell Survival," *Cell* 2007; 130: 1095

175 *Journal of the American Medical Association* 2007; 298: 505

176 *Cell Metabolism* 2007; 5: 415, 426

177 "Small Molecule Activators of Sirtuins Extend Saccaromyces Cerevisiae Lifespan," *Nature* 2003; 425: 191

178 *Nutrition Journal* 2007; 137: 2668

179 *Metabolism—Clinical & Experimental* 2008; 57: s32

180 *Nutrition Journal* 2008; 138: 1602

181 *New York Times,* July 8, 2007

182 "Resveratrol Improves Mitochondrial Function and Protects Against Metabolic Disease by Activating SRT1 and PGC-1 Alpha," *Cell* 2006; 127: 1109

183 *Nature,* November 2006; 444: 337

184 *Nature,* Sept. 13, 2007

185 *American Journal of Clinical Nutrition* 2009; 89: 27

186 *Cell Metabolism,* November 2007

187 Comparative Biochemistry and Physiology Biochemistry & Molecular Biology 2004; 139: 543

188 Utah State University Biology Department; June 20, 2006, *Salt Lake Tribune*

189 *Journal of the American Medical Association* 2006; 296: 1577

190 *Science* 2008; 322: 449

191 Brigham Young University, Nov. 18, 2005

192 Brigham Young University, December 2005

193 *American Journal of Clinical Nutrition* 2005; 82: 236S

194 J. American Geriatric Society 2007;55:49

195 *Diabetes Care* 2008; 31: 2050

196 *New England Journal of Medicine* 2003; 349: 1966

197 Imperial College, London. *Salt Lake Tribune,* May 11, 2007

198 *Circulation* 2007; 116: 1234

199 *Diabetes Care* 2007; 30: 343

200 *Archives of Internal Medicine* 2007; 167: 11518

201 *Archives Internal Medicine* 2007; 167: 886, 875

202 *American Journal of Clinical Nutrition* 2006; 84: 789

203 *Nutrition,* 2003; 133: 4260

[204] *New England Journal of Medicine* 2003; 349: 9236

[205] *Journal of the American Medical Association* 2005; 293: 2200

[206] *American Journal Physiololgy – Endocrinology and Metabolism* 2000; 279: E1286

[207] *Journal of Clinical Endocrinology & Metabolism* 2003; 88: 469

[208] *Nature Neuroscience* 2005; 8: 579

[209] "The Effects of Insulin on the Central Nervous System: Focus on Appetite Regulation," *Hormone and Metabolism Research,* 2006; 38: 442

[210] *American Journal of Clinical Nutrition,* 2008: 87: 303

[211] *Nutrition* 2006; 136: 2131

[212] *Nature Medicine* 2004; 10: 727

[213] *Journal of Alternative and Complementary Medicine* 2008; 14: 139

[214] American Chemical Society National Meeting and Exposition, Atlanta, Ga., 2006

[215] *British Journal of Nutrition* 1994; 72: 775

[216] *Lipids* 2004; 39: 383

[217] *Diabetes, Technology & Therapeutics* 2008; 10: 405

[218] *British Journal of Nutrition* 2008; Aug. 19: 1 e-pub

[219] *Journal of the American Medical Association* 2007; 297: 1819

[220] "Diabetes, Obesity, and the Brain," *Science* 2005; 307: 375

[221] *Female Patient* 2004; 29: 23

[222] *Science,* July 13, 2007

[223] Joseph Mercola, *Sweet Deception* (Nelson Books: 2006)

[224] *American Journal of Clinical Nutrition,* 2009; 89: 1

[225] "What Role Has Nutrition Been Playing in Our Health? The Xenohormesis Connection," *Integrative Medicine,* 2007; 6: 22

[226] *Chemische Berichte* 1879; 12: 469

[227] *American Journal of Epidemiology* 2008; 167: 1235

[228] *Food and Chemical Toxicology* 1985; 23: 491

[229] International Agency for Research on Cancer, supp 1987

[230] *British Medical Journal* 1996; 313; 386

[231] *New York Times,* Feb. 12, 2006

[232] *Biology Psychiatry* 1993; 34: 13

[233] University of Virginia Health System Website; accessed December 5th 2009

[234] American Association for Cancer Research; April 5, 2006, *Salt Lake Tribune*

[235] *Seminars in Cancer Biology* 1998; 8: 255

[236] Web site: www.epa.gov

[237] *Toxicology and Applied Pharmacology* 1978; 45: 201

[238] United States Food and Drug Administration, April 20, 1995

[239] H. J. Roberts, *Aspartame Disease: An Ignored Epidemic* (Sunshine Sentinel Press: 2001)

[240] *Food and Chemical Toxicology* 2000; 38: s91

[241] *Food and Chemical Toxicology* 2000; 38: s111

[242] *Food and Chemical Toxicology* 2000; 38: s1

[243] *Journal of Reproduction and Fertility* 1978; 52: 153

[244] *Food and Chemical Toxicology* 2002; 38: s43

[245] *Mutation Research* 2002; 519: 103

[246] *Salt Lake Tribune*, May 12, 2007

[247] Richard K. Bernstein, *Diabetes Solution* (Little Brown and Company: 2003)

[248] *Drug Chemistry Toxicity* 1997; 20: 3

[249] *Clinical Therapeutics* 2003; 11: 2797

[250] *USA Today*, Dec. 21, 2008

[251] David Richard, *Stevia Rebaudiana: Nature's Sweet Secret* (Vital Health Publishing: 1996)

[252] *National Geographic*, May 2008

[253] *Nutrition Journal* 2008; 138: 171

[254] *Nutrition Journal* 2007; 137: 2121

[255] *Journal of Pediatrics* 2006; 118: 2066

[256] *Nutrition Research Reviews* 2006; 16: 163

[257] *Annals of Oncology* 2001; 10: 1460

[258] *J. Behavioral Neuroscience*, 2008, Vol. 122, No. 1.

[259] "The Bush White House: Science Advice Still Out in the Cold," *Lancet* 2001; 357: 1773

[260] *New York Times*, July 12, 2007

[261] "What if Fat Doesn't Make You Fat?" *New York Times Magazine*, July 7, 2002

[262] *Science* 2001; 291: 2536

[263] Gary Taubes, *Good Calories, Bad Calories* (Anchor: 2008)

[264] "What if Fat Doesn't Make You Fat?" *The New York Times Magazine*, July 7, 2002

[265] *Nutrition Journal* 2002; 132: 329

[266] *British Journal of Nutrition* 2004; 92: 895

[267] *American Journal of Clinical Nutrition* 2003; 78: 65

[268] *Journal of the American Medical Association* 2008; 300;1508

[269] *Lancet* 2003; 362: 1593

270 *Circulation* 2002; 10: 1161

271 *Lancet* 2004; 264: 662

272 *New England Journal of Medicine* 2001; 344: 1959

273 *New England Journal of Medicine* 2005; 352: 20

274 "Food Industry and Health: Mostly Promises, Little Action," *Lancet* 2006; 368: 562

275 *American Journal of Clinical Medicine* 2004; 79: 774

276 *American Journal of Clinical Nutrition* 1999; 70: 221

277 *Critical Reviews in Food Science and Nutrition* 2007; 47: 561

278 *American Journal of Clinical Nutrition* 2008; 87: 1194

279 Joseph Ellis, *Founding Brothers* (Vintage Books: 2002)

280 *Science* 2002; 296: 1243

281 Adam Smith, *The Wealth of Nations* (Prometheus Books: 1991)

282 Adam Smith, *The Theory of Moral Sentiments* (Kessinger Publishing, LLC: 2004)

283 Barbara Kingsolver, *Animal, Vegetable, Mineral* (HarperCollins: 2007)

284 Marion Nestle, *Food Politics* (University of California Press: 2002)

285 *Science* 2002; 297: 198

286 *Lancet* 2003; 362: 808

287 *Lancet* 2002; 360: 473

288 *Nutrition Reviews* 1999; 57: s2

289 *New York Times*, Sept. 14, 2008

290 *Archives of Internal Medicine* 2004; 164: 1873

291 Marion Nestle, *Food Politics* (University of California Press: 2002)

292 *New York Times*, Nov. 15, 1995

293 Lester Brown, Earth Policy Institute; June 2007

294 James Kuntsler, *The Great Emergency* (Atlantic Monthly Press: 2005)

295 *Salt Lake Tribune*, July 11, 2007

296 *New York Times Magazine*, Oct. 12, 2003

297 *New England Journal of Medicine* 2005; 352: 1138

298 *Environmental Health Perspectives* 2004; 112: A821

299 Book "2004 Annual Review of Nutrition."

300 *Salt Lake Tribune*, Oct. 16, 2007

301 Neal Barnard, Physicians Committee for Responsible Med; *Salt Lake Tribune*, Oct. 28, 2007

302 Jeffrey E. Garten, *The Politics of Fortune* (HBS Press: 2002)

[303] *New York Times Magazine*, April 22, 2007, page 15

[304] Barbara Kingsolver, *Animal, Vegetable, Mineral* (HarperCollins: 2007)

[305] *Annals of Internal Medicine* 1999; 130: 1034

[306] *British Journal of Nutrition* 2000; 83s: 181

[307] *Journal of the American Medical Association* 2000; 284: 820, 2002; 288: 2178

[308] *New York Times*, Dec. 18, 2008

[309] *Nutrition Journal* 2007; 137: 453

[310] *Journal of the American Medical Association* 2002; 288: 2179

[311] *New York Times*, July 4, 2007

[312] *American Journal of Public Health* 2001; 91: 689

[313] *New York Times*, Oct. 25, 2006

[314] *New York Times*, July 17, 2007

[315] *Journal of the American Medical Association* 2007; 297: 1132

[316] "Physician-Citizen: Public Roles and Professional Obligations," Journal of the American Medical Association 2004; 291: 94

[317] "Health and Development," *Lancet* 2003; 362: 678

[318] *Salt Lake Tribune*, June 20, 2006

[319] Richard P. Feynman, Ralph Leighton, and Edward Hutchings, *Surely You're Joking, Mr. Feynman!* (W.W. Norton & Company, Inc.: 1985)

[320] *Diabetes Care* 2001; 24: 1936

[321] California Center for Public Health Advocacy, April 30, 2008

[322] Louisiana State University study, Oct. 22, 2002

[323] Diabetologia 1991; 34: 891

[324] "Glycemic Load Comes of Age," *Nutrition Journal* 2003; 133: 2695

[325] *American Journal of Clinical Nutrition* 2007; 86: 1331

[326] *New York Times*, July 22, 2007

[327] *Salt Lake Tribune*, July 29, 2008

[328] Center for Science, 1999; Washington, D.C.

[329] *New York Times*, April 11, 2006

[330] European Association for the Study of Diabetes Annual Meeting, Amsterdam, 2007

[331] *American Journal of Preventive Medicine*, October 2006

[332] Childhood Obesity Conference, Anaheim, Calif., 2007; *Salt Lake Tribune*, Jan. 26, 2007

[333] *New York Times*, Nov. 26, 2007

[334] *American Journal of Clinical Nutrition* 2005; 82: 1011

[335] Annual Meeting American Psychological Society, Toronto, Canada, 2001

[336] *American Journal of Clinical Nutrition* 2005; 82: 1011

[337] *Society for Neuroscience's annual meeting; October 2009, Chicago*

[338] John Hopkins study; *Salt Lake Tribune*, Feb. 17, 2007

[339] Romans 12:2

[340] John Bradshaw, *Homecoming* (Bantam: 1990)

[341] *Proceedings of the National Academy of Science, July 2007*

[342] *New England Journal of Medicine* 2007; 357: 370

[343] *Journal of Alternative and Complementary Medicine* 2002; 8: 185

[344] *Psychosomatic Medicine* 2002; 64: 563

[345] "Hidden Disruptions in Metabolic Syndrome: Drug-Induced Nutrient Depletion as a Pathway to Accelerated Pathophysiology of Metabolic Syndrome," *Alternative Therapies*, March/April 2006; 12 #2: 26

[346] *American Journal of Health Promotion*, August 2003

[347] *Journal of the American Medical Association* 2003; 289: 187

[348] "Can Cities Be Designed to Fight Obesity?" *Lancet* 2003; 362: 1046

[349] *Salt Lake Tribune*, Jan. 26, 2008

[350] "Health Disparities and Access to Health," *Journal of the American Medical Association* 2007; 297: 1118

[351] *American Journal of Clinical Nutrition* 2008: 87: 310

[352] "Sleepless in America," *Archives of Internal Medicine* 2005; 165: 15

[353] *American Journal of Clinical Nutrition* 2009; 89: 126

[354] *Archives of Internal Medicine* 2006; 166: 1701; *European Journal of Endocrinology* 2008; 159: s59

[355] *Obesity Research* (now called *Obesity*) 2007; 8: 119

[356] *Sleep* 2008; 31: 619

[357] Forty-third Annual Conference on Cardiovascular Disease, Epidemiology, and Prevention, New York, 2003

[358] *American Journal of Clinical Nutrition* 2004; 80: 243

[359] *Clinical Endocrinology* 2004; 59: 374

[360] *Cardiovascular Diabetology* 2006; 5: 22

[361] *Diabetes Care* 207; 30: 1233

[362] *Respiratory Medicine* 2006; 100: 980

[363] International Conference of the American Thoracic Society, San Francisco, Calif., 2007

[364] "Chemical Toxins: Hypothesis to Explain the Global Obesity Epidemic," *Journal of Alternative and Complementary Medicine* 2002; 8: 185

[365] *Journal of the American Medical Association* 2002; 283: 2253

366 Environmental Protection Agency, Nov. 1, 2001; *Journal of the American Medical Association* 2008; 300: 814

367 "The Chemicals Within Us," *National Geographic,* October 2006; page 116

368 *New England Journal of Medicine* 2000; 342: 1441

369 *New England Journal of Medicine* 2000; 342: 1441

370 *New England Journal of Medicine* 2000; 342: 1392

371 *Family Practice News,* Dec. 15, 2007, page 25

372 *American Journal of Clinical Nutrition* 2006; 84: 551

373 *British Medical Journal,* October 2001, page 7319

374 Daniel 1:5-16

375 "Clinical Update: The Low-Glycemic Index Diet," *Lancet* 2007; 369: 890

376 *Diabetes Care* 2008; 31: 2281

377 *Journal of the American Medical Association* 2002; 287: 2114; *American Journal of Clinical Nutrition* 2009; 89: 97

378 *Hormone and Metabolic Research* 2006; 38: 465

379 *American Journal of Clinical Nutrition* 2007; 85: 724

380 *American Journal of Clinical Nutrition* 2007; 85: 724

381 *"Clinical Update: The Low-Glycemic Index Diet,"* Lancet 2007; 369: 890

382 Lipids 2003; 38: 117; American Journal of Clinical Nutrition 2005; 82: 547

383 "Effects of Dietary Glycemic Index on Adiposity, Glucose Homeostasis and Plasma Lipids in Animals," *Lancet* 2004; 364: 778, 736

384 *Family Practice Recertification* 2006; 28 #4: 32

385 *American Journal of Clinical Nutrition* 2002; 76: supp 266-290s

386 "High Sensitivity CRP: A Useful Marker for Cardiovascular Disease and the Metabolic Syndrome," *Clinical Chemistry* 2005; 51: 504

387 *American Journal of Clinical Nutrition* 2002; 75: 492

388 *Diabetes Care* 2005; 28: 2497

389 *American Journal of Clinical Nutrition* 2006; 84: 70

390 *Archives of Internal Medicine* 2007; 167: 31

391 *American Journal of Clinical Nutrition* 2002; 75: 343, 344

392 *American Journal of Epidemiology,* Feb. 15, 2005

393 *American Journal of Clinical Nutrition* 2006; 83: 124

394 *Journal of the American Dietetic Association* 2006; 106: 1380

395 *Journal of the American Medical Association* 2007; 297: 969

396 *Family Practice News,* Feb. 1, 2007, page 11

397 *Atherosclerosis, Thrombosis, and Vascular Biology* 2006; 26: 1958

398 *Journal of Clinical Investigation* 2007; 117: 746

[399] *Journal of the American Medical Association* 2007; 297: 2092

[400] *Journal of the American Medical Association,* May 2004

[401] "How Safe is Fructose For Persons With or Without Diabetes?" American Journal of Clinical Nutrition 2008; 88: 1189

[402] *American Journal of Clinical Nutrition* 2008; 88: 1419

[403] *Diabetes* 2005; 54: 609

[404] *American Journal of Clinical Nutrition* 2007; 298: 895

[405] *Atherosclerosis, Thrombosis, and Vascular Biology* 2006; 26: 1958

[406] *Journal of Hepatology* 2008; 48: 993

[407] *Nutrition Reviews* 2005; 63: 133; Diabetes 2005; 54: 1907

[408] *Diabetes Care* 2007; 30: 1406

[409] "A 4-Week High Fructose Diet Alters Lipid Metabolism Without Affecting Insulin Sensitivity or Ectopic Lipids in Healthy Human," *American Journal of Clinical Nutrition* 2006; 84: 1374

[410] *Pediatrics* 2005; 115: 736

[411] 2007 California Childhood Obesity Conference, Anaheim, Calif.; *Salt Lake Tribune,* Jan. 26, 2007

[412] "The Metabolic Syndrome, a Post-Prandial Disease?" *Hormone and Metabolic Research* 2006; 38: 435

[413] *British Medical Journal* 2008; 337: 1091

[414] *Journal of the American Medical Association* 2003; 289: 1837

[415] *American Journal of Clinical Nutrition* 2003; 78: 957

[416] *American Journal of Clinical Nutrition* 2003; 78: 965

[417] *Diabetes Care* 2006; 29: 245

[418] *New England Journal of Medicine* 2008; 359: 26

[419] *Scandinavian Gastroenterology* 2007; 42: 48

[420] *Scandinavian Gastroenterology* 2007; 42: 60

[421] *Journal of the American Medical Association* 2003; 289: 1969

[422] *Salt Lake Tribune,* July 16, 2007

[423] *New England Journal of Medicine* 2003; 348: 2161

[424] *Journal of the American College of Nutrition* 2001; 20: 32

[425] Reuters News, July 4, 2002

[426] *Journal of Endocrinology Investigation* 2003; 26: 265

[427] "Dairy Products Do Not Lead to Alterations in Body Weight or Fat Mass," *American Journal of Clinical Nutrition* 2005; 81: 751; *Obesity Research* (now called *Obesity*) 2005; 13: 1720

[428] *Obesity Research* (now called *Obesity*), April 2004

[429] *American Journal of Clinical Nutrition* 2008; 88: 877

[430] *New York Times,* Feb. 12, 2006

[431] Center for Science in the Public Interest, July 2003

[432] *Metabolism—Clinical and Experimental* 2007; 56: 280

[433] *American Journal of Preventive Medicine* 2005; 29: 320

[434] *British Journal of Nutrition* 2006; 95: 539

[435] *Journal of the American Geriatric Society* 2007; 55: 49

[436] *Metabolism—Clinical and Experimental* 2005; 54: 306; *Diabetes Care* 2007; 30: 3011

[437] *Metabolism—Clinical and Experimental* 2007; 56: 599

[438] *Family Practice News,* April 1, 2007, page 1

[439] *Annals of Nutrition & Metabolism* 2006; 50: 407

[440] *Endocrinology Practice* 2007; 13: 239

[441] *Journal of the American Medical Association* 2006; 295: 1135

[442] *British Journal of Nutrition* 2005; 93: 773

[443] -Scranton University Report, August 29, 2005. *Reuters News*

[444] -"Is Coffee a Functional Food?", British J. Nutrition 2005;93:773

[445] *American Journal of Clinical Nutrition* 2007; 86: 604

[446] *Nutrition Journal* 2008; 138: 167

[447] *Nutrition Journal* 2008; 138: 725

[448] *American Journal of Clinical Nutrition* 2008; 88: 58

[449] *American Journal of Clinical Nutrition* 2008; 87: 872

[450] "Effects of Low Habitual Cocoa Intake on Blood Pressure and Bioactive Nitric Oxide," *Journal of the American Medical Association* 2007; 298: 49

[451] *General Dentistry,* May/June 2005

[452] "Studies Probe Oral Health-Diabetes Link," *Journal of the American Medical Association* 2008; 300; 2471

[453] *Journal of the National Cancer Institute* 2006; 98: 644

[454] *British Medical Journal* 2008; 336: 309

[455] *Arthritis & Rheumatism* 2008; 59: 109

[456] *Arthritis & Rheumatism* 2007; 57: 816

[457] *Obesity Research,* July 2005

[458] *Journal of the American Medical Association* 2004; 292: 927

[459] *American Journal of Clinical Nutrition* 2008; 88: 1487

[460] *Circulation* 2007; 116: 480

[461] Journal of the Medical Association 2008; 299: 2137

462 *Salt Lake Tribune,* July 24, 2007

463 *Wall Street Journal,* March 13, 2008

464 *American Journal of Clinical Nutrition* 2006; 84: 274

465 *American Journal of Clinical Nutrition* 2006; 84: 274

466 *American Journal of Clinical Nutrition* 2008; 87: 1662

467 *Nutrition Journal* 2007; 137: 1447

468 *American Journal of Clinical Nutrition* 2007; 85: 651

469 *Risk Analysis: An International Journal,* October 2005

470 *Salt Lake Tribune,* July 24, 2007

471 *Journal of the American Medical Association* 2008; 299: 2137

472 *American Journal of Clinical Nutrition* 2006; 84: 274

473 *Salt Lake Tribune,* June 13, 2006

474 *New England Journal of Medicine* 2000; 342: 1441

475 *British Medical Journal/USA* 2002; 2: 543

476 *Hormone and Metabolic Research* 2006; 38: 435

477 *British Medical Journal* 2002; 324: 1190

478 "How Should Hamsters Run? Some Observations About Sufficient Patient Time in Primary Care," *British Medical Journal* 2001; 323: 266

479 *Preventive Medicine* 2003; 36: 41

480 *Salt Lake Tribune,* May 27, 2007

481 "Effects of Improved Glycemic Control on Health Care Costs and Utilization," *Journal of the American Medical Association* 2001; 285: 182

482 *Diabetes Care* 2007; 30: 228

483 *American Medical News,* July 28, 2008, page 14

484 *American Journal of Clinical Nutrition* 2006; 83 supp: 929s

485 Journal of the American Medical Association 2002; 287: 2945

486 Dr. Hannah Sahud, pediatrician at Allegheny General Hospital in Pittsburgh, Penn.; *Salt Lake Tribune,* Dec. 5, 2006

487 *American Journal of Clinical Nutrition* 2004; 80: 348

488 *American Journal of Clinical Nutrition* 2004; 80: 337

489 *Journal of the American Medical Association* 2007; 297: 1362

490 *Salt Lake Tribune,* June 13, 2006

491 *Nutrition Reviews* 2000; 58: 154

492 *Journal of the American Medical Association* 2001; 285: 182

493 *Health Affairs,* March 2007

494 www.american-heart.org/nutrition/sugar, Aug 25th 2009-10-05

495 *Lancet* 2007; 369: 2059

496 *Annals of Internal Medicine* 2006; 145: 91

497 *Journal of the American Medical Association* 2003; 290: 1884

498 *Journal of the American Medical Association* 2007; 298: 920

499 *Archives of Pediatrics & Adolescent Medicine* 2008; 162: 981; *Pediatrics* 2008; 153: 839

500 "Childhood Obesity," A New Pandemic of the New Millennium," *Pediatrics* 2002; 110: 1003

501 *Pediatrics,* February 1995

502 *European Journal of Pediatrics* 1997; 156: 557

503 *Journal of the American Medical Association* 2007; 298: 874

504 *Diabetes Care* 2003; 26: 433

505 *Family Practice News,* August 2005, page 24

506 Annual Meeting Primary Care Research, Tucson, Ariz., 2007

507 *American Journal of Clinical Nutrition* 2007; 86: 33

508 *Diabetes Care* 2007; 30: 2091

509 Annual Meeting of the Pediatric Academy Societies, Toronto, Canada, 2007

510 *Family Practice News,* Feb. 1, 2009, page 29

511 *Clinical Endocrinology & Metabolism* 2007; 92: 4753

512 American Assocociation for the Study of Liver Diseases; *Family Practice News,* Aug. 1, 2005, page 39

513 *Archives of Pediatrics & Adolescent Medicine* 2008; 162: 764

514 *Salt Lake Tribune,* Feb. 27, 2007

515 *Pediatrics,* April 2006

516 *Pediatric and Adolescent Surgery,* February 2007

517 *Lancet* 2002; 360: 473

518 *Pediatrics,* September 2007

519 *Family Practice News,* Feb. 1, 2009, page 29

520 *Psychology Bulletin,* July 2007

521 *Archives of Pediatrics & Adolescent Medicine* 2008; 162: 929

522 *Archives of Pediatrics & Adolescent Medicine,* August 2007

523 *Lancet* 2005; 366: 2064

524 *Pediatrics,* December 2006

525 *American Journal of Public Health* 2002; 92: 1475

526 The Center for Science in the Public Interest; CBS News, Aug. 4, 2008

527 "Food Marketing and Childhood Obesity, a Matter of Policy," *New England Journal of Medicine* 2006; 354: 2527

[528] "Food Marketing and Childhood Obesity, a Matter of Policy," *New England Journal of Medicine* 2006; 354: 2527

[529] *New York Times,* July 18, 2007

[530] *Salt Lake Tribune,* Sept. 24, 2006

[531] *Preventive Medicine* 2002; 35: 376

[532] *Salt Lake Tribune,* March 26, 2007

[533] *Salt Lake Tribune,* June 5, 2008

[534] *New York Times,* Dec. 2, 2007

[535] *Archives of Pediatrics & Adolescent Medicine* 2007; 161: 553

[536] *Archives Pediatrics & Adolescent Medicine* 2006; 160: 411, 436; *American Journal of Clinical Nutrition* 2009; 89: 37

[537] *Lancet* 2004;364:257

[538] *Salt Lake Tribune,* April 24, 2008

[539] *Pediatrics,* October 2006

[540] *Salt Lake Tribune,* July 8, 2007

[541] *Archives of Pediatrics & Adolescent Medicine* 2006; 160: 363

[542] *Nutrition Journal* 2001; 17: 952

[543] *International Journal of Obesity* 2002; 26: 1310

[544] *Pediatrics* 2007; 150: 383

[545] *Archives of Pediatrics & Adolescent Medicine* 2008; 162: 305

[546] *Archives of Pediatrics & Adolescent Medicine* 2008; 162: 313

[547] *Pediatrics* 1999;104:341

[548] *American Journal of Clinical Nutrition* 2007; 85: 355

[549] *Diabetes Care* 2007; 30: 1567

[550] *Archives of Pediatrics & Adolescent Medicine* 2008; 162: 239

[551] *Archives of Pediatrics & Adolescent Medicine* 2007; 161: 480

[552] Brigham Young University study; *Salt Lake Tribune,* July 2, 2008

[553] *Archives of Pediatrics & Adolescent Medicine* 2006; 160: 411

[554] *Salt Lake Tribune,* March 15, 2007

[555] American Medical Association report; Chicago, Ill., June 2007

[556] *Archives of Pediatrics & Adolescent Medicine* 2007; 160: 411

[557] *American Journal of Preventive Medicine,* August 2007

[558] *Journal of the American Medical Association* 2008; 300: 295

[559] Kaiser Permanente study in California; *Salt Lake Tribune,* April 28, 2008

[560] *Nutrition Journal* 2005; 21: 773

[561] *Nutrition Today* 2007; 42: 6

562 *Journal of the American Medical Association* 2007; 298: 613

563 *Family Practice News,* June 1, 2008, page 23

564 Annual Clinical Meeting of the Society of Obstetricians and Gynaecologists of Ottawa, Canada, 2007

565 *Diabetes Care* 2007; 30: s112

566 *Diabetes Care* 2008; 31: 2362

567 *Salt Lake Tribune,* Feb. 4, 2008

568 "A Prospective Study of Dietary Patterns, Meat intake and the Risk of Gestational Diabetes   Mellitus," Diabetologia 2006; 49: 2604

569 *Diabetes Care* 2007; 30: 348

570 "Gestational Diabetes Increases the Risk of Cardiovascular Disease in Women with a Family History of Type II Diabetes," *Diabetes Care* 2006; 29: 2078

571 *Diabetes Care* 2007; 30: 1968

572 *Diabetes Care* 2007; 30: s188, s206

573 *Diabetes Care* 2007; 30: s246, s242

574 *Family Practice News,* May 15, 2007, page 32

575 Annual Meeting of the Pediatric Academic Societies, Seattle, Wash., 2003

576 *Circulation* 2007; 115: 2931

577 *Journal of the American Medical Association* 2008; 300: 2886

578 *American Journal of Public Health* 2007; 97: 157

579 *American Journal of Clinical Nutrition* 2003; 78: 972

580 *Journal of the American Medical Association* 2009; 301: 636

581 *American Journal of Clinical Nutrition* 2003; 78: 1024

582 *American Journal of Clinical Nutrition* 2008; 87: 887

583 *American Journal of Clinical Nutrition* 2008; 87: 912

584 Utah Department of Health, February 2008

585 Annual Meeting of the American Diabetic Society, Washington, D.C., 2006

586 -J. Nature; Online publication December 6th 2009

587 *Salt Lake Tribune,* April 16, 2007

588 *New York Times,* Dec. 20, 2007

589 *Journal of the American Medical Association* 2007; 297: 2684

590 *Journal of the American Medical Association* 2007; 297: 2697

591 *Salt Lake Tribune,* April 26, 2007

592 *Archives of Pediatric & Adolescent Medicine* 2008; 162: 232

593 *Diabetologia* 2007; 50: 1401

594 *New York Times,* April 30, 2007

595 *British Medical Journal* 2006; 333: 1041

596 *Salt Lake Tribune,* June 25, 2007

597 *Pediatrics,* January 2005

598 The Center for Science in the Public Interest, Washington, D.C., June 2006

599 *American Journal of Clinical Nutrition* 2007; 86: 428

600 *Lancet* 1998; 317: 1683

601 "The Growing Political Movement Against Soft Drinks in School," *Journal of the American Medical Association* 2002; 288: 2181

602 *British Medical Journal/USA* 2004; 4: 410

603 *Journal of the American Medical Association* 2004; 292: 927

604 *International Journal of Obesity,* July 2004

605 "The School Lunch Test," *New York Times Magazine,* Aug. 20, 2006, page 30

606 "Type 2 Diabetes in Children and Young Adults: A New Epidemic," *Clinical Diabetes* 2002; 20: 217

607 *American Family Physician* 2008; 78: 1052

608 Annual Meeting at the American College of Sports Medicine, New Orleans, La., 2007

609 *American Journal of Clinical Nutrition* 2003; 78: 199

610 *Archives of Pediatrics & Adolescent Medicine* 2007; 161: 865

611 "Researchers Address Childhood Obesity Through Community-Based Programs," *Journal of the American Medical Association* 2007; 298: 2728

612 "Pediatric Obesity Guidelines Released," *Journal of the American Medical Association* 2008; 300: 2238

613 "The Thermodynamics of Healing, Health and Love," *Journal of Alternative & Complementary Medicine* 2007; 13: 5

614 Graham Hancock, *The Supernatural* (The Disinformation Company: 2006)

615 Candace Pert, *Molecules of Emotion* (Touchstone Books: 1997)

616 *Biology* 1997; 40: 187

617 Lynne McTaggart, *The Intention Experiment* (Free Press: 2008)

618 James Gardner, *The Intelligent Universe* (Career Press: 2007)

619 Erwin Schrodinger, *What is Life?* (Cambridge University Press: 1996)

620 "A Global Perspective on Energy: Health Effects and Injustices," *Lancet* 2007; 370: 965; "Electricity Generation and Health," *Lancet* 2007; 370: 979

621 P. C. W. Davies and Julian R. Brown, *The Ghost in the Atom* (Cambridge University Press: 1986)

622 Jeremy Narby, *The Cosmic Serpent* (Tarcher: 1998)

623 "Do We Have to Spell It Out?" *New Scientist* 2004; 183: 30

624 Ray Kurzweil, *The Singularity Is Near* (Viking Penguin: 2005)

625 Time Life Editiors, *Cosmic Connections* (Time Life Education: 1973)

626 "2001 Replayed," *Astronomy News* 2006; 20: 21

627 David Bohm, *Wholeness and the Implicate Order* (Ark Press: 1980)

628 Desiderius Erasmus, *Praise of Folly* (Penguin Books: 1971)

629 Bruce Lipton, *The Biology of Belief* (Mountain of Love Books: 2005)

630 "Are You a Hologram?" *Scientific American*, July 14, 2003

631 "Information in the Holographic Universe," *Scientific American*, Jan. 1, 2006

632 Michael Talbot, *The Holographic Universe* (Harper Perennial: 1991)

633 "The Thermodynamics of Healing, Health and Love," *Journal of Alternative & Complementary Medicine* 2007; 13: 5

634 Jeremy Narby *The Cosmic Serpent* (Tarcher: 1998)

635 "Energy Cardiology: A Dynamical Energy Systems Approach for Integrating Conventional and Alternative Medicine," *Advances* 1996; 12: 4

636 David Deutsch, *The Fabric of Reality* (Penguin Books: 1997)

637 "Quantum Cellular Biology," *Medical Hypotheses* 2001; 57: 358

638 Lynne McTaggart, *The Field* (HarperCollins: 2002)

639 *Science and Technology* 2001; 79: 29

640 *Trends in Immunology* 2006; 27: 32

641 *Diabetologia* 2007; 50: 1523

642 Dean Radin, *The Conscious Universe* (Herped Edge: 1997)

643 *Proceedings of the National Academy of Science* 2008; 105: 16242

644 *Journal of the American Medical Association* 2001; 286: 327

645 *Journal of Clinical Endocrinology & Metabolism* 2007; 92: 2041

646 "High Glycemic Load Increases C- Reactive Protein," *American Journal of Clinical Nutrition* 2002; 75: 492

647 *Metabolism — Clinical and Experimental* 2008; 57: 1221, 1232

648 *Diabetes* 2003; 52: 2097

649 *Metabolism — Clinical and Experimental* 2007; 56: 662; *American Journal of Clinical Nutrition* 2009; 89: 85

650 *American Journal of Clinical Nutrition* 2008; 87: 30

651 *Arteriosclerosis, Thrombosis, and Vascular Biology* 2003; 23: 1042

652 *Endocrinology* 2006; 147: 4550

653 Current Opinion in Clinical Nutrition & Metabolic Care 2002; 5: 551

654 *Metabolism — Clinical and Experimental* 2008; 57: 1375

655 *Endocrine Reviews* 2003; 88: 2399

656 *Family Practice News*, March 2004, page 11

657 *Clinical Chemistry* 2007; 53: 456

[658] *Diabetes/Metabolism Research and Reviews* 2006; 22: 257

[659] *Diabetes* 2007; 56: 1783

[660] *Arteriosclerosis, Thrombosis, and Vascular Biology* 2004; 24: 823

[661] "Mortality in Randomized Trials of Antioxidant Supplementation for Primary and Secondary   Prevention," *Journal of the American Medical Association* 2007; 297: 842

[662] *Journal of the American Medical Association* 2007; 297: 842

[663] *American Journal of Clinical Nutrition* 2009; 89: 773

[664] "Energy Expenditure and Substrate Oxidation Predicts Changes in Body Fat in Children," *American Journal of Clinical Nutrition* 2006; 84: 862

[665] *Circulation* 2008; 117: 2431, 2492

[666] Medical Hypotheses 2006: 66: 832

[667] Book "The Heart's Code," Paul Pearsall. Broadway Books, 1998

[668] "Mitochondrial Dynamics in Disease," *New England Journal of Medicine* 2007; 356: 1707

[669] "Mitochondrial Energetics and Insulin Resistance," *Endocrinology* 2008; 49: 950

[670] "Mild Mitochondrial Uncoupling Impacts Cellular Aging in Human Muscles in Vivo," *Proceedings of the National Academy of Science* (USA):2007;104: 1057

[671] "Mitochondrial Dysfunction and Oxidative Stress: Cause and Consequence of Epileptic Seizures," *Free Radical Biology Medicine* 2004: 37: 1951

[672] "Mitochondrial DNA Modifies Cognition in Interaction with the Nuclear Genome and Age in Mice," *Nature Genetics* 2003: 35: 65

[673] *Annals of Neurology* 2008: 63: 35

[674] "Mitochondrial Disease," *Lancet* 2006; 368: 70; *Diabetologia* 2007; 50: 2085

[675] *American Journal of Clinical Nutrition* 2007; 85: 662

[676] *Journal of the Royal Society Medicine* 2006; 99: 506

[677] *Journal of Clinical Endocrinology & Metabolism* 2007; 92: 880

[678] *Nutrition Journal* 2007; 137: 1835

[679] *Circulation* 2008; 117: 2431

[680] *Diabetes Care* 2008; 57: 3222

[681] "Does High Sucrose Diet Alter Skeletal Muscle and Liver Mitochondrial Respiration?" *Hormonal Metabolism Research* 2003: 35: 546

[682] *Medicine & Science in Sports & Exercise* 2001; 33: s167

[683] *Neurology Reviews* 2005; 13: 1

[684] Federation of American Societies for Experimental Biology (*FASEB*) 2005; 19: 638

431

685 *British Journal of Nutrition* 2007; 97: 855

686 "Neuroprotection in Parkinson's Disease," *Journal of the American Medical Association* 2004; 291: 358

687 *Atherosclerosis, Thrombosis, and Vascular Biology* 2007; 27: 1375

688 New England Journal of Medicine 2004: 350: 664; Science 2003: 300: 1140

689 *Science* 1998; 282: 642

690 *Functional Medicine* 2007; 27 #4

691 *Journal of the American Medical Association* 2004; 292: 2823

692 *Diabetes* 2007; 56: 1376

693 *Diabetes Research & Clinical Practice* 1998; 42: 161

694 "Mitochondria DNA Mutations, Oxidative Stress, and Apoptosis in Mammalian Aging," *Science* 2005; 309: 481

695 Archives of Internal Medicine 2008; 14: 1487

696 *Journal of the American Dietetic Association* 2003: 103: 1029; *Nutrition Journal* 2006: 22: 136

697 "A Role for Supplements in Optimizing Health: The Metabolic Tune-up," *Archives of Biochemistry and Biophysics* 2004: 423: 227

698 *Diabetes* 2004; 53: 2861

699 "A Cluster of Metabolic Defects Caused by Mutations in Mitochondrial tRNA," *Science* 2004; 306: 1190

700 *Nutrition* 2001; 131: 924

701 "Mitochondrial Medicine: A Metabolic Perspective on the Pathology of Oxidative Phosphorylation Disorders," *Cell Metabolism* 2006; 3: 9

702 *Lipids* 1979; 14: 727

703 *Bollettino-Societa Italiana Biologia Sperimentale* (Napoli) 1984; 60: 1029

704 Federation of American Societies for Experimental Biology (*FASEB*) 1997; 13: a163

705 *Journal of Allergy and Clinical Immunology* 1997; 99: S175

706 Journal of Clinical Endocrinology & Metabolism 2007; 92: 1229, 1467

707 *Metabolism* 2001; 50: 868; *European Journal of Clinical Nutrition* 2002; 56: 1137

708 "Mitochondrial Diabetes," *Journal of Endocrinology Investigation* 2002; 25: 477

709 "Human Disease Classification in the Postgenomic Era: A Complex Systems Approach to Human Pathobiology," *Molecular Systems Biology* 2007; 3: 124 e-pub July 10, 2007

710 *Diabetes* 1993; 42: 966

711 *Science* 2001; 291: 2263-25

712 Emil Mondoa and Mindy Kitea, *Sugars That Heal* (Ballantine Books: 2001)

[713] *American Journal of Clinical Nutrition* 2006; 83: 1082

[714] *Medical Hypotheses* 2008: 70: 265

[715] *Science* 2008; 319: 1402

[716] "Searching for Medicine's Sweet Spot," *Science* 2001; 291: 2263-25

[717] *Scientific American,* July 2002, cover story; page 40

[718] *Science* 2001; 291: 2263-25

[719] *Biotechnology* 1990; 8: 108

[720] *Cellular Microbiology* 2006; 8: 923

[721] *Science* 2002; 297: 1795

[722] "Bent Out of Shape," *Science* 2001; 291: 2263-25

[723] *Medical Hypotheses* 2007; 69: 166

[724] *Science* 2001; 291: 2263-25

[725] *Acta Anatomica* 1998; 161: 1

[726] *Glycoscience and Nutrition* 2001; 2 #14

[727] "Dietary Specific Sugars for Serum Protein Enzymatic Glycosylation in Man," *Metabolism* 1998; 47: 1499-1503

[728] *Glycobiology* 1998; 8: 285

[729] *Drug Chemistry Toxicity* 1997; 20: 3

[730] *Archives of Pediatrics & Adolescent Medicine* 2005; 12: 6

[731] Academy of General Dentistry

[732] *British Journal of Nutrition* 2005; 93: 911

[733] *Journal of Dermatological Science* 2005; 38: 207

[734] Institute of Dentistry, Finland, 2005

[735] Institute of Dentistry, Finland, 2005

[736] *Journal of Tokyo Medical and Dental University* 2005; 72: 106

[737] *Current Allergy and Asthma Reports* 2005; 5: 313

[738] *European Archives of Psychiatry and Clinical Neuroscience* 1999; 249: s68

[739] *Science* 1999; 285: 1390

[740] *American College of Nutrition* 1997; 16: 397

[741] *Genetica* 1993; 91: 239

[742] Annual Meeting for Pharmagenomics, 2004

[743] *Endocrinology* 2003; 26: 42

[744] *Journal of Internal Medicine* 2002; 251: 87

[745] *Endocrinology* 2007;193:269

[746] *Proceedings of the National Academy of Science,* Nov. 12, 2002

[747] *Circulation* 2004; 110: 285

748   *Diabetes Care* 2008; 31: 539

749   *Hormone and Metabolic Research* 2008; 40: 614

750   *Arteriosclerosis, Thrombosis, and Vascular Biology* 2005; 25: 815

751   *Proceedings of the National Academy of Science* 1994; 91: 4766

752   *Medical Hypotheses* 2005; 65: 953

753   *Hepato-Gastroenterology* 2002; 49: 928

754   *Clinical Diabetes* 2003;21:186

755   *Arteriovascular, Thrombosis, and Vascular Biology* 2005; 25: 879, 1042

756   *Circulation* 2006; 113: 1226

757   *Clinical Endocrinology & Metabolism* 2006;91:4628

758   *Arthritis & Rheumatism* 2002; 46: 114, 3212

759   *The Journal of Clinical Investigation* 1993; 93: 421

760   "Advanced Glycation End Products [are] a Potential Target for Treatment of Cardiovascular   Disease" *Hypertension* 2002; 20: 1483

761   *Medical Hypotheses* 2002; 59: 297

762   *Diabetologia* 2002; 11: 1515

763   *Metabolism — Clinical and Experimental* 2008; 57: 1465

764   *Endocrinology* 2005; 146: 5561

765   *Metabolism — Clinical and Experimental* 2006; 55: 1155

766   "The Endocrine System in Chronic Nitric Oxide Deficiency," *European Journal of Endocrinology* 2007; 156: 1

767   "Mental Stress Induces Prolonged Endothelial Dysfunction Via Endothelin-A Receptors," *Circulation* 2002; 105: 2817

768   *Family Practice News, Feb. 15, 2009, page 17*

769   *Archives of Internal Medicine* 2008; 168: 33

770   *Diabetes Care* 2003; 26: 702

771   *Pediatrics* 2007; 150: 608

772   *Journal of Allergy and Clinical Immunology* 2003; 111: 3

773   *Trends in Immunology* 2003; 24: 444

774   *Journal of the American Medical Association* 2002; 287: 2505

775   *Internal Medicine Journal* 2003; 253: 225

776   *Journal of Clinical Endocrinology & Metabolism* 2002; 87: 998

777   *Diabetes Care* 2002; 255: 30

778   ABC News, July 2, 2007

779   *American Journal of Reproductive Immunology* 2005; 54: 63

780   *Diabetes* 2007; 56: 1382

781 *Neuroscience* 2006; 26: 2434

782 University of Pittsburgh, Sept. 26, 2002

783 *Psychoneuroendocrinology* 2006; 31: 325

784 "Nutritional Hormesis," *European Journal of Clinical Nutrition* 2007; 61: 147

785 *British Medical Journal* 2008; 336: 1144

786 "Hormesis: Why it is Important to Toxicology and Toxicologists," *Environmental Toxicology and Chemistry* 2008; 27: 1451

787 *Medical Hypotheses* 2006; 67: 36

788 "Unhappy Meal: How Our Need to Detect Stress May Have Shaped Our Preferences for Taste," *Medical Hypotheses* 2007; 69: 746

789 *Hormone and Metabolic Research* 2008; 40: 848

790 Bruce Lipton, *The Biology of Belief* (Mountain of Love Books: 2005)

791 Antoine de Saint-Exupery, *The Little Prince* (Harcourt: 1945)

792 *Clinical Endocrinology* 2004; 59: 314

793 *Diabetes Care* 2006; 29: 1638

794 "Relationship Between Serum Concentratons of Persistent Organic Pollutants and the Prevalence of Metabolic syndrome Among Non-Diabetic Adults," *Diabetologia* 207; 50: 1841

795 *Lancet* 2006; 368: 558

796 "The Chemicas Within Us," *National Geographic*, October 2006, page 116

797 "A Strong Dose-Response Relation Between Serum Concentrations of Persistent Organic Pollutants and Diabetes," *Diabetes Care* 1996; 29: 1638

798 *Environmental Health Perspectives* 2001; 109: 871

799 *Epidemiology* 2006; 17: 352

800 *Diabetes Care* 2008; 31: 1574

801 J. Lancet 2006;368:558

802 "Association Between Serum Concentrations of Persistent Organic Pollutants and Insulin Resistance Among Non-Diabetic Adults," *Diabetes Care* 2007; 30: 622

803 "Environmental Chemicals and Thyroid Function," *European Journal of Endocrinology* 2006; 154: 599

804 J. Diabetes 2007; 56: 1761

805 *American Journal of Clinical Nutrition* 2008; 87;L1219

806 *Journal of the American Medical Association* 2008; 300: 1303, 1353

807 Devra Davis, *The Secret History of the War on Cancer* (Basic Books: 2008)

808 *Journal of the American Medical Association* 2008; 300: 1353

809 Randall Fitzgerald, *The Hundred-Year Lie: How Food and Drugs are Ruining Your Health* (Plume: 2006)

810 *Medical Hypotheses* 2006; 66: 263

811 *Integrative Medicine* 2007; 6: 22

812 *Medical Hypotheses* 2006; 67: 36

813 *New England Journal of Medicine* 2000; 342: 301

814 United States Environmental Protection Agency, 2001

815 "European Union Shifts ED Research into Overdrive," *Science* 2003; 300: 1069

816 *Environmental Health Perspectives* 2003; 111: 155

817 *Environmental Health Perspectives* 2001; 109: 245

818 *Diabetes Care* 2002; 25: 1534

819 *Toxicology Letters* 2002; 133: 69

820 *Toxicology Letters* 2002; 133: 69

821 *Journal of the American Medical Association* 2007; 298: 2654

822 *Circulation* 2005; 112: 862

823 *American Journal of Medicine* 2000; 109: 538

824 *British Medical Journal* 2002; 324: 26

825 *American Journal of Respiratory and Critical Care Medicine* 2001; 164: 831

826 *Epidemiology* 2002; 13: 588

827 *Annals of Rheumatologic Diseases* 2001;60:934

828 *Occupational and Environmental Medicine* 2006; 63: 844

829 *Medical Hypotheses* 2004; 64: 14

830 "Energy Balance and Pollution by Organochlorides and Polychlorinated Bi-phenyls," *Obesity Reviews* 2003; 4: 17

831 Devra Davis, *The Secret History of the War on Cancer* (Basic Books: 2007)

832 *Archives of Environmental Contamination and Toxicology* 2002; 42: 93

833 Organic Consumer Association, March 3, 2003; a_byrum@acs.org; American Chemical Society

834 *Bioscience* 2005; 55: 573

835 *American Journal of Alternative Agriculture* 2002; 18: 59

836 Jeffrey Smith, *Seeds of Deception: Exposing Industry and Government Lies About the Safety of the Genetically-Modified Foods You Are Eating* (Yes! Books: 2003)

837 *Diabetología* 2002; 5: 625

838 *Family Practice Recertification* 2005; 27 #2: 49

839 Childhood Obesity Conference, Anaheim, Calif., 2007; *Salt Lake Tribune,* Jan. 26, 2007

840 *New York Times,* July 17, 2007

841 *Journal of the American Medical Association* 2007; 298: 1625

842   *Nutrition & Environmental Medicine* 2001; 11: 275

843   *American Journal of Clinical Nutrition* 2006; 84: 694

844   *Endocrinology* 2009; 150: 555

845   *Clinical Endocrinology* 2006; 65: 593

846   *Family Practice News,* June 15, 2008, page 13

847   *Diabetes Care* 2007; 30: 2569

848   "Supplementation with Calcium and Vitamin D Enhances the Beneficial Effect of Weight Loss on Plasma Lipid and Lipoprotein Concentrations,"*American Journal of Clinical Nutrition* 2007; 85: 54

849   *European Journal of Endocrinology* 2008; 159: 41

850   *Archives of Internal Medicine* 2007; 167: 1730; *National Cancer Institute* 2007; 99: 1594

851   *Family Practice News,* Feb. 1, 2008, page 39

852   *Family Practice News,* Aug. 15, 2007, page 34

853   *National Cancer Institute,* January 2005

854   *American Journal of Clinical Nutrition* 2000; 71: 795

855   Dr. Hollick, Boston U. School of Medicine, reporting at Institute of Functional Medicine Symposium, Palm Springs, 2005

856   *Salt Lake Tribune,* May 29, 2007

857   *New England Journal of Medicine* 2007; 357: 266

858   *Journal of Clinical Endocrinology & Metabolism* 1988; 67: 373

859   "Vitamin D Update," *Functional Medicine Update,* 2004; 24, No. 8

860   *Journal of Clinical Endocrinology & Metabolism* 2007; 92: 2130

861   *Skin and Allergy News* 2006; 37 #4: 1

862   *American Journal of Clinical Nutrition* 2007; 298: 959

863   J. Lancet Oncology July 29th 2009

864   *Lancet* 2006; 368: 83

865   *Archives of Internal Medicine* 2007; 167: 1159; *Circulation* 2008; 117:503

866   *Archives of Internal Medicine* 2008; 168: 1174

867   *Journal of Endocrinology* 2008; 149: 6336

868   *American Journal of Clinical Nutrition* 2006; 84: 18

869   Annual Meeting International Society for Clinical Densitometry, Tampa, Fla., 2007

870   Journal of Nutrition 2006; 136: 1117

871   *Journal of Nutrition* 2007; 137: 2437

872   "Vitamin D Receptor Gene Polymorphisms, Dietary Promotion of Insulin Resistance, and Colon Rectal Cancer," *Nutrition and Cancer* 2006; 55: 35

437

873 *Journal of Endocrinology* 2007; 148: 1396

874 *American Journal of Clinical Nutrition* 2006; 84: 616

875 *Alternative Therapies* 2008; 14: 75

876 *New England Journal of Medicine* 2007; 357: 266

877 *Archives of Internal Medicine* 2006; 166: 424

878 *Journal of Clinical Investigation* 2006; 116: 2062

879 *Proceedings of the National Academy of Science* 2007; 104: 15087

880 *Archives of General Psychiatry* 2008; 65: 508

881 "Vitamin D Update," *Functional Medicine Update,* 2004; 24, No. 8

882 *Archives of Neurology* 2008; 65: 1348

883 *New England Journal of Medicine* 2007; 357: 266

884 "Vitamin D and Autoimmune Disease: Implications for Practice from the Multiple Sclerosis   Literature," *Journal of the American Dietetic Association* 2006; 106: 418

885 *Neurology* 2004; 62: 60

886 *British Medical Journal* 2003; 327: 316

887 *Annals of Neurology* 2000; 48: 271

888 *Lancet* 2001; 358: 1500

889 *New England Journal of Medicine* 2007; 357: 266

890 *Arthritis & Rheumatism* 2004; 50: 72

891 "*Vitamin D Update,*" *Functional Medicine Update,* 2004; 24, No. 8

892 *Mayo Clinic Proceedings* 2003; 78: 1463

893 *Spine* 2003; 28: 177

894 *Epidemiology & Infection* 2006; 134: 1129

895 *Archives of Internal Medicine* 2009; 169: 384

896 *Science,* March 24, 2006, page 1770

897 "Vitamin D and Health in the 21st Century," *American Journal of Clinical Nutrition* (supp) 2004; 80(6S)

898 *American Journal of Clinical Nutrition,* June 2007

899 *Scandinavian Journal of Gastroenterology* 2006; 41: 673

900 *Carcinogenesis* 2005; 27: 32

901 *American Journal of Public Health* 2006; 96: 252

902 *Diabetes Care* 2001; 24: 2065

903 *New England Journal of Medicine* 2003; 349: 1966

904 *Diabetes Care* 2007; 30: 343

905 *Metabolism — Clinical and Experimental* 2007; 56: 106

906 *Pediatrics* 2007; 150: 535

907 *New England Journal of Medicine* 2003; 349: 1966

908 *New England Journal of Medicine* 2005; 353: 1454

909 *Journal of Endocrinology Investigation* 2006; 29: 528

910 *Diabetes Care* 2007; 30: 228

911 *Doc News*, November 2006, page 6

912 *Annals of Internal Medicine* 2004; 141: 413

913 *Archives of Internal Medicine* 2004; 164: 1627

914 *Journal of the American Medical Association* 2006; 295: 1707

915 *Diabetes Care* 2008; 31: 1991

916 *Diabetes Care* 2005; 28: 1981

917 *Journal of General Internal Medicine* 2004; 19: 1175

918 *British Medical Journal* 2001; 322: 15

919 Forty-second Annual Meeting for the European Association for the Study of Diabetes, Copenhagen, Denmark, 2006

920 *Diabetes Care* 2008; 31: 1473

921 *Diabetes Care* 2008; 31: 381; Journal of the American Medical Association 2009; 301: 1528

922 *Journal of Internal Medicine* 2006; 260: 263

923 *Archives of Internal Medicine* 2001; 161: 397

924 *Diabetes Care* 2008; 31: 884

925 *Family Practice News*, April 1, 2007, page 1

926 *Lancet* 2003; 361: 544

927 *Journal of Internal Medicine* 2003; 253: 136

928 *Diabetologia* 2005; 48: 732

929 *Pediatrics* 2007; 150: 31

930 *Medical Hypotheses* 2004; 62: 53

931 *Diabetes Care* 2007; 30: 38

932 *Diabetes Care* 1999; 22: 883

933 Annual Meeting of the American Association for Clinical Chemistry, Orlando, Fla., 2003

934 *Metabolism — Clinical and Experimental* 2006; 55: 143

935 *Diabetes Care* 2008; 31: 1026

936 *Family Practice*, Oct. 15, 2003, page 11

937 *American Journal of Cardiology* 2003; 92: 606

938 *Journal of Clinical Endocrinology* 2004; 59: 756

939   *Diabetes Care* 2007; 30: 1544

940   *Annals of Internal Medicine* 2003; 139: 802

941   *Family Practice Review,* Dec. 15, 2003, page 6

942   *Journal of Clinical Endocrinology & Metabolism* 2002; 11: 5092

943   *Family Practice News,* April 1, 2006

944   *Family Practice News,* May 1, 2007, page 21

945   *Journal of Endocrine Investigation* 2003; 25: 74

946   *American Journal of Physiology – Endocrine and Metabolism* 2004; 286: 102

947   *Journal of the American Medical Association* 2001; 286: 241

948   *Diabetes Care* 2003; 26: 2426; *International Journal of Obesity-Related Metabolism Disorders* 2004; 28: 222

949   *Family Practice Recertification* 2000; 22: 25

950   *Clinical Diabetes* 2000; 18: 81

951   *Journal of Clinical Endocrinology & Metabolism* 2007; 92: 399

952   "Does a Diagnosis of Metabolic Syndrome Have Value in Clinical Practice?" *American Journal of Clinical Nutrition* 2006; 83: 1248

953   *Journal of Alternative and Complementary Medicine* 2007; 13: 11

954   American College of Endocrinology, National Harbor, MD, 2008; *Family Practice News,* Aug. 15, 2008, page 1

955   World Health Organization, 1999

956   *Comparative Biochemistry and Physiology and Molecular and Integrative Physiology* 2003; 136: 95

957   *Journal of the American Medical Association* 2002; 288: 2709

958   "Insulin and Endothelin: An Interplay Contributing to Hypertension Development?" *Journal of Clinical Endocrinology & Metabolism* 2007; 92: 379

959   *Hypertension* 2002; 10: 509

960   *Journal of the American Medical Association* 2001; 285: 2055

961   *Journal of the American Medical Association* 2003; 240: 2945

962   *Metabolism—Clinical and Experimental* 2006; 55: 143

963   *Hormone Metabolism Research* 2006; 38: 469

964   *Arteriosclerosis, Thrombosis, and Vascular Biology* 2007; 192: 169

965   *Diabetes Care* 2007; 30: 1255

966   *Journal of Clinical Endocrinology & Metabolism* 2003; 88: 2399

967   *Journal of Rheumatology* 2002; 29: 7

968   *American Journal of Hypertension* 2002; 15: 927

969   *Journal of the American Medical Association* 2004; 292: 2227

970   *Journal of Clinical Endocrinology & Metabolism* 2002; 12: 5503

971 *New England Journal of Medicine* 2001; 345: 1291

972 *Archives of Internal Medicine* 2008; 168: 571

973 *Lipids* 2002; 37: 231

974 *Metabolism — Clinical and Experimental* 2007; 56: 245

975 "Oxidative Stress and its Association with Coronary Artery Disease and Different Atherogenic Risk Factors," *Journal of Internal Medicine* 2004; 256: 308

976 *Journal of the American Medical Association* 2007; 297: 2092

977 *Journal of Clinical Endocrinology & Metabolism* 2007; 92: 2292

978 *Diabetes Research and Clinical Practice* 2002; 55: 159

979 *Arteriosclerosis, Thrombosis, and Vascular Biology* 2005; 25: 1026

980 *Free Radical Biology & Medicine* 2000; 28: 1707

981 *Circulation* 2004; 110: 285

982 *Arteriosclerosis, Thrombosis, and Vascular Biology* 2003; 23: 1437

983 *Journal of the American Medical Association* 2002; 287: 598

984 *British Journal of Nutrition* 2002; 88: 335

985 *Diabetes/Metabolism Research and Reviews* 2007; 23: 35

986 *Nature Medicine* 2007; 13: 1015

987 *Diabetes Care* 2007; 30: 1789

988 *Journal of the American Medical Association* 2008; 299: 2287

989 *Archives of Internal Medicine* 2007;167:1195; *American Journal of Clinical Nutrition* 2009; 89: 71

990 Atherosclerosis (2007) Epub, doi:10.1016/j.atherosclerosis.2007.05.012

991 *New England Journal of Medicine* 2002; 346: 1221

992 *American Journal of Clinical Nutrition* 2003; 78: 928

993 *Journal of the American Medical Association* 2007; 298: 308

994 *Trends in Immunology,* July 2006, volume 27

995 "Is Oxidative Stress the Pathogenic Mechanism Underlying Insulin Resistance, Diabetes and Cardiovascular Disease? The Common Soil Hypothesis Revisited," *Arteriosclerosis, Thrombosis, and Vascular Biology* 2004; 24: 823

996 *Journal of Clinical Investigation* 2007; 117: 746

997 *Archives of Internal Medicine* 2007; 167: 1195

998 *American Journal of Clinical Nutrition* 2008: 87: 424

999 *Journal of the American Medical Association* 2007; 292; 1490

1000 *British Medical Journal* 2002; 2: 339

1001 *British Journal of Clinical Pharmacology* 2004; 58: 326

1002 *Trends in Molecular Medicine* 2008; 14: 37

[1003] "Endothelial Dysfunction, Oxidative Stress and Inflammation in Atherosclerosis: Beneficial Effects of Statins," *Current Medicinal Chemistry* 2007; 14: 243

[1004] *Annals of Neurology* 2006; 60: 45

[1005] *Family Practice News*, May 25, 2008, page 16

[1006] "Are Lipid-Lowering Guidelines Evidence-Based?" *Lancet* 2007; 369: 168

[1007] *Nature Neuroscience* 2005; 8: 468

[1008] "Effects of Olive Oils on Biomarkers of Oxidative DNA Stress in Northern and Southern Europeans," Federation of American Societies for Experimental Biology (*FASEB*) 2007; 21: 45

[1009] "High Total Cholesterol Levels in Late Life [are] Associated with a Reduced Risk of Dementia," *Neurology* 2005; 64: 2689

[1010] Federation of American Societies for Experimental Biology (*FASEB*) 2009; 23: 58

[1011] *Journal of the American Geriatric Society* 2005; 53: 219

[1012] *American Journal of Clinical Nutrition* 2006; 84: 37

[1013] *Family Practice News*, Sept. 15 2005, page 12

[1014] *Science* 2008; 322: 220

[1015] "The Metabolic Syndrome: A New Focus for Lifestyle Modification," *Patient Care*, November 2002, page 74

[1016] "Selling Sickness: The Pharmaceutical Industry and Disease Mongering," *British Medical Journal* 2002; 2: 339

[1017] American Society of Bariatric Physicians Symposium, San Diego, Calif., 2006; *Family Practice News*, Jan. 1, 2007, page 34

[1018] *Family Practice News*, Jan. 1, 2007, page 34

[1019] *Journal of the American Medical Association* 2001; 286: 2421

[1020] "Irregular Menses Linked to Increased Heart Risk," Annual Scientific Sessions of the American Heart Association, Orlando, Fla., 2007

[1021] *Diabetes Care* 2008; 31: 2013

[1022] *Family Practice News*, Nov. 15, 2007, page 15

[1023] *Journal of Clinical Endocrinology & Metabolism* 2007; 92: 4637

[1024] *Journal of Clinical Endocrinology & Metabolism* 2007; 92: 2066

[1025] Annual Meeting Endocrine Society, Toronto, Canada, 2007

[1026] *Journal of Endocrinology Investigation* 2006; 28: 882

[1027] *Journal of Clinical Endocrinology & Metabolism* 2007; 92: 4609

[1028] *Fertility & Sterility* 2002; 77: 1128

[1029] "The Metabolic Syndrome in PCOS," *Endocrinology* 2006; 29: 270

[1030] *Journal of Clinical Endocrinology* 2006; 65: 655

[1031] *Circulation*, June 18, 2002

[1032] *Archives of Pediatrics & Adolescent Medicine* 2006; 160: 933

[1033] *Journal of Clinical Endocrinology* 2004; 60: 560

[1034] *American Journal of Clinical Nutrition* 2007; 85: 231

[1035] *Science* 2005; 308: 1392

[1036] Annual Meeting of the Androgen Excess Society, Boston, Mass., 2006

[1037] *Lancet* 2007; 369: 597

[1038] *American Journal of Obstetrics & Gynecology* 1998; 179: 94

[1039] International Conference on Women, Heart Disease, and Stroke, Orlando, Fla., 2005

[1040] *Journal of Clinical Endocrinology & Metabolism* 2002; 87: 1017

[1041] *Journal of Clinical Endocrinology & Metabolism* 2003; 88: 3626

[1042] *Journal of Clinical Endocrinology & Metabolism* 2005; 90: 6014

[1043] *Journal of Clinical Endocrinology & Metabolism* 2005, page 2693

[1044] *Journal of Clinical Endocrinology & Metabolism* 2006; 91: 1660

[1045] *Journal of Clinical Endocrinology & Metabolism* 2007; 92: 430

[1046] *British Medical Journal* 2006; 333: 1159

[1047] *Journal of the American Medical Association* 2008; 299: 279

[1048] *Family Practice News*, Aug. 15, 2007, page 23

[1049] *Endocrinology Metabolism Clinics of North America* 1999; 28: 397

[1050] *Family Practice News*, Aug. 1, 2006; page 20

[1051] *Skin and Allergy News*, March 2007, page 68

[1052] Annual Experimental Biology Conference, New Orleans, La., 2002

[1053] *Free Radical Biology & Medicine* 2006; 40: 3

[1054] *New England Journal of Medicine* 1999; 340: 1314

[1055] *New England Journal of Medicine*, May 30, 2007

[1056] *Endocrinology* 2007; 148: 2669

[1057] *Metabolism—Clinical and Experimental* 2007; 56: 129

[1058] Annual Meeting of the American Heart Association, Chicago, Ill., 2002

[1059] *Archives of Internal Medicine* 2006; 166: 1975

[1060] *Acta Obstetricia et Gynecologica Scandinavica* 2007; 137: 973

[1061] *European Journal of Obstetrics, Gynecology, and Reproductive Biology*, Nov. 16, 2006

[1062] *Fertility & Sterility* 2006;86: 1688

[1063] Annual Meeting American College of Ob-Gyn, Washington, 2006

[1064] Annual Meeting Society for Adolescent Medicine, Boston, Mass., 2006

[1065] National Center for Health Statistics, Aug. 24, 2007; *Salt Lake Tribune,* Aug. 25, 2007

[1066] *Journal of the American Medical Association* 2001; 285: 1607

[1067] *Family Practice News,* April 1, 2008, page 28

[1068] World Congress of the International Society for the Study of Hypertension in Pregnancy, Vienna, 2005

[1069] *Diabetologia* 2007; 50: 523

[1070] *European Journal of Endocrinology* 2008: 158: 101

[1071] *Annals of Internal Medicine* 2008; 149: 461

[1072] *Free Radical Biology & Medicine* 2003; 35: 1453

[1073] *Diabetes Care* 2008; 149: 2026

[1074] Annual Scientific Sessions of the American Diabetes Association, Orlando, Fla., 2004

[1075] *Diabetes Care* 2008; 31: 1275

[1076] *Doc News,* May 2007

[1077] *Diabetes Care* 2008; 31: 1386

[1078] *Diabetes Care* 2005; 28: 1995

[1079] *Diabetes Care* 2007; 30: 348

[1080] *Journal of Clinical Endocrinology & Metabolism* 2003; 88: 2393

[1081] *Diabetes Care* 2008; 31: e30

[1082] *Journal of Endocrinology Investigation* 2004; 27: 629

[1083] *Diabetes Care* 2008; 31: 1037

[1084] *Family Practice News,* July 15, 2007, page 1

[1085] *Diabetologia* 2001; 8: 972

[1086] *American Journal of Public Health* 2007; 97: 157

[1087] *Diabetes Care* 2008; 31: 483

[1088] *New England Journal of Medicine* 2007; 356: 2053

[1089] *Lancet* 2003; 362: 1777

[1090] World Congress International Society for the Study of Hypertension in Pregnancy, Vienna, Austria, 2005

[1091] Federation of American Societies for Experimental Biology (*FASEB*) 2007; 21: 366

[1092] *Nutrition Journal* 2008; 138: 753

[1093] National Institutes of Health publication 1995; page 703

[1094] *American Journal of Clinical Nutrition* 2006; 84: 807

[1095] *American Journal of Obstetrics and Gynecology,* April 2007

[1096] *British Medical Journal,* February 2008

[1097] "Improvement of Glutathione and Total Antioxidant Status with Yoga," *Journal of Alternative and Complementary Medicine* 2007; 13: 1085

[1098] *Journal of Clinical Endocrinology & Metabolism* 2003; 88: 4904

[1099] *Journal of Clinical Oncology* 2002; 20: 1436

[1100] *Journal of Clinical Endocrinology & Metabolism* 2003; 88: 2404

[1101] *Archives of Internal Medicine* 2008; 168: 1568

[1102] *Clinical Diabetes* 2000; 18: 38

[1103] *Medical Hypotheses* 2002; 59: 660

[1104] "Thyroid Function is Intrinsically Linked to Insulin Sensitivity and Endothelium Dependent   Vasodilatation in Healthy Euthyroid Subjects," *Journal of Clinical Endocrinology & Metabolism* 2006; 91: 3337

[1105] *Journal of Clinical Endocrinology & Metabolism* 2007; 92: 491

[1106] *Journal of Clinical Endocrinology & Metabolism* 2007; 92: 491

[1107] *Lancet* 2002; 360: 353

[1108] *Diabetes Care* 2005; 28: 2073

[1109] *Endocrinology* 2005; 146: 5425

[1110] *Diabetes Care* 2005; 28: 2073

[1111] *Annals of Internal Medicine* 2000; 132: 270

[1112] *Metabolism — Clinical and Experimental* 2005; 54: 1524

[1113] *European Journal of Endocrinology* 2006; 154: 599

[1114] *Journal of Endocrinological Investigation* 2001; 24: supp #7, R12, page 5

[1115] *Endocrinology* 2005; 146: 5128

[1116] "Estrogen-Related Receptors as Emerging Targets in Cancer and Metabolic Disorders," *Current Topics in Medicinal Chemistry* 2006; 6: 181

[1117] *Journal of Internal Medicine* 2006; 260: 53

[1118] *Endocrinology* 2005; 146: 5176

[1119] *European Journal of Endocrinology* 2006; 155: 593

[1120] **"Effect of Dehydroepiandrosterone Replacement on Lipoprotein Profile in Hypoadrenal** Women," *Journal of Clinical Endocrinology & Metabolism* 2009; 94: 761-764

[1121] *Atherosclerosis* 2007; 181: 39

[1122] *Endocrinology* 2008; 149: 889

[1123] *Journal of the American Medical Association* 2002; 287: 2505

[1124] *New England Journal of Medicine* 1999; 341: 248, 1013

[1125] *American Journal of Hypertension* 1999; 12: 747

[1126] "Pituitary-Adrenal and Autonomic Responses to Stress in Women After Sexual and Physical Abuse in Childhood," *Journal of the American Medical Association* 2000; 284

[1127] *Endocrinology* 2008; 149: 2724

[1128] *Diabetologia* 1994; 37: 247

[1129] *Journal of the American Medical Association* 1999; 281: 1328

[1130] J. Hormone and Metabolism Research 2006;38:437

[1131] J. Hormone and Metabolism Research 2006;38;437

[1132] *Female Patient Magazine* 2004; 29: 23

[1133] "Increased Levels of Multiple Types of Childhood Trauma in CFS," *Archives of General Pschiatry* 2006; 63: 1258

[1134] *Journal of the American Medical Association* 2006; 295: 1304

[1135] *Scientific American,* December 2005, page 92

[1136] JAMA 2001; 286: 1897

[1137] "Plasma Ghrelin, Obesity, and the PCOS: Correlation with Insulin Resistance and Androgen Levels," *Journal of Clinical Endocrinology & Metabolism* 2002; 87: 5625

[1138] *Annals of Internal Medicine* 2008; 149: 601

[1139] *Journal of Clinical Endocrinology & Metabolism* 2000; 85: 4481

[1140] *Diabetes Care* 2008; 31: 397

[1141] "Time for Creative Thinking About Men's Health," *Lancet* 2001; 357: 1813

[1142] *Endocrinology* 2006; 147: 4160

[1143] *Journal of the American Medical Association* 2001;286: 1206, 1230

[1144] *Diabetes Care* 2007; 30: 1507

[1145] *Neurology* 2002; 59: 1674

[1146] *Journal of Clinical Endocrinology & Metabolism* 2000; 85: 4481

[1147] "Sex Hormones, Inflammation and the Metabolic Syndrome," *European Journal of Endocrinology* 2003; 149: 601

[1148] *Family Practice Recertification* 2005; 27 #11: 74

[1149] *Family Practice News,* March 15, 2007, page 12

[1150] *Family Practice News,* April 2007, page 34

[1151] *Diabetologia* 2001; 9: 1155

[1152] *Diabetologia,* October 2001, page 7319

[1153] *Metabolism — Clinical and Experimental* 2006; 55: 1564

[1154] *Journal of Sex & Marital Therapy* 2003; 29: 207

[1155] *Journal of Urology* 2002; 168: 2070

[1156] *Diabetes Care* 2008; 31: 940

[1157] Journal of the American Medical Association 2004; 291: 2978, 3011

[1158] *Lancet* 2000; 356: 1165

[1159] "Androgens and Diabetes in Men," *Diabetes Care* 2007; 30: 234

1160 *Diabetes* 2005; 54: 765

1161 *Diabetes Care* 2007; 30: 1972

1162 *American Family Physician* 2005; 72: 1107

1163 *Nutrition Biochemistry,* April 4, 2007

1164 *Nutrition Journal* 2008; 138: 167

1165 *Nutrition Journal* 2009; 139: 264

1166 Eleventh International Symposium of Functional Medicine, Vancouver, Canada 2004

1167 *Journal of the American Medical Association* 2006; 295: 1288

1168 "Hypogonadism and Metabolic Syndrome: Implications for Testosterone Therapy," *Journal of Urology* 2005; 174: 827

1169 *Journal of Endocrinology Investigation* 2004; 27: 353

1170 *Journal of the National Cancer Institute* 2003; 95: 1086

1171 *American Journal of Epidemiology* 2006; 164: 769

1172 "Endocrine Disrupting Chemicals Probed as Potential Pathways to Illness," *British Journal of Nutrition* 2006; 95: 539

1173 *American Journal of Preventive Medicine* 2005; 29: 320

1174 *Menopause* 2004; 11: 531

1175 *Lancet* 2002; 359: 1740

1176 "Low Dose of Insulin-Like Growth Factor-1 Improves Insulin Resistance, Lipid Metabolism, and Oxidative Damage in Aging Rats," *Endocrinology* 2008; 149: 2433

1177 *Arteriosclerosis, Thrombosis, and Vascular Biology* 2007; 27: 2684

1178 *Endocrinology* 2002; 174: 335

1179 *European Journal of Endocrinology* 2008; 159: 585

1180 *Annals of Nutrition & Metabolism* 2007; 2006; 50: 499

1181 *Lancet* 2002; 359: 46

1182 *American Journal of Clinical Nutrition* 2008; 88: 1187

1183 *Hormone and Metabolism Research* 2008; 40: 794

1184 *Circulation* 2008: 117: 798

1185 *Endocrinology* 2007; 148: 921

1186 *Journal of the American Medical Association* 2007; 298: 1506

1187 *Diabetes Care* 2008; 31: 1170

1188 *Diabetes* 2003; 52: 1204

1189 *American Journal of Hypertension* 2002; 15: 773

1190 *Diabetes Care* 2008; 31: 2357

1191 Annual Meeting American College of Nutrition, Reno, Nev., 2007

[1192] *Family Pactice News,* March 15, 2008, page 44

[1193] *American Journal of Clinical Nutrition* 2007; 298: 899

[1194] *Journal of the American Society of Nephrology,* 2007

[1195] *Family Practice News,* Feb. 1, 2007, page 17

[1196] *Mayo Clinic Proceedings* 2007; 82: 822

[1197] *American Journal of Clinical Nutrition* 2007; 86: 633

[1198] *Metabolism—Clinical and Experimental* 2007; 56: 153

[1199] Annual European Congress of Rheumatology, Vienna, Austria, 2006

[1200] *Rheumatology* 2005; 32: 774

[1201] *Arthritis & Rheumatism* 2007; 57: 109

[1202] *Family Practice News,* Sept. 1, 2005

[1203] Annual Meeting European Congress of Rheumatology, Vienna, Austria, 2005

[1204] *Rheumatology* 2002; 29: 7

[1205] *Hypertension* 2003; 41: 1183

[1206] *Journal of the American Geriatric Society* 2001; 49: 1679

[1207] *Archives of Internal Medicine* 2008; 168: 1104

[1208] *Circulation* 2007; 115: 2526

[1209] *Journal of the American Medical Association* 2008; 300: 924

[1210] *Metabolism—Clinical and Experimental* 2006; 55: 1293

[1211] *Journal of the American Medical Association* 2005; 293: 477

[1212] *Arthritis & Rheumatism* 2007; 57: 816

[1213] *Surgical Obstetric & Gynecology* 1990; 171: 493

[1214] Annual Meeting of the European Association for the Study of Diabetes, Amsterdam, 2007

[1215] *Clinical Obstetrics & Gynecology* 2002; 45: 259

[1216] Urology 1988; 140: 36

[1217] *International Journal of Urogynecology* 2001; 12: 271

[1218] "Prostate Enlargement: The Canary in the Coal Mine?" *American Journal of Clinical Nutrition* 2002; 75: 605

[1219] *Diabetes Care* 2008; 31: 476

[1220] Annual Meeting of the American Urology Association, Anaheim, Calif., 2007

[1221] *Family Practice News,* July 1, 2007

[1222] *Journal of the American Medical Association* 2001; 286: 1882

[1223] *Journal of Pharmacy and Pharmacology* 1991; 1; 15

[1224] *Planta Medica* 2007; 73: 6

[1225] *Metabolism — Clinical and Experimental* 2007; 56: 160

[1226] *Scientific American,* July 2002, page 40

[1227] *Metabolism — Clinical and Experimental* 2007; 56: 998

[1228] *Archives of Surgery* 1999; 134: 1229

[1229] *Antimicrobial Agents and Chemotherapy* 1994; 38: 1

[1230] *Molecular Psychiatry* 1997; 2: 99

[1231] *Trends in Immunology* 2004; 25: 193

[1232] "Hormetic Dose-Response Relationships in Immunology," *Critical Reviews in Toxicology* 2005; 35: 89

[1233] "Mucosal Immunity: Its Role in Defense and Allergy" *International Archives of Allergy and Immunology* 2002; 128: 77

[1234] *National Geographic,* November 2005

[1235] Stephen Jay Gould, *The Planet of Bacteria* (Crown Press: 1996)

[1236] "Yale Probiotics Workshop," *Clinical Gastroenterology* 2006; 40: 231

[1237] "The Danger Model: A Renewed Sense of Self," *Science* 2002; 296: 301

[1238] *Gut* 2002; 50: 32

[1239] *Journal of the American Medical Association* 2007; 297: 2339

[1240] "The Terrain Concept in Microbiology: The Cellular Basis of Immunity," *Presse Medicale* 1964: 72: 2105

[1241] "Nutrigenomics and Gut Health," *Mutation Research* 2007; 622: 1

[1242] "The Nature vs. Nurture Debate on Bioactive Phytochemicals: The Genome vs. Terroir," *Science of Food and Agriculture* 2006; 86: 2510

[1243] *Digestive Diseases and Sciences* 2007; 52: 103

[1244] *Clinical Endocrinology* 2003; 58: 20

[1245] *Medical Hypotheses* 2001; 57: 532

[1246] New England Journal of Medicine; H1N1 Influenza Center. Accessed Deember 12th 2009

[1247] USA Today, September 29th 2009

[1248] J. Skin Allergy News 2009;40:23

[1249] British Nespaper, The Guardian October 28th 2009

[1250] "Factors Associated with Death or Hospitalization Due to Pandemic 2009 Influenza A(H1N1) Infection in California," JAMA 2009;302:1896

[1251] *Biotechnology* 1990; 8: 108

[1252] *American Journal of Clinical Nutrition* 2002; 75: 49

[1253] *British Medical Journal* 2007; 335: 897

[1254] *Journal of the American Medical Association* 2008; 300: 2754

[1255] *Lancet* 2006; 367: 618

1256 *Muder by Injection,* Eustace Mullins; page 351

1257 *Journal of Science* 2007; 316: 1

1258 *Lancet* 2001; 357: 539

1259 *Journal of the National Cancer Institute* 2003; 95: 1086

1260 *Journal of the National Cancer Institute* 2002; 94: 1293

1261 *International Journal of Cancer* 1999; 81: 539

1262 *Diabetologia* 2006; 49: 2819

1263 "Increased Telomere Activity and Comprehensive Lifestyle Changes," *Lancet Oncology* 2008; 9: 1048; "Multivitamin Use and Telomere Length in Women," *American Journal of Clinical Nutrition* 2009; 89: 1857

1264 *Diabetologia* 2006; 49: 945

1265 *American Journal of Epidemiology* 2003; 157: 1092

1266 *New England Journal of Medicine* 2003; 348: 1625

1267 Endocrine Reviews 2007; 28: 763

1268 *Environmental Health Perspectives* 2003; 101: a691

1269 *Endocrine Reviews* 2007; 28: 20

1270 *Clinical Gastroenterology* 2007; 41: 285

1271 *Nutrition and Cancer* 2007; 56: 158

1272 *Journal of Clinical Endocrinology & Metabolism* 2006; 91: 4401

1273 *American Journal of Epidemiology* 2006; 164: 769

1274 "Obesity and Cancer," *British Medical Journal* 2006; 333: 1109

1275 "The Glycemic Index of Foods Influences Postprandial IGF-1 Binding Protein Responses in Lean Young Subjects," *American Journal of Clinical Nutrition* 2005; 82: 350

1276 American Association for Cancer Research Annual Meeting, National Harbor, Md., 2008

1277 *Nutrition Journal* 2008: 138: 250

1278 *Journal of the American Medical Association* 2006; 295: 1577

1279 *Journal of the American Medical Association* 2001; 286: 921

1280 *Journal of the American Medical Association* 2003; 290: 1323

1281 *American Journal of Clinical Nutrition* 2007; 86: 817s

1282 *Americal Journal of Clinical Nutrition* 2007; 86: 817s

1283 *American Journal of Clinical Nutrition* 2007; 86: 858s

1284 *American Journal of Clinical Nutrition* 2007; 86: 872s

1285 "Colon Cancer Associated with Coronay Artery Disease: Common Denominator, Metabolic Syndrome," *Journal of the American Medical Association* 2007; 298: 1412

[1286] *American Journal of Clinical Nutrition* 2007; 86: 878s

[1287] *American Journal of Clinical Nutrition* 2007; 86: 889s

[1288] *American Journal of Clinical Nutrition* 2007; 86: 882s

[1289] *Food and Chemical Toxicology* 2008; 46: 1365

[1290] *Carcinogenesis* 2007; 28: 233

[1291] Book review in the *Journal of the American Medical Association* 2006; 295: 2891

[1292] "Futile Cancer Treatments on the Rise," American Society of Clinical Oncology, Atlanta, Ga., 2006

[1293] Devra Davies, *The Secret History of the War on Cancer* (Basic Books: 2007)

[1294] "Obesity in Middle-Age and Future Risk of Dementia," *British Medical Journal* 2006; 330: 1360

[1295] "The Metabolic Syndrome and Alzheimer's Disease," *Archives of Neurology* 2007; 64: 93

[1296] *Neurology* 2006; 67: 843; 2007; 69: 1094

[1297] *Functional Medicine Update*, May 2007

[1298] *Archives of Neurology* 2007; 64: 984

[1299] *Diabetes Care* 2007; 30: 2001; *Archives of Neurology* 2008; 65: 1066

[1300] *Neurology* (online), April 9, 2008

[1301] International Conference on AD, Madrid, Spain, 2006

[1302] "Impaired Insulin and Insulin-Like Growth Factor Expression and Signaling Mechanisms in AD: Is This Type III Diabetes?" *Journal of Alzheimer's Disease* 2005; 7: 63

[1303] *Archives of Neurology* 2005; 62: 1728

[1304] *Current Alzheimer Research* 2007; 4: 117

[1305] *Archives of Neurology* 2005; 62: 1734; "Receptor for AGE Activation Injures Primary Sensory Neurons Via Oxidative Stress," *Endocrinology Reviews* 2007; 148: 548

[1306] *Family Practice News*, June 1, 2003, page 1

[1307] *Neurobiology of Aging* 2005; supp: 80

[1308] *Psychosomatic Medicine* 2005; supp: s26

[1309] *Journal of Clinical Endocrinology & Metabolism* 2007; 92: 2439

[1310] "Stress, Aging, and Neurodegenerative Disease," *New England Journal of Medicine* 2006; 355: 2254

[1311] *Diabetologia* 2006; 49: 855

[1312] *Family Practice News*, Nov. 15, 2003, page 5; "The Metabolic Syndrome, Inflammation, and Risk of Cognitive Decline," *Journal of the American Medical Association* 2004; 292: 2237

1313 *Neurology* 2007; 69: 951

1314 *Journal of the American Medical Association* 2004; 292: 2237

1315 *Archives of Neurology* 2007; 64: 570

1316 *Neurology, Neurosurgery & Psychiatry* 2003; 74: 70

1317 *Neurology* 2007; 68: 1809

1318 *Proceedings of the National Academy of Science,* Feb. 1, 2003

1319 *Nature Neuroscience,* April 2008

1320 *Lipids* 2007; 42: 5

1321 *Neurology News,* January 2007, page 4

1322 *Archives of Neurology* 2007; 64: 103

1323 *British Journal of Nutrition* 2006; 96: supp #2

1324 *American Journal of Clinical Nutrition* 2003; 78: 647

1325 *Journal of the American Medical Association* 2007; 297: 2339

1326 *Journal of Neuroinflammation,* April 2008

1327 *Neurology* 1994; 36: 333

1328 *Neurology,* May 2007

1329 *Archives of Medical Research* 2008; 39: 1

1330 Federation of American Societies for Experimental Biology (*FASEB*) 2002; 16: 1738

1331 *Neurology Reviews* 2002; 7: 39

1332 Annual Experimental Biology Conference, New Orleans, La., 2002

1333 "Insulin Effects Weigh Heavily on the Brain," *Journal of the American Medical Association* 2006; 296: 1717

1334 Annual Meeting Endocrine Society, Boston, Mass., 2006

1335 *Journal of the American Medical Association* 2006; 296: 1717

1336 Annual Meeting American Academy of Neurology, Chicago, Ill., 2008

1337 *Journal of the American Medical Association* 2006; 296: 1717

1338 *Psychiatric Practice* 2005; 11: 302

1339 *Metabolism* 2007; 56: 1652

1340 *Family Practice News* 2006; 36 #16: 1

1341 *Proceedings of the National Academy of Science* 2003; 100: 6221

1342 *Archives of Neurology* 2005; 62: 1043

1343 *Endocrinology* 2008; 149: 5951

1344 *Medical Hypotheses* 2006; 66: 263

1345 *Journal of the American Medical Association* 1995; 274: 1617

1346 *International Journal of Biosocial and Medical Research* 1982; 3: 1

[1347] "Apathy Tied to Poor Glycemic Control," Annual Meeting of the Academy of Psychosomatic Medicine, Tucson, Ariz., 2006; *Family Practice News*, Jan. 1, 2007, page 20

[1348] *Diabetologia* 2006; 49: 855

[1349] *Nutrition Report* 1991; 3: 17

[1350] *Abnormal Psychology* 1985; 94: 565

[1351] "Outcome-Based Comparison of Ritalin Versus Food-Supplement Treated Children with AD/HD," *Alternative Medicine Review* 2003; 8: 319

[1352] *Archives of Pediatrics & Adolescent Medicine* 2008; 162: 612

[1353] *New England Journal of Medicine* 2006; 354: 1445; United States Food and Drug Administration announcement, Feb. 2, 2006

[1354] *Cancer Letters*, March 2005

[1355] *American Academy Child & Adolescent Psychiatry*, November 2006

[1356] *New York Times*, November 1st, 2007

[1357] *Immunology* 2001; 166: 2831

[1358] *Archives of Neurology*, July 2006

[1359] *Neurology* 1999; 53: 772

[1360] *Archives of Neurology* 2008; 65: 476

[1361] *Diabetes Care* 2007; 30: 842

[1362] *Neurology Reviews*, June 2003, page 10

[1363] *Annals of Neurology* 2006; 60: 197

[1364] *Neuroscience*, June 27, 2007

[1365] *Optometry* 2000; 71: 755

[1366] "Neuroprotection in Parkinson's Disease," *Journal of the American Medical Association* 2004; 291: 358

[1367] Shambhala, 1987

[1368] *Science and Consciousness*, June 2004

[1369] *Lancet* 2001; 358: 1174

[1370] Norman Doidge, *The Brain that Changes Itself* (Viking: 2007)

[1371] *Science* 1968; 160: 265

[1372] Jim Marrs, *The Rise of the Fourth Reich* (William Morrow Publishers: 2008)

[1373] "Brain Foods: The Effects of Nutrients on Brain Function," *National Review of Neuroscience* 2008; 9: 568

[1374] Annual Meeting of the American Clinical Neurophysiology Society; Atlantic City, NJ 2005

[1375] *British Journal of Nutrition* 2001; 86: 117

[1376] *Lancet* 1979; 1: 955

[1377] *Neurology* 2007; 68: 1851

[1378] Annual Meeting of the American Headache Society, Chicago, Ill., 2007

[1379] Annual Meeting of the American Psychiatric Association, San Diego, Calif., 2007

[1380] *Archives of General Psychiatry* 2008; 65: 1386

[1381] *Journal of the American Medical Association* 2008; 299: 2751; *Diabetes Care* 2008; 31: 2368

[1382] *American Journal of Psychiatry* 2001; 10: 1612

[1383] *Scientific American* 1989; 260: 68

[1384] *Molecular Pharmacology* 1996; 50: 266

[1385] *Drug Metabolism and Disposition* 2000; 28: 1038

[1386] *Archives of Internal Medicine* 2007; 167: 1137

[1387] *American Journal of Clinical Nutrition* 2003; 77: 1112

[1388] *Diabetologia* 2002; 2: 242

[1389] *Diabetologia* 2006; 49: 2959

[1390] International Stroke Conference, New Orleans, La., 2008

[1391] *Salt Lake Tribune*, Feb. 20, 2008

[1392] *Neurology* 2003; 60: 1447

[1393] *Archives of Internal Medicine* 2005; 165: 227

[1394] *Journal of the American Medical Association* 2005; 294; 557

[1395] "Impaired Neuronal Glucose Uptake in Pathogenesis of Schizophrenia," *Medical Hypotheses* 2005; 65: 1076

[1396] Fifty-second Annual Meeting Association Neuromuscular and Electrodiagnostic Medicine, Monterey, Calif., 2005; *Neurology Reviews*, October 2005, page 27

[1397] "The Metabolic Anatomy of Tourette's Syndrome," *Neurology* 1997; 48: 927

[1398] - "Confectionary Consumption in Childhood and Adult Violence," British J. Psychiatry 2009;195:366

[1399] - British J. Psy 2009;195:366

[1400] *Neuropsy* 1982; 8: 30

[1401] "The effect of sugar on behavior or cognition in children. A meta-analysis," **Journal of the American Medical Association 1995 Nov 22-29;274(20):1617-21.**

[1402] *Applied Nutrition* 1991; 43: 131

[1403] *International Journal of Biosocial Research* 1982; 3: 1

[1404] *International Journal of Biosocial Research* 1986; 8: 185

[1405] *Journal of Alternative & Complementary Medicine* 1999; 5: 125

[1406] "Does Eating Salmon Lower the Murder Rate?" *New York Times,* April 16, 2006

[1407] "Potential Roles of Insulin and Insulin Growth Factor-1" *Trends in Neuroscience* 2003; 26: 404

[1408] *European Journal of Endocrinology* 2004; 151: 39

[1409] *Diabetologia* 1994; 37: 247

[1410] *Neuroscience* 2003; 23: 9687

[1411] *Neurology Reviews* 2002; 7: 1

[1412] *Journal of Occupational and Environmental Medicine* 2001; 58: 569

[1413] *American Journal of Respiratory and Critical Care Medicine* 2002; 165: 677

[1414] *Neuropsychopharmacology* 2001; 25: s74

[1415] *Archives of Internal Medicine* 2005; 165: 1022

[1416] *Endocrinology* 2004; 154: 1042

[1417] "DHEA: Is There a Role for Replacement?" *Mayo Clinic Proceedings* 2003; 78: 1257

[1418] *Annals of Neurology,* May 2007

[1419] *Neurology* 2007; 69: 108

[1420] *Neurology* 2007; 69: 1418

[1421] *Neurology News,* July 2007, page 58

[1422] *Neurobiology of Aging* 2004; 25: 311

[1423] Alzheimer's Association International Conference on Preventing Alzheimer's; Washington, D.C., 2005

[1424] J. Neurology News, December 2005, page 44

[1425] "Metabolic Learning in the Intestines: Adaptation to Nutrition and Luminal Factors," *Hormone Metabolism Research* 2006; 38: 452

[1426] Michio Kaku, *Hyperspace* (Anchor Books: 1994)

[1427] *Lancet,* July 11, 2001

[1428] *American Journal of Gastroenterology* 2000; 95: 2698

[1429] Michael Gershon, *The Second Brain: New Understanding of Nervous Disorders of the Stomach and Intestine* (HarperCollins: 1998)

[1430] *American Journal of Clinical Nutrition* 2003; 78: 675

[1431] *Endocrinology* 2008; 149: 4765

[1432] *Endocrinology* 2008; 149: 4768

[1433] *Digestive Diseases and Sciences* 2007; 52: 103

[1434] *Medical Microbiolology* 2003; 52: 169

[1435] *Infections and Immunology* 1993; 61: 619

[1436] "Serotonergic Neuroenteric Modulators," *Lancet* 2001; 358: 2061

[1437] *Neurology* 2003; 60: 1308

[1438] *Journal of Clinical Psychiatry* 2001; 27: 10

[1439] "Effectiveness of Antipsychotic Drugs in Patients with Chronic Schizophrenia," *New England Journal of Medicine* 2005; 353: 1209

[1440] *Family Practice News,* July 1, 2007

[1441] "Gut Derived Signaling Molecules and Vagal Afferents in the Control of Glucose and Energy Homeostasis," *Current Opinion in Clinical Nutrition & Metabolic Care* 2004; 7: 471

[1442] *Experimental Medicine* 2005; 202: 1023

[1443] *Lancet* 2002; 359: 1360

[1444] *Journal of Gastroenterology* 2003; 124: 1532

[1445] *Lancet* 2002; 359: 1740

[1446] *Scandinavian Journal of Gastroenterology* 2007; 42: 464

[1447] *Endocrine Reviews* 2006; 27: 719

[1448] *International Archives of Allergy and Immunology* 2002; 128: 77

[1449] "Close Encounters: Good, Bad, and the Ugly," *Science* 2000; 290: 1491

[1450] *Nutrition Journal* 1998; 128: 1099

[1451] "The Transmutation of Species in Bacteriology," *Journal of the American Medical Association* 2006; 295: 226

[1452] *Rheumatology* 2003; 30: 11

[1453] *Nutrition Journal* 2007; 137: 433

[1454] *Pediatrics* 2002; 109: 833

[1455] *Journal of Clinical Endocrinology & Metabolism* 2003; 1: 162

[1456] *Family Practice News,* Sept. 1, 2008, page 18

[1457] *Diabetes Care* 2006; 29: 2452

[1458] *Pediatrics* 2007; 150: 461

[1459] *Scandinavian Journal of Gastroenterology* 2007; 42: 60

[1460] *Scandinavian Journal of Gastroenterology* 2007; 42; 48

[1461] *Neurology* 2001; 56: 385

[1462] *Journal of Gastroenterology* 2006; 41: 10

[1463] *Gut* 2005; 54: 935

[1464] "Changes in Gut Microbiota Control Inflammation in Obese Mice Through a Mechanism Involving GLP-2 Driven Improvement of Gut Permeability," *Gut* 2009; 58: 1091

[1465] *Diabetologia* 2006; 49: 2824

[1466] *Current Opinion in Clinical Nutrition & Metabolic Care* 2004; 7: 479

[1467] *Gut* 2005; 54: 823

[1468] *American Journal of Clinical Nutrition* 2004; 80: 38

[1469] *Hepatology* 2007; 45: 1261

[1470] *American Journal of Epidemiology* 2004; 160: 11

[1471] *Scandinavian Journal of Gastroenterology* 2008; 43: 1483

[1472] *American Journal of Medicine* 2006; 119: 760

[1473] *American Journal of Gastroenterology* 2006; 101: 2247

[1474] *Arteriosclerosis, Thrombosis, and Vascular Biology* 2008; 28: 27

[1475] "Comparative Review of Diets for the Metabolic Syndrome," *American Journal of Clinical Nutrition* 2007; 86: 285

[1476] American Liver Foundation report in *Salt Lake Tribune*, Sept. 8, 2008

[1477] *Science*, Sept. 18, 2008

[1478] *Family Practice News*, May 15, 2007, page 39

[1479] Annual Meeting of the American Society for Bariatric Surgery, San Diego, Calif., 2007

[1480] *Family Practice News*, July 1, 2004, 1

[1481] *Journal of Clinical Gastroenterology* 2006; 40: 930

[1482] *Journal of Gastroenterology* 2007; 133: 496

[1483] *American Journal of Gastroenterology* 2006; 101: 2247

[1484] *American Journal of Clinical Nutrition* 2008; 88: 257

[1485] *Metabolism—Clinical and Experimental* 2008; 57: 1190

[1486] *American Journal of Clinical Nutrition* 2006; 84: 136

[1487] *Diabetes Care* 2007; 30: 1212

[1488] *American Journal of Clinical Nutrition* 2008: 87: 295

[1489] *Archives of Internal Medicine* 2008; 168: 1609

[1490] *Gut* 2005; 54: 1003

[1491] *Nature Medicine* 2005; 11: 183

[1492] *Journal of Gastroenterology* 2008: 134: 416

[1493] *American Journal of Clinical Nutrition* 2007; 86: 285

[1494] *New England Journal of Medicine* 2006; 355: 2297

[1495] *Nutrition Journal* 2008; 138: 1872

[1496] *Nutrition Journal* 2009; 139: 63

[1497] *Alimentary Pharmacology & Therapeutics* 2006; 24: 1553

[1498] "The Sunshine Deficit and Cardiovascular Disease," *Circulation* 2008; 118: 1476

[1499] "The Role of Inflammation in Vascular Insulin Resistance," *Hormone and Metabolic Research* 2008; 40: 635

[1500] *Diabetes Care* 2007; 30: 318, 325, 332, 337

[1501] *Archives of Internal Medicine* 2007; 167: 642

[1502] *Diabetologia* 2007; 50: 1409

[1503] *Endocrine Reviews* 2007; 28: 463

[1504] *Circulation* 2008; 118: 33

[1505] *Nature Medicine* 2002; 8: 1218

[1506] Annual Meeting for the European Association for the Study of Diabetes, Rome 2008; *Metabolism—Clinical and Experimental* 2008; 57: 1487

[1507] *Townsend Letter,* May 2007, page 72

[1508] "The Metabolic Syndrome and Preventive Cardiology: Working Together to Reduce Cardiometabolic Risks," *Metabolic Syndrome and Related Disorders* 2006; 4:233

[1509] *Journal of Clinical Endocrinology & Metabolism* 2007; 92: 399

[1510] *Diabetes Care* 2007; 30: 1206

[1511] *Circulation* 2007; 116: 151

[1512] *Journal of the American College of Cardiology* 2007; 50: 843

[1513] *American Journal of Clinical Nutrition* 2007; 86: 48

[1514] *Diabetes Care* 2007; 30: 1647

[1515] "Abnormal Glucose Tolerance, a Common Risk Factor in Patients with Acute Myocardial Infarction in Comparison with Population-Based Controls," *Journal of Internal Medicine* 2004; 256: 288

[1516] Annual Scientific Session of the American Heart Association, New Orleans, La., 2008

[1517] *Clinical Cornerstone* 2006; 8 supp: S21

[1518] *Circulation* 2008; 117: 1018

[1519] *Diabetologia* 2002; 2: 210

[1520] *Psychophysiology* 2007; 44: 154

[1521] *Diabetes Care* 2008; 31: 576

[1522] *Clinical Chemistry* 2007; 53: 456

[1523] *Diabetes* 1995; 44: 369

[1524] *Journal of the American Medical Association* 2008; 299: 1265

[1525] *Cardiology Review* 2002; 19: supp: 13

[1526] "Cardiovascular Death and the Metabolic Syndrome," *Diabetes Care* 2006; 29: 1363

[1527] *Atherosclerosis* 2007; 181: 215

[1528] *Mayo Clinic Proceedings* 2008; 83: 1350

[1529] "Metabolic Syndrome and Salt Sensitive High Blood Pressure Linked," International Society on Hypertension in Blacks, Atlanta, Ga., 2006

[1530] *Journal of the American Medical Association* 2007; 298: 1300

[1531] *Journal of the American Medical Association* 2008; 300: 2389

[1532] *Circulation* 1996; 94: 1

[1533] *Circualtion* 2007; 116: 375

[1534] *New England Journal of Medicine* 1996; 334: 952

[1535] *Archives of Internal Medicine* 2004; 164: 1066, 982

[1536] *Diabetes Care* 1991; 14: 173

[1537] *Lancet* 2007; 370: 667

[1538] *Archives of Internal Medicine* 2006; 166; 444

[1539] *New York Times Magazine,* June 25, 2006, page 17

[1540] "Insulin Resistance and Atherosclerosis," *Endocrine Reviews* 2006; 27: 242; *Diabetes Care* 2008; 57: 3307

[1541] Annual Scientific Sessionof the American Heart Association, New Orleans, La., 2008

[1542] Book review in the *Journal of the American Medical Association* 2008; 299: 2328

[1543] *Annual Review of Physiology* 1995; 57: 171

[1544] *Journal of Clinical Endocrinology & Metabolism* 2001; 11: 5491; *Journal of the American Medical Association* 2004; 291: 1978

[1545] *Lancet* 2001; 358: 1400

[1546] American Heart Association conference, New Orleans, La., 2008

[1547] J. Clinical Endocrinology & Metabolism 2007;92:491

[1548] "Association Between Serum Uric Acid, Metabolic Syndrome, and Carotid Atherosclerosis," *Arteriosclerosis, Thrombosis, and Vascular Biology* 2005; 25: 1038

[1549] *Diabetes Care* 2007; 30: 649

[1550] "Metformin Increases Blood Flow in Non-Obese Type II Diabetes Patients," *Hormone and Metabolic Research* 2006; 38: 513

[1551] Annual Congress of European Society of Cardiology, Munich 2008

[1552] "Endothelial Dysfunction Varies According to IR," *Diabetes Care* 2007; 30: 1226

[1553] *"Effects of Antioxidant Supplementation on Insulin Sensitivity, Endothelial Adhesion Molecules, and Oxidative Stress in Normal Weight and Overweight Adults," Metabolism—Clinical and Experimental 2009; 58: 254*

[1554] "Insulin Resistance, ADMA Levels and Cardiovascular Disease," *Journal of the American Medical Association* 2002; 287: 1451

[1555] *American Journal of Clinical Nutrition* 2008; 88: 1018

[1556] *Vascular Medicine* 1999; 4: 27

[1557] *Arteriosclerosis, Thrombosis, and Vascular Biology* 2006; 26: 1419

1558 *Clinical Chemistry* 2007; 53: 273

1559 *Endocrinology* 2007; 148: 4548

1560 "Dietary L-Arginine Supplementation Reduces Fat Mass in Diabetic Rats," *Nutrition Journal* 2005; 135: 714

1561 "ADMA, an Endogenous Inhibitor of Nitric Oxide Synthase Explains the 'L-Arginine Paradox' and Acts as a Novel Cardiovascular Risk Factor," *Nutrition Journal* 2004; 134 #10

1562 *Nature Medicine* 2003; 9: 653

1563 *Diabetes Care* 2008; 57: 3247

1564 *Journal of the American Medical Association* 2007; 297: 1344, 1376

1565 *Journal of the American Medical Association* 2007; 297: 1255

1566 *Business Week,* May 29, 2006, cover issue

1567 *Journal of the American Medical Association* 2008; 299; 885

1568 "Controversies Surround Heart Drug Study," *Journal of the American Medical Association* 2008; 299: 885

1569 *New York Times,* March 31, 2008

1570 *The Medical Letter,* August 2008; study available at www.escardio.org

1571 *Science* 2008; 322: 220

1572 *New York Times,* Jan. 17 and Jan. 27, 2008

1573 Walter C. Willett and P. J. Skerrett, *Eat, Drink, and Be Healthy* (Harvard Press: 2002)

1574 *Nutrition Journal* 2009; 139: 1

1575 Dean Ornish, *Reversing Heart Disease* (Ballantine Books: 1990)

1576 *Cardiology Review* 2003; 20: 10

1577 *New England Journal of Medicine,* Nov. 9, 2008 (10.1056/NEJMoa0807646)

1578 *American Journal of Medicine* 2008; 121: 1002

1579 "Is Oxidative Stress the Pathogenic Mechanism Underlying Insulin Resistance, Diabetes and Cardiovascular Disease? The Common Soil Hypothesis Revisited," *Arteriosclerosis, Thrombosis, and Vascular Biology* 2004; 24: 823

1580 Annual Meeting of the American Heart Association, Chicago, Ill., 2003

1581 *Journal of the Royal Society of Medicine* 2002; 96: symposium

1582 *Family Practice News,* August 15, 2006, page 12

1583 *Diabetologia* 2005; 48: 741

1584 *Journal of the American Medical Association* 2007; 298: 299, 309, 336

1585 *Diabetes Care* 2008; 149: 2032

1586 *Nature Medicine* 2002; 8: 1211

1587 *Lancet* 2007; 369: 1090

[1588] *American Journal of Preventive Medicine* 2006; 31: 316

[1589] American Heart Association, January 2003

[1590] *Lancet* 2003; 361: 477

[1591] *American Journal of Cardiology* 2006; 98: 61i

[1592] "Mechanisms by Which Dietary Fatty Acids Modulate Plasma Lipids," *Nutrition Journal* 2005; 135: 2075

[1593] *American Journal of Cardiology* 2006; 98: 34i

[1594] *Nutrition Journal* 2008: 138: 287

[1595] *Nutrition Journal* 2008: 138: 272

[1596] *American Journal of Cardiology* 2006; 98: 1369

[1597] *Journal of the American Medical Association* 2007; 298: 776

[1598] *Journal of Internal Medicine* 2006; 259: 493

[1599] *Archives of Internal Medicine* 2004; 164: 2156; *Journal of the American Medical Association* 2005; 293: 2641

[1600] *British Medical Journal* 2000; 321: 199

[1601] *Atherosclerosis* 2002; 163: 149; *Metabolism — Clinical and Experimental* 2008; 57: 1760

[1602] *Journal of Clinical Endocrinology & Metabolism* 2007; 92: 2532

[1603] *Lancet* 2002; 359: 133

[1604] *Arteriosclerosis, Thrombosis, and Vascular Biology* 2005; 25: 1629; *Blood* 2004; 104: 323

[1605] *American Journal of Clinical Nutrition* 2008; 88: 356

[1606] *Diabetes Care* 2008; 31: 2092

[1607] *Blood*, April 15, 2007

[1608] *Journal of Bone and Mineral Metabolism* 2001; 19: 146

[1609] *Agro Food Industry Hi-Tech* 2002; 13: 11

[1610] *Nutrition Journal* 2004; 134: 3100

[1611] "Periodontal Microbiota and Intima Media Thickness," *Circulation* 2005; 111: 576

[1612] "Effect of Lactobacillus Plantarun 299v on Cardiovascular Disease," *American Journal of Clinical Nutrition* 2002; 76: 1249

[1613] *Diabetes Care* 1998; 21: 2116

[1614] *Hypertension* 2003; 21: 371

[1615] *Endocrinology and Metabolism* 2001; 86: 1403

[1616] *American Journal of Cardiology* 2003; 1: 108

[1617] *Yonsei Medical Journal* 2004; 45: 838

[1618] *Environmental Health Perspectives* 2006; 114: 1718

[1619] *"Fruits, Vegetables and Fish Consumption and Heart Rate Variability," American Journal of Clinical Nutrition 2009; 89: 773*

[1620] *Hormone and Metabolic Research 2008; 40: 583*

[1621] *Circulation 2008; 117: 1255*

[1622] Annual Meeting for the European Society of Cardiology, Barcelona, Spain, 2006

[1623] *Journal of the American Medical Association 2004; 292: 2471*

[1624] *Circulation 2008; 117: 1130*

[1625] *Medical Hypotheses 2002; 59: 537*

[1626] "Associations Between Depressive Symptoms and Insulin Resistance," *Diabetologia 2006; 49: 2974*

[1627] Dean Ornish, *Love and Survival* (HarperCollins: 1997)

[1628] *Diabetes Care 2007; 30: 1520*

[1629] *Circulation 2007; 116: 434*

[1630] "Hyperglycemia and Heart Dysfunction: An Oxidant Mechanism Contributing to Heart Failure in Diabetes," *Journal of Endocrinology Investigation 2002; 25: 485*

[1631] *American Journal of Cardiology,* Nov. 1, 2008

[1632] "Left Ventricular Diastolic Function is Related to Glucose in a Middle-Age Population," *Journal of Internal Medicine 2002; 251: 415*

[1633] *Archives of Internal Medicine 2006; 166: 1613; Circulation 2007; 115: 1371*

[1634] *Diabetes Care 2008; 31: 1502*

[1635] *Medicine & Science in Sports & Exercise 2001; 33: s167*

[1636] *Journal of Toxicology Sciences 2008; 33: 459*

[1637] *European Heart Journal,* July 2007

[1638] *Archives of Internal Medicine,* August 2008

[1639] J. Hormonal Metabolism Research 2008; 40:583

[1640] "Metabolic Syndrome in Women with Chronic Pain," *Metabolism — Clinical and Experimental 2007; 56: 87*

[1641] *Metabolism — Clinical and Experimental 2008; 57: 1691*

[1642] *Diabetes Care 2006; 9: 1929*

[1643] *New England Journal of Medicine 2001; 345: 1785*

[1644] *International Journal Integrative Medicine 2000; 2: 7*

[1645] *American Journal of Clinical Nutrition 1999; 70s: 539*

[1646] *American Journal of Clinical Nutrition 1976; 70: 236*

[1647] *Archives of Pediatrics & Adolescent Medicine 2000; 154: 610*

[1648] *Journal of the American College of Nutrition 2000; 19: 715*

[1649] *Clinical Diabetes* 2004; 22: 10

[1650] *Medical Hypotheses* 2007; 69: 860

[1651] J. Rheumatology 2002; 29:7

[1652] *Metabolism — Clinical and Experimental* 2007; 56: 623

[1653] *Journal of Clinical Endocrinology & Metabolism* 2002; 87: 3324

[1654] *Journal of Endocrinology Investigation* 2007; 30: 126

[1655] *Journal of Clinical Endorinology & Metabolism* 2002; 87: 3324

[1656] *PloS Medicine* (online journal), July 2007

[1657] Annual Meeting of the American Society for Bone and Mineral Research, Honolulu, Hawaii, 2008; reported in *Skin and Allergy News*, February 2008, page 57

[1658] *Journal of the American Medical Association* 2005; 294: 2336

[1659] *New England Journal of Medicine* 2007; 357: 266

[1660] *Nutrition Journal* 2008: 138: 277

[1661] *Nutrition Journal* 2009; 139: 329

[1662] *American Journal of Clinical Nutrition* 2008; 88: 356

[1663] *Journal of the American Medical Association* 2005; 294: 113

[1664] Annual Meeting of the Canadian Diabetes Association; *Family Practice News*, Dec. 1, 2006, page 16

[1665] "A Possible Role of Osteocalcin in the Regulation of Insulin Secretion," *Endocrinology* 2008; 199: 151

[1666] *Pediatrics* 2005; 115: 736

[1667] "Industry Manipulation of Medical Science," *Journal of the American Medical Association* 2008; 299: 1800, 1813, 1833

[1668] *Journal of the American Medical Association* 2007; 298: 413

[1669] *Salt Lake Tribune*, July 25, 2007

[1670] *New England Journal of Medicine* 2007; 357: 266

[1671] "Shifting the Focus in Fracture Prevention From Osteoporosis to Falls," *British Medical Journal* 2008; 337: 124

[1672] *Journal of the American Medical Association* 2002; 288: 321

[1673] *Archives of Internal Medicine* 2008; 168: 826

[1674] *Journal of the American Medical Association* 2006; 296: 2927

[1675] *Journal of the American Medical Association* 2006; 296: 2947

[1676] *Journal of the American Medical Association* 2005; 294; 2989

[1677] *Endocrinology* 2008; 149: 4799

[1678] *Archives of Internal Medicine* 2007; 167: 1240, 1246

[1679] *American Journal of Epidemiology* 2004; 160: 521

[1680] British Medical Journal 2008: 336: 126

[1681] *New England Journal of Medicine* 2006; 355: 1647

[1682] *Archives of General Psychiatry* 2005; 62: 154

[1683] *Rheumatology* 2007; 34: 460

[1684] *American Journal of Medicine* 2003; 114: 753

[1685] *Medical Hypotheses* 2002; 59: 577

[1686] *Rheumatology* 2003; 30: 1402

[1687] "Insulin Resistance in Rheumatoid Arthritis Underlies Cardiovascular Risk," Annual Meeting for the British Society for Rheumatology, Glasgow, 2006

[1688] "Etanercept Cuts CRP in Metabolic Syndrome," *Family Practice News*, June 1, 2006, page 20

[1689] *Journal of the American Medical Association* 2007; 297: 1645

[1690] *Gastroenterology* 2005; 129: 827

[1691] "The Gut in Ankylosing Spondylitis and Other Arthropathies: Inflammation Beneath the Surface," *Rheumatology* 2003; 30: 11

[1692] *Toxicology Letters* 2003; 140: 105

[1693] *Gut* 2006; 55: 1240

[1694] *Gastroenterology* 2005; 129: 827

[1695] "Small Intestinal Bacterial Overgrowth," *Journal of the American Medical Association* 2004; 292: 852

[1696] "A Vegan Diet Free of Gluten Improves the Signs and Symptoms of Rheumatoid Arthritis: The Effects on Arthritis Correlate with a Reduction in Antibodies to Food Allergens," *Rheumatology* 2001; 40: 1175

[1697] *Lancet* 2007; 369: 946

[1698] *Diabetes Care* 2008; 31: 2312

[1699] *Archives of Opthalmogy* 2008; 126: 1554

[1700] *American Journal of Clinical Nutrition* 2008; 88: 886

[1701] *Family Practice News*, Sept. 1, 2008, page 16

[1702] *Diabetes Care* 2008; 31: 1590

[1703] *Archives of Internal Medicine* 2008; 168: 1678

[1704] *Archives of Internal Medicine* 2008; 168: 1678

[1705] Annual Meeting for the American Academy of Orthopedic Surgeons, San Francisco, Calif., 2008

[1706] *Diabetes Care* 2008; 31: 1373

[1707] *Family Practice News*, July 1, 2008, page 14

[1708] Annual Meeting for the European Society of Human Reproduction and Embryology, Barcelona, Spain, 2008

[1709] *Journal of Allergy and Clinical Immunology* 2008; 121: 1075, 1087

[1710] *Metabolism — Clinical and Experimental* 2008; 57: 522

[1711] *Diabetes Care* 2008; 31: 1001

[1712] *Journal of Allergy and Clinical Immunology* 2008; 121: 1096

[1713] *Skin & Allergy News,* May 2008, page 9; *American Academy of Dermatology* 2008; 58: 787

[1714] *Diabetes Care* 2007; 30: 842

[1715] *American Academy of Dermatology* 2007; 57: 247

[1716] *American Academy of Dermatology* 2007; 57: 1092

[1717] *Skin & Allergy News,* April 2008, page 49

[1718] *Neurology Reviews,* April 2008, page 1

[1719] *Diabetes Care* 2008; 31: 464

[1720] *Journal of Clinical Endocrinology & Metabolism* 2007; 92: 4623

[1721] *Orv Hetil* 2007; 148: 2259 (Hungarian: use of CoQ10, L-carnitine)

[1722] *Gut* 2007; 56: 1503

[1723] *Circulation* 2007; 116: 2275

[1724] Annual Meeting for the American Association of Diabetes Educators, St. Louis, Mo., 2007

[1725] *American Journal of Clinical Nutrition* 2007; 86: 556

[1726] *Gut* 2007; 56: 1296

[1727] *Archives of Internal Medicine* 2007; 167: 1670

[1728] *Skin & Allergy News,* October 2007, page 8

[1729] *Diabetes Care* 2007; 30: 1964

[1730] *Archives of Internal Medicine* 2007; 167: 1670

[1731] *Archives of Dermatology* 2008; 144: 1571

[1732] *Diabetes Care* 2007; 30: 1795

[1733] *Gastroenterology* 2007; 133: 34

[1734] *American Journal of Clinical Nutrition* 2007; 86: 5

[1735] *Family Practice News,* July 1, 2007

[1736] *Journal of Clinical Endocrinology & Metabolism* 2007; 92: 2046

[1737] *Diabetes Care* 2007; 30: 1187

[1738] *Journal of the American Medical Association* 2007; 298: 2275

[1739] *Journal of Clinical Endocrinology & Metabolism* 2007; 92: 1430

[1740] *Archives of Internal Medicine,* April 2007

[1741] *American Journal of Clinical Nutrition* 2007; 85: 35

[1742] *Current Pain and Headache Reports* 2006; 10: 363

[1743] *Archives of Neurology* 2006; 63: 1075

[1744] *Journal of Nutrition* 2009; 139: 96

[1745] *American Journal of Clinical Nutrition* 2006; 83: 880, 733

[1746] *Journal of the American Medical Association* 2006; 294: 2872

[1747] Annual Meeting for the American College of Osteopathy, Grapevine, Texas, 2006

[1748] *Archives of Dermatology* 2006; 141: 1527

[1749] *American Journal of Gastroenterology* 2006; 101: 70

[1750] *Journal of Endocrinology Investigation* 2005; 28: 940

[1751] *Americal Journal of Clinical Nutrition* 2005; 82: 504

[1752] *American Journal of Epidemiology* 2005; 161: 546

[1753] *Heart* 2003; 89: 1217

[1754] *Journal of Internal Medicine* 2003; 253: 574

[1755] *Pediatrics* 2001; 138: 474; *Clinical Diabetes* 2002; 20: 217

[1756] *Metabolism — Clinical and Experimental* 2007; 56: 670

[1757] *Ophthalmologica* 2003; 217: 302

[1758] *New Scientist,* December 2002 (study from the University of Melbourne, Australia)

[1759] *Archives of Dermatology* 2002; 138: 1584

[1760] *Journal of the American Nutraceutical Association* 1997; 1: 24

[1761] *Acta Ophtalmologica Scandinavica* 2002; 48: 25

[1762] *Caries Research* 1998; 32: 107

[1763] *Essence* 1992; 23: 79

[1764] *Diabetes* 1999; 48: 7991

[1765] *Diabetes* 1999; 48: 7991

[1766] *Nutrition Reviews* 2007; 65: s173

[1767] *Archives Internal Medicine* 2007; 167: 1145

[1768] *Archives of Internal Medicine* 2007; 167: 635

[1769] "Aging, Natural Death and the Compression of Mortality" *New England Journal of Medicine* 1980; 303: 130

[1770] *New England Journal of Medicine* 1998; 338: 1035

[1771] James Gardner, *The Intelligent Universe,* (New Page Books: 2007)

[1772] "Like Parent, Like Child," *Archives of Pediatrics & Adolescent Medicine* 2008; 162: 1063

[1773] Gina Kolata, *Rethinking Thin: The New Science of Weight Loss — and the Myths and Realities of Dieting* (Farrar Straus Books: 2007)

[1774] *Journal of the American Medical Association* 2007; 298: 617

[1775] Book "The Secret History of the American Empire", John Perkins; Dutton Bools, 2007

[1776] "Experts Weigh Pros and Cons of Screening and Treatment for Childhood Obesity," *Journal of the American Medical Association* 2008; 300: 1401

[1777] Jeffrey Garten, *The Politics of Fortune* (Harvard Business School Press: 2002

[1778] John Perkins, *The Secret History of the American Empire*, (Dutton Books: 2007)

[1779] Richard Sennett, *The Corrosion of Character: Personal Consequences of Work in the New Capitalism* (Norton: 1998)

[1780] "Why Business is Bad for Your Health," *Lancet* 2004; 363: 1173, 1193

[1781] *Archives of Internal Medicine* 2007; 167: 766

[1782] "Corporate Health and Wellness Programs: A Business Necessity," *Business Week*, Jan. 2, 2006

[1783] "The Health of the People is the Supreme Law of the Land," *American Journal of Public Health* 2001; 91: 689

[1784] "More Calling for Single-Payer System," *Managed Care Magazine*, May 2003, page 20

[1785] *Salt Lake Tribune*, July 29, 2007

[1786] Steven Hiatt and John Perkins, *A Game as Old as Empire* (Berrett-Koehler Publishers: 2007)

[1787] Joseph Ellis, *Founding Brothers* (Vintage Books: 2000)

[1788] *Salt Lake Tribune*, July 8, 2007

[1789] *Public Library of Science Medicine*, February 2008; *Salt Lake Tribune*, Feb. 5, 2008

[1790] *New York Times*, July 4, 2007

[1791] "Swarm Theory," *National Geographic*, July 2007, page 126

[1792] *Journal of the American Medical Association* 2001; 285: 182

[1793] *Archives of Internal Medicine*, Oct. 28, 2008

[1794] *Journal of the American Medical Association* 2009; 301: 865

[1795] *Lancet* 2006; 368: 1673

[1796] *American College of Physicians Foundation*, July 31, 2007

[1797] *American College of Endocrinology*, 2007

[1798] *Journal of the American Medical Association* 2002; 288: 1909

[1799] *New York Times*, August 4, 2007

[1800] *Lancet* 2007; 369: 71

[1801] *Annals of Internal Medicine* 2006; 145: 81

[1802] *Archives of Internal Medicine* 2002; 162: 484

[1803] *Journal of Clinical Endocrinology & Metabolism* 2006; 91: 2074

[1804] *Journal of Family Practice* 2008; 57: 526

[1805] *British Journal of Nutrition* 2006; 96: 326

[1806] Annual Scientific Session of the American Diabetic Association, San Diego, Calif., 2005

[1807] *Diabetes Care* 2003; 26: 251

[1808] *Diabetes Care* 2006; 29: 1997

[1809] *Diabetologia* 2006; 49: 930

[1810] *Family Practice News,* Sept. 15, 2007, page 20

[1811] *Diabetologia* 1999; 42: 1033

[1812] *American Journal of Cardiology* 2002; 90: 34g

[1813] *Science* 1999; 27: 1409

[1814] *Diabetes* 2002; 51: 2796

[1815] Forty-second Annual Meeting European Association for the Study of Diabetes, Copenhagen, Denmark, 2006

[1816] *New England Journal of Medicine* 2006; 355: 2427

[1817] *Lancet* 2008; 372: 1520

[1818] *Family Practice News,* Dec. 15, 2008, page 8

[1819] *New England Journal of Medicine,* May 21, 2007

[1820] *New York Times,* June 7, 2007

[1821] Associated Press report, July 13, 2007

[1822] United States Food and Drug Administration, July 27, 2007

[1823] *Family Practice News,* June 1, 2007, page 22

[1824] *Family Practice News,* Sept. 1, 2008, page 1

[1825] *Journal of the American Medical Association* 2007; 298: 187

[1826] *Diabetes Care* 2006; 29: 435

[1827] *Journal of the American Medical Association* 2007; 298: 194

[1828] United States Food and Drug Administration, December 2008

[1829] *Journal of the American Medical Association* 2002; 287: 598

[1830] "Vitamin A Depletion Causes Oxidative Stress, Mitochondrial Dysfunction, and PARP-1 Dependent Energy Deprivation," *FASEB* (Federation of American Societies for Experimental Biology) 2008; 22: 3878

[1831] *Lancet* 2007; 369: 168

[1832] *British Medical Journal* 2007; 334: 983

[1833] *Journal of Chinese Medicine* 2007; 1: 4; *European Journal of Cardiovascular Rehabilitation* 2007; 14: 438; *American Journal of Cardiology,* June 8, 2008

[1834] *Diabetes Care* 2007; 30: 1945

[1835] Annual Scientific Sessions of the American Diabetes Association, Chicago, Ill., 2007

[1836] *Metabolism — Clinical and Experimental* 2006; 55: 1619

[1837] *Family Practice News,* March 2004, page 20

[1838] *Planta Medica* 2007; 73: 6

[1839] European Association for the Study of Diebetes Annual Meeting, Amsterdam, 2007

[1840] *Diabetes Care* 2007; 30: 1694

[1841] *Family Practice News,* Dec. 1, 2008

[1842] *Family Practice News* 2006; 36 #19: 1

[1843] *Archives of Internal Medicine* 2006; 166: 902

[1844] Annual Meeting of the British Society for Rheumatology, Glasgow, 2006

[1845] Annual Interscience Conference on Antimicrobial Agents and Chemotherapy,
San Francisco, Calif., 2006; *Skin & Allergy News,* December 2006, page 25

[1846] *New York Times,* July 22, 2007

[1847] Dateline NBC, July 29, 2007

[1848] *Alternative Therapies in Health and Medicine,* March/April 2006; 12 #2: 26

[1849] *Toxicology and Applied Pharmacology* 2007; 223: 173

[1850] *Experimental Neurology* 2005; 196: 112

[1851] *Molecular Aspects of Medicine* 1994; 15: s265

[1852] *European Journal of Endocrinology* 2008: 158: 47

[1853] *American Family Physician* 2004; 69: 1961

[1854] *Science* 2002; 296: 698

[1855] *Nature Medicine,* July 29, 2007

[1856] Annual Meeting of the Diabetes Association, Chicago, Ill., 2007

[1857] *Journal of the American Medical Association* 2005; 294: 1861

[1858] Agency for Healthcare Research and Quality, branch of Public Health Service, July 23, 2006

[1859] *New England Journal of Medicine* 2007; 357: 753

[1860] *Journal of the American Medical Association* 2008; 299: 316

[1861] *Family Practice News, Feb. 15, 2009, page 23*

[1862] *New York Times Magazine,* Nov. 18, 2007

[1863] *Pediatric and Adolescent Surgery,* February 2007

[1864] *Annals of Internal Medicine* 2009; 150: 94; *Pediatrics,* January 2009

[1865] *New England Journal of Medicine* 2004; 350: 2549

[1866] *Family Practice News,* Aug. 1, page 4

[1867] *Diabetes Care* 2004; 27: 2887

[1868] *Metabolism—Clinical & Experimental* 2007; 56: 245

[1869] *Circulation* 1999; 99: 733, 779

[1870] *Journal of the American Medical Association* 2007; 297: 2092

[1871] *New England Journal of Medicine* 2007; 356: 212

[1872] *Nutrition Reviews* 2006; 64: 403

[1873] *Circulation* 2008; 117: 169

[1874] *American Journal of Clinical Nutrition* 2008; 87: 8

[1875] "Dietary Treatment of Diabetes Mellitus in the Pre-Insulin Era," *Perspectives in Biology and Medicine* 2006; 49: 77

[1876] *British Medical Journal* 2007; 334: 299

[1877] *Family Practice News*, Jan. 1, 2008, page 17

[1878] *Journal of the American Medical Association* 2007; 298: 1661

[1879] "The Metabolic Syndrome: May Be a Guidepost or Detour to Preventing Type 2 Diabetes and Cardiovascular Disease," *British Medical Journal* 2003; 327: 61

[1880] "Effect of Weight Loss with Lifestyle Intervention on Risk of Diabetes," *Diabetes Care* 2006; 29: 2102

[1881] *American Journal of Clinical Nutrition* 2007; 86: 276

[1882] *Family Practice News*, April 15, 2008, page 12

[1883] *American Association of Clinical Endocrinologists*, 2007

[1884] *Family Practice News*, Jan. 1, 2008, page 17

[1885] *New England Journal of Medicine* 2006; 355: 1563

[1886] *Science* 2007; 334: 819

[1887] *Lancet* 2003; 361: 544

[1888] *New England Journal of Medicine* 2005; 353: 1009

[1889] *Archives of Pediatrics & Adolescent Medicine* 2007; 161: 495

[1890] Caroline M. Apovian and Carine M. Lenders, *A Clinical Guide for Management of Overweight and Obese Children and Adults* (CRC: 2006)

[1891] *Journal of the American Medical Association* 2007; 298: 463

[1892] "An Evidence-Based Approach to Medical Nutrition Education," *American Journal of Clinical Nutrition* 2006; 83 supp: 929s

[1893] *Journal of the American Medical Association* 2004; 293: 43, 96

[1894] "Experts Charge New US Dietary Guidelines Pose Daunting Challenge for the Public," *Journal of the American Medical Association* 2005; 293: 918

[1895] Marion Nestle, *Food Politics*, (University of California Press: 2002)

[1896] *The Sunday Mail*, Brisbane, Australia; June 17, 2007

[1897] *American Journal of Clinical Nutrition* 2007; 86: 542

[1898] *American Journal of Clinical Nutrition* 2007; 86: 542

[1899] *Current Opinion in Lipidology* 2008; 19: 63

[1900] "Mediterranean Diet, Lifestyle Factors and 10-Year Mortality in Elderly European Men and Women," *Journal of the American Medical Association* 2004; 292: 1433

[1901] *Journal of the American Medical Association* 2004; 292: 1440

[1902] *Annals of Nutrition and Metabolism* 2006; 50: 20

[1903] *American Journal of Clinical Nutrition* 2006; 84: 328

[1904] *American Journal of Clinical Nutrition* 2006; 84: 1043

[1905] *International Journal of Obesity,* May 2007

[1906] "Xenohormesis: Sensing the Chemical Cues of Other Species," *Cell* 2008; 133: 387

[1907] Michael Pollan, *In Defense of Food,* (Penguin Press: 2008)

[1908] Proceedings of the National Academy of Sciences, Nov. 12, 2002

[1909] Clinical Diabetes 2003; 21: 186

[1910] "The Soft Science of Dietary Fat," *Science* 2001; 291: 2536

[1911] *Family Practice Recertification* 2005; 27 #2: 49

[1912] *Lancet* 2003; 362: 1593

[1913] "The (Agri) Cultural Contradictions of Obesity," *New York Times Magazine,* Oct. 12, 2003

[1914] "The Fat of the Land," *Environmental Health Perspectives* 2004; 112: A821

[1915] University of Utah School of Medicine, *Salt Lake Tribune,* Dec. 11, 2007

[1916] "To Eat or Not to Eat: How the Gut Talks to the Brain," New England Journal of Medicine 2003; 349: 9236.

[1917] *Journal of Nutraceuticals, Functional & Medical Foods* 2006; 9: 49

[1918] *Journal of Nutrition 2009; 139: 335*

[1919] *Journal of the American Medical Association* 2000; 284: 592

[1920] Albert Bandura, *Self-Efficacy: The Exercise of Control,* (Worth Publishers: 1997)

[1921] British Journal of Nutrition 2006; 95: 496

[1922] Journal of the American Medical Association 2004; 293: 43, 96

[1923] "The Influence of Food Portion Size and Energy Density on Energy Intake: Implications for Weight Management," American Journal of Clinical Nutrition 2005; 82: 236S

[1924] American Journal of Clinical Nutrition 2002; 75 supp: 365

[1925] Annual Scientific Section of the American Diabetes Association, Washington, DC, 2006

[1926] Western Journal of Medicine 1999; 171: 25

471

[1927] American Journal of Clinical Nutrition 2007; 86: 531

[1928] New England Journal of Medicine 2000; 342: 1441

[1929] *"Mastication of Almonds: Effects of Lipid Bioaccessibility, Appetite and Hormone Response," American Journal of Clinical Nutrition 2009; 89: 793*

[1930] *American Journal of Clinical Nutrition 2008; 87: 855*

[1931] *Lancet 2008: 371: 411*

[1932] "Inadequate Dietary Protein Increases Hunger and Desire to Eat," *Nutrition Journal* 2007; 137: 1478

[1933] "A High-Protein Diet Induces Sustained Reductions in Appetite, Ad Libitum Caloric Intake, and Body Weight," American Journal of Clinical Nutrition 2005; 82 #1(s); "The Satiating Power of Protein-a Key to Obesity Prevention?" American Journal of Clinical Nutrition 2005;82:1

[1934] *Longevity Journal,* June 1990

[1935] American Journal of Clinical Nutrition 2008; 87: 846

[1936] *Archives of Internal Medicine 2007; 167: 956*

[1937] *Nutrition Journal 2008; 138: 439*

[1938] *Archives of Internal Medicine 2007; 167: 2304*

[1939] *Journal of the American Medical Association 2008; 300: 2742*

[1940] *Archives of Internal Medicine 2007; 167: 502*

[1941] *Nutrition Journal 2008; 138: 775*

[1942] "Effects of Probiotics and Prebiotics," *Nutrition Journal* 2007; 137# 3S-II

[1943] J. K. Rowling, *Harry Potter and the Half-Blood Prince* (A. Levine Books: 2005)

[1944] *Critical Reviews in Food Science and Nutrition 2008; 48: 905*

[1945] *Archives of Internal Medicine 2007; 167: 956*

[1946] Critical Reviews in Food Science and Nutrition 2007; 47: 389

[1947] "Insoluble Cereal Fiber Reduces Appetite and ShorttTerm Food Intake and Glycemic Response to Food Consumed 75 Minutes Later by Healthy Men," *American Journal of Clinical Nutrition 2007; 86: 972*

[1948] Journal of Nutrition 2008; 138: 732

[1949] Honolulu Star Bulletin, Nov. 19, 1999

[1950] *Journal of Neuroscience,* December 2004

[1951] *Endocrinology* 2002; 173: 415& "Targeted Metabolomics Identifies Glucuronides of Dietary Phytoestrogens as a Major Class of MRP3 Substrates In Vivo", J. Gastroenterology 2009;137:1725

[1952] *Environmental Health Perspectives 2002; 110: 743*

[1953] Annual Meeting of American Society of Clinical Oncology, Atlanta, Ga., 2006

[1954] JAMA 2009;302:2437

[1955] *American Journal of Clinical Nutrition* 2006; 83: 103

[1956] Orlando, Fla., 2003; Loma Linda University; published in the *Journal of Nutrition* 2004; 134: 1205s

[1957] *Townsend Letter,* October 2000, page 105

[1958] *Metabolism — Clinical & Experimental* 2008; 57: s16

[1959] *Journal of Nutrition* 2008; 138: 1360

[1960] Journal of Nutrition 2008; 138: 1288

[1961] Journal of Nutrition and Cancer 2008; 60: 145

[1962] Journal of Nutrition 2008: 138: 462

[1963] Journal of Nutrition and Cancer 2008: 60: 7

[1964] Journal of Nutrition 2008: 138: 332

[1965] Journal of Nutrition 2008: 138: 297

[1966] Endocrinology 2007; 148: 5396

[1967] *American Journal of Clinical Nutrition* 2007; 86: 938

[1968] *Diabetes Care* 2007; 30: 1871

[1969] *Atherosclerosis* 2007; 192: 184

[1970] *American Journal of Clinical Nutrition* 2007; 85: 735

[1971] *British Journal of Nutrition* 2006; 96: 249

[1972] *International Journal of Obesity* 2004; 28: 1349

[1973] *Endocrine Research* 2004; 30: 215

[1974] *Endocrinology* 2003; 144: 3315

[1975] "Glycosylation and the Immune System," J. Science 2001; 291: 2370-2375

[1976] "Effect of a Mediterrranean Diet Supplemented with Nuts on Metabolic Syndrome Status," *Archives of Internal Medicine* 2008; 168: 2449

[1977] *Nutrition Journal* 2007; 137: 1846

[1978] *Annals of Nutrition & Metabolism* 2006; 50: 425

[1979] *American Heart Association* 2008; 155: 175

[1980] Jeffrey E. Garten, *The Politics of Fortune* (Harvard Business Press: 2002)

[1981] "Sunshine Laws and the Pharmaceutical Companies," *Journal of the American Medical Association* 2007; 297: 1255

[1982] "From Blockbuster Medicine to Personalized Medicine," *Personalized Medicine* 2008; 5: 55

[1983] United States Food and Drug Administration, Sept. 18, 2008

[1984] Barbara Kingsolver, *Animal, Vegetable, Mineral* (HarperCollins: 2007)

[1985] "High Dose Vitamin Therapy Stimulates Variant Enzymes with Decreased Coenzyme Binding Affinity," *American Journal of Clinical Nutrition* 2002; 75: 616

[1986] Michael Pollan, *In Defense of Food* (Penguin Press: 2008)

[1987] T. Colin Campbell and Thomas M. Campbell, II., *The China Study,* (BenBella Books: 2004)

[1988] *Family Practice News,* Aug. 1, 2007, page 13

[1989] *Journal of the American Medical Association* 2007; 298: 164

[1990] Archives of Internal Medicine 2008; 168: 713

[1991] *Journal of the American Medical Association* 2007; 298: 272

[1992] *American Journal of Preventive Medicine* 2007; 33: 34

[1993] *American Journal of Clinical Nutrition* 2000; 72: 1088

[1994] *New York Times,* May 13, 2008

[1995] *Journal of the American Medical Association* 2002; 288: 3095

[1996] *Family Practice Recertification* 2000; 22: 32 #9

[1997] *Family Practice News,* March 2004, page 30

[1998] *Women's Health in Primary Care* 2005; 8: 325

[1999] *Hormone and Metabolic Research* 2007; 39: 347

[2000] *Journal of Ethnopharmacology* 2001; 75: 101

[2001] *British Medical Journal* 1981; 282: 1823

[2002] *Indian Journal of Experimental Biology* 1997; 35: 841

[2003] *Pancreas* 2003; 26: 292

[2004] Ira Wolisnky and Judy A. Driskell, *Nutrition: Energy Metabolism and Exercise* (CRC Press: 2007); reviewed in *Journal of American Medical Association* 2008; 299: 2330

[2005] *Cell,* July 31, 2008; *New England Journal of Medicine* 2008; 359: 1842

[2006] *Diabetes Care,* February 2007

[2007] *American Journal of Clinical Nutrition* 2008; 88: 51

[2008] *Annals of Internal Medicine* 2007; 147: 357

[2009] *Archives of Internal Medicine* 2004; 164: 1092; *Archives of Pediatrics and Adolescent Medicine* 2006; 160: 573; *Atherosclerosis, Thrombosis, and Vascular Biology* 2007; 27: 2650

[2010] *Journal of the American Medical Association* 2008; 300: 1027

[2011] *Diabetes Care* 2007; 2101

[2012] *Archives of Internal Medicine* 2003; 163: 1440

[2013] *Salt Lake Tribune,* July 6, 2007

[2014] *Circulation,* October 2002

[2015] *Journal of the American Medical Association* 2003; 290: 3092

[2016] *Diabetes Care* 2005: page 1295

[2017] *Archives of Pediatrics & Adolescent Medicine* 2007; 161: 677

[2018] Quote by Henry David Thoreau

[2019] Lau Tzu, *Tao Te Ching* (HarperCollins: 1988)

[2020] Jeffrey Moussaieff Masson, *When Elephants Weep: The Emotional Lives of Animals*, (Delta Books: 1995)

[2021] *New England Journal of Medicine* 2007; 357: 328

[2022] "Swarm Theory," *National Geographic*, July 2007, page 126

[2023] David C. Johnston, *Free Lunch: How the Wealthiest Americans Enrich Themselves at Government Expense (and Stick You with the Bill)* (Penguin Press: 2007)

[2024] Vicki Robin, Joe Dominguez, Monique Tilford, *Your Money or Your Life* (Penguin Books: 1992)

[2025] *British Medical Journal*, January 2006

[2026] *Diabetes Care* 2002; 255: 30

[2027] *Lancet* 2004; 363: 1589

[2028] "Transcendental Meditation on Components of the Metabolic Syndrome with Coronary Heart Disease," *Archives of Internal Medicine* 2006; 166: 1218

[2029] *Family Practice News*, Dec. 15, 2006, page 14

[2030] *New York Times*, Feb. 28, 2008

[2031] *Lancet* 2007; 368: cover story

[2032] Norman Cousins, *Anatomy of an Illness* (Bantam Books: 1979)

[2033] *British Medical Journal*, Dec. 4, 2008

[2034] Frank Tipler, *Physics of Immortality* (Doubleday Books: 1994)

[2035] *Lancet* 2009: 373: 68 and Jan. 3, 2009, cover issue

[2036] John Bradshaw, *Homecoming* (Bantam Books: 1990)

[2037] *Epidemiology and Community Health*, May 2007

[2038] *Diabetes Care* 2008; 31: 1293

[2039] Annual Meeting of the Academy of Psychosomatic Medicine, Tucson, Ariz., 2006; *Family Practice News*, Jan. 1, 2007, page 20

[2040] Byram Karasu, MD, *The Art of Serenity* (Simon & Schuster: 2003)

[2041] *American Journal of Public Health* 1992; 82: 1089

[2042] National Institutes of Health study, *Salt Lake Tribune*, May 29, 2007

[2043] Byram Karasu, MD, *The Art of Serenity* (Simons & Schuster: 2003)

[2044] Michael Murphy, *The Future of the Body* (Tarcher Books: 1992)

[2045] *Maui News*, Aug. 17, 1997, page A6

[2046] *Diabetes Care* 2003; 26: 1651

[2047] *New Scientist*, June 2007

[2048] *Journal of Allergy and Clinical Immunology* 2007; 119: 1019

[2049] Book "*The Upanishads*," Eknath Easwaran; Nalgiri Press, 1987

[2050] Antoine de Saint-Exupery, *The Little Prince* (Harcourt: 1943)

[2051] *New York Times,* July 22, 2007

[2052] Paul Reps and Nyogen Senzaki, *Zen Flesh, Zen Bones* (Tuttle Publishing: 1998)

[2053] Matthew, 6: 25-29

[2054] Robert Sapolsky, *Why Zebras Don't Get Ulcers* (Freeman and Company: 1994)

[2055] Bruce Lipton, *The Biology of Belief* (Mountain of Love Books: 2005)

[2056] Lynne McTaggart, *The Intention Experiment* (Free Press: 2007)

[2057] Joyce Whiteley Hawkes, *Cell-Level Healing* (Atria Books: 2006)

[2058] Jon Kabat-Zinn, *Full Catastrophe Living* (Delta Books: 1990)

[2059] M.K. Gandhi, *Living from the Heart* (Siftsoft: 1985)

[2060] Larry Dossey, *Space, Time, & Medicine* (Shambala: 1985)

[2061] Dean Ornish, MD, *Love & Survival* (Harper Collins: 1998)

[2062] Albert Bandura, *Self-Efficacy: The Exercise of Control* (W.H. Freeman and Co.: 1997)

[2063] Victor Hugo, *Les Miserables* (Gallimar: 1963)

[2064] Antoine de Saint-Exupery, *The Little Prince* (Harcourt: 1943)

[2065] Tom Robbins, *Jitterbug Perfume* (Bantam Books: 1984)

[2066] *Occupational & Environmental Medicine,* May 2007

[2067] *Archives of Internal Medicine,* February 2007

[2068] *Journal of the American Medical Association* 1996; 275: 1405

[2069] *New York Times,* July 3, 2007

[2070] *Family Practice News,* June 15, 2007, page 19

[2071] *Journal of the American Medical Association* 2007; 297: 1599

[2072] *Salt Lake Tribune,* Nov. 26, 2007

[2073] *Journal of the American Medical Association* 2006; 296: 1458

[2074] *American Journal of Clinical Nutrition* 2000; 72: 2 supp

[2075] *New York Times,* Sept. 20, 2007

[2076] "Hereditary Variation of Liver Enzymes Involved with Detoxification and Neurodegenerative Diseases," *Journal of Inherited Metabolic Disease* 1991; 14: 431

[2077] *Food Technology* 2005; 5: 18

[2078] *Current Drug Metabolism* 2006; 7: 67

[2079] *Journal of Nutritional & Environmental Medicine* 1996; 6: 141

[2080] *Annals Clinical Research* 1988; 20: 267

[2081] *Cardiology* 1994; 83: 562

[2082] *Journal of the American College of Cardiology* 2002; 39: 5

[2083] *Eating and Weight Disorders* 2001; 6: 49

[2084] *New England Journal of Medicine* 1999; 341: 924

[2085] *Journal of Carcinogenesis* 2007; 28: 233

[2086] *Science* 2007; 316: 1

[2087] *Journal of Nutrition* 2001; 131: 3121

[2088] *Nature Clinical Practice Oncology* 2005; 2: 518

[2089] "Clinical Decisions: From Art to Science and Back Again," *Lancet* 2001; 358: 523

[2090] "Dumbing Down," *Journal of the American Medical Association* 2003; 289: 1349

[2091] "To Inform or Persuade? Direct to Consumer Advertising of Prescription Drugs," *New England Journal of Medicine* 2005; 352: 325

[2092] "Blood Pressure Regulation and Vegetarian Diets," *Nutrition Review* 2005: 63: 1; "Dietary Intervention for Blood Pressure Control: A Call to Action!" *American Journal of Clinical Nutrition* 2009; 89: 734

[2093] Web site: www.ourhealthcoop.com

[2094] "Environmental Chemicals and Thyroid Function," *European Journal of Endocrinology* 2006; 154: 599

[2095] Tracy Kidder, *Mountains Beyond Mountains*, (Random House: 2003)

[2096] *Family Practice News*, Sept. 1, 2008, page 42

[2097] Doris Kearns Goodwin, *Team of Rivals* (Simon & Schuster: 2005)

[2098] *Journal of the American Medical Association* 2002; 287: 1909

[2099] "A Systems Approach to Patient-Centered Care," *Journal of the American Medical Association* 2006; 296: 2848

[2100] "Inside the Presidency," *National Geographic,* January 2009, page 131, 144

[2101] *Archives of Pediatrics & Adolescent Medicine* 2008; 162: 1063

9 781608 604753